Forensic Imaging of Trauma

Silke Grabherr · Sarah Heinze
Tony Fracasso
Editors

Forensic Imaging of Trauma

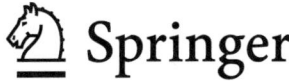 Springer

Editors
Silke Grabherr
Geneva University Hospitals
and University of Geneva
University Hospital of Vaud
University of Lausanne
University Center of Legal Medicine
Lausanne-Geneva
Geneva, Switzerland

Sarah Heinze
Diagnostic & Research Institute
of Forensic Medicine
Medical University Graz
Graz, Austria

Tony Fracasso
Geneva University Hospitals
and University of Geneva
University Hospital of Vaud
University of Lausanne
University Center of Legal Medicine
Lausanne-Geneva
Geneva, Switzerland

ISBN 978-3-031-48383-7   ISBN 978-3-031-48381-3   (eBook)
https://doi.org/10.1007/978-3-031-48381-3

This Springer imprint is published by the registered company Springer Nature Switzerland AG
The registered company address is: Gewerbestrasse 11, 6330 Cham, Switzerland

If disposing of this product, please recycle the paper.

Foreword

It is an honour for me to write this foreword and introduce this book that, I think, is going to become the reference in forensic imaging. It is a field with a long history, but that has seen rapid changes linked to the explosion of technologies.

The first forensic application of X-rays occurred in 1895, immediately after its discovery. It was used to localize projectiles. Over the ensuing years, radiographs were fully integrated into the daily practice of forensic pathology and led to numerous clinical applications. X-ray computed tomography (CT) and magnetic resonance imaging were developed in the 1970s. While these techniques were integrated into the practice of medicine very early, forensic pathology was slower to adopt them. This was probably a consequence of the false perception that autopsy was the only gold standard and that other techniques carried too high price with too little added value.

The introduction of the concept of Virtual Autopsy and the creation of the Centre of Forensic Imaging and Virtopsy® in Berne were the cornerstones in realizing the importance of forensic imaging and in the development of the field. In Europe, the University Center of Legal Medicine Lausanne-Geneva (CURML), located in Switzerland, is among the most active in using the latest technology advances. The role of imaging in forensic applications had an important impact in the field especially over the last 20 years. In fact, image technologies had an extremely fast evolution and, accordingly, new forensic applications became reality.

This book allows forensic practitioners to update their knowledge, from emerging technologies to their applications. It is specially orientated to forensic radiologists and pathologists, but it also serves as an excellent go to source for all multidisciplinary teams working on forensic caseworks.

Penned by some of the leading international experts, this is the first book that addresses the topic of forensic imaging of trauma, which is a key element in our field. The interpretation of image data in the context of forensic imaging requires knowledge, experience and special training. This book is an opportunity to share the updated knowledge in a quickly evolving field.

University of Santiago de Compostela, Spain   A. Carracedo

Acknowledgement

The editors want to thank all the authors that contributed to this book. We all know how hard it is, on top of daily casework, to find time for scientific writing. Their investment in this work is highly appreciated.

A special thanks to Melody Gut, secretary at the head office of the University Center of Legal Medicine Lausanne-Geneva who guaranteed the administrative workload of this project.

We also want to thank the numerous professionals working in the Institutes of Legal Medicine: you all indirectly contributed to this book. Indeed, every case shows the complex interaction among specialists of different fields that are necessary to build a medico-legal investigation. This essential aspect of our work is at the heart of the scientific outputs detailed in this book.

Contents

Introduction

1

Silke Grabherr, Sarah Heinze, and Tony Fracasso

Since the discovery of X-rays by Wilhelm Conrad Röntgen in 1895, medicine has lived a revolution that influenced all of its disciplines. The sudden possibility to have a glimpse inside of the human body without incising it opened new ways in medical examining and diagnostics. Today, modern medicine without imaging has become unthinkable. Radiological methods are used to perform diagnosis, to prepare surgical interventions, to follow the state of a patient and even for treatment in the context of radiotherapy and angiographic interventions.

It is evident that radiology has also influenced forensic and legal medicine. Already 1 year after Röntgen's discovery, first post-mortem images were made, and Charles Thurstan Holland, a pioneer in the early days of radiology, started to collect radiographs of hands of idividuals at the age form 1 year upwards to obtain knowledge of skeletal age and the observable changes on X-rays. He also used X-rays for the non-invasive exami-

nation of ancient Egyptian mummies and of stillborn babies and foetuses [1].

Although X-rays were used regularly in forensic medicine, especially to detect foreign bodies such as projectiles, most authors agree that the era of modern forensic imaging started with the development of multi-detector computed tomography and its use in 'virtual autopsy', especially the with the creation of the Center of Forensic Imaging and Virtopsy in Bern, Switzerland [2]. Although it is clear that this group did not invent forensic Imaging, it was the first time that a specific research group consisting of radiologists and forensic pathologists was dedicated specifically to the systematic investigation of advantages and limitations of conventional autopsy and modern imaging methods. Additionally to techniques of medical imaging, other methods of digital imaging were applied with the aim to digitalise the body of deceased and render it accessible for digital treatment. Therefore, techniques such as digital photogrammetry and 3D-surface scanning including structured light techniques or laser scanning techniques were added as tools to the forensic imaging set-up.

As medicine and techniques are developing rapidly, the science of forensic imaging is subject to regular upgrade of knowledge. Many developments are in accordance with clinical imaging or at least similar to it. But the use of technology coming from industrial developments leads to

S. Grabherr (✉) · T. Fracasso
Geneva University Hospitals and University of Geneva, University hospital of Vaud, University of Lausanne, University Center of Legal Medicine Lausanne-Geneva, Geneva, Switzerland
e-mail: silke.grabherr@chuv.ch;
tony.fracasso@hcuge.ch

S. Heinze
Diagnostic and Research Institute of Forensic Medicine, Medical University of Graz, Graz, Austria
e-mail: sarah.heinze@medunigraz.at

significant difference in knowledge concerning the methodology applied.

Also in terms of investigated cases, important difference can be seen between clinical and forensic imaging. Indeed, the question asked in forensic cases differs very much from those in clinical radiology. This leads to the fact that for the analysis of the obtained images, the interest is different between the two fields. While clinical radiology is focused to answer questions of diagnosis and treatment, forensic radiology has a reconstructive question. By analysing the images, the physician wants to know what has happed to a person and when, what could be the mechanism of a trauma, and in which circumstances lesions were created. By viewing the images, the investigator wants to get answers concerning what has happed in the past and not to what shall be the future of a patient. Therefore, we can say that forensic radiology is a kind of retrospective analysis, while clinical radiology aims a prospective evaluation of a patient (Fig. 1.1).

Additionally to the difference of the temporal approach for the reading (retrospective or prospective analysis), the focus of the interest differs between forensic and clinical interpretation of the images. Indeed, as the clinical investigation aims to orientate treatment, clinical radiologists are essentially focused on findings that indicate a necessary treatment. They are not used to report findings of no or small medical interest, such as small infiltrations in the subcutaneous tissue. For the forensic pathologist however, such findings may be of utmost interest, as such a finding can indicate an impact in the context of a blunt trauma, for example. Therefore, it is important to report and recognise as the location of an impact helps to reconstruct the event (impact of a hit during a physical aggression, impact of the vehicle on a pedestrian in a case of traffic accident, etc.).

The focus of the forensic radiological reading is orientated according to the forensically relevant questions, which are in general those indicated in Fig. 1.1 (What? Who? When? How?), but which can also vary depending on the investigated case. For example, if the identity of the examined corpses is unknown or unclear, a special attention has to be given to parameters that might allow its identification (such as specific pathologies, medical implants, stigmata of surgery, anatomical variants). Also, a special regard to bone structures allowing age estimation might be indicated and those might even need special scanning protocols in order to display them in a resolution high enough for anthropological analysis.

Specific questions also need knowledge in forensic medicine. For example, in order to

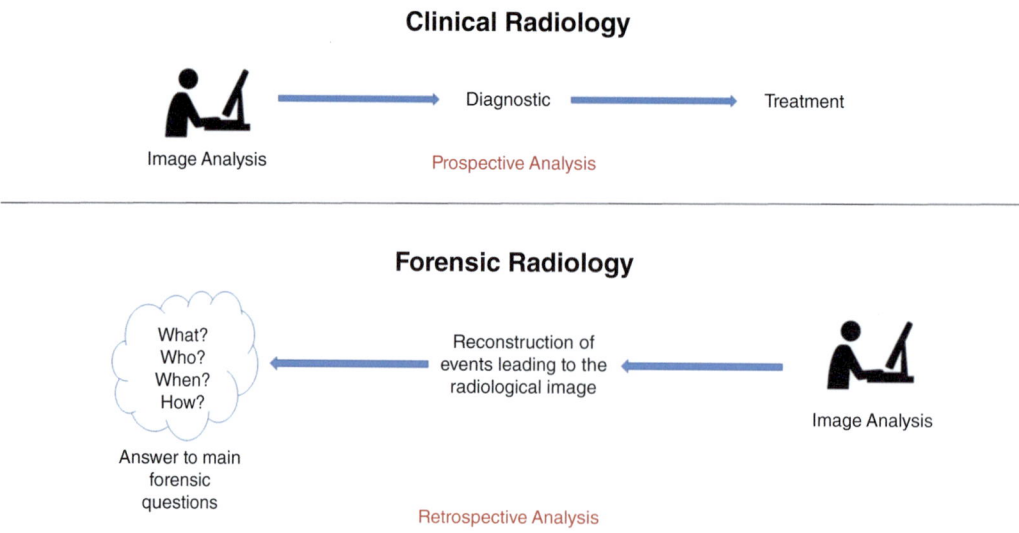

Fig. 1.1 Difference of the clinical approach and the forensic approach of radiological image analysis

examine a case of lethal gunshot trauma, it is important to know basics about wound ballistic, to be able to recognise entry and exit wound and to reconstruct the bullet trajectory.

For some questions, specific scanning protocols might be necessary, which imply high resolution of specific structures (e.g. cranial sutures for anthropological investigations), or the visualisation of regions that might normally not be necessarily in the focus of the radiological image (e.g. skin of the back in a case of stabbing to reconstruct the trajectory of the knife). In order to visualise regions or structures that are normally not of interest in clinical radiology, it is important to adapt not only the technical parameters of the imaging unit but also the position of the examined corpse or person (e.g. ventral positioning). In some cases, even the application of radiologically visible markers may be necessary, especially if a link should be achieved between internal lesions and marks that are visible on the skin without seeing them in the radiological image (e.g. traces of wheels in a person that was run over by a car).

The need of specific protocols for the image acquisition is therefore the biggest limitation in cases when clinically performed images should be reinterpreted for medico-legal questions. Here we often see cases in which the forensically most interesting part is not registered on the images (e.g. the scalp in cases of blunt trauma to the head). Still, a reinterpretation of such clinically acquired images by forensically trained experts is of high benefit as it permits to obtain additional information. An example is the reinterpretation of a CT scan of the facial bones in case of blunt trauma to the head. The orientation of fragments of a nasal bone fracture or other fractions of the face may allow the forensic expert to differentiate between a fall and a punch when confronting the fracture's morphology to the description of the victim and/or the supposed perpetrator. The use of CT data acquired in the emergency department is also essential for examining survived sharp and ballistic trauma. Often these images are the only data that are available before any manipulation of the lesions during emergency surgery.

The most evident reason why forensic radiology needs specific experience and knowledge is the fact that post-mortem changes appear rapidly after death. As scientific papers recently have shown, first artefacts due to the appearance of gas bubbles happen already some hours after death [3]. Although the presence of gas is the most striking and evident post-mortem artefact, many other artefacts due to post-mortem changes have been described in the literature [4]. Some cases are especially sensitive to post-mortem changes, and they need clearly specific knowledge in order to recognise them as such. Best examples are cases of putrefied bodies [5] and charred bodies [6].

For all these reasons, the interpretation of image data in the context of forensic imaging needs experience and special training. Most centres have created collaborations between forensic pathologists and radiologists in order to organise common reading sessions, or use the help of radiologists with specific training. In some centres and countries, forensic pathologists are used to read forensic imaging data since the very beginning of their postgraduate training, and platforms exist that shall help to allow such training even if the centre does not have access to own imaging units [7]. Whatever the solution is, knowledge of the specific aspects of forensic imaging is important. An overview of major specificities of forensic radiology compared to clinical radiology is given in Table 1.1.

As forensic medicine is the discipline investigating violent death or sudden death that might be suspected to be violent, a main interest of forensic imaging is the analysis of cases of trauma. This applies not only to deceased persons but also to victims that survived such trauma. The interpretation of radiological data of trauma victims needs not only knowledge in radiological reading but also some basic knowledge of different specialities related to forensic medicine such as traumatology, biomechanics, ballistics, etc. For this reason, this book, which is dedicated to forensic imaging in trauma, is structured in a way that it allows the reader to obtain knowledge of these important elements.

Table 1.1 Aspects specific for forensic radiology that are not common in clinical radiology

Specificity	In which case	Consequence
No motion artefacts	All post-mortem cases	Less artefacts and increase in image quality
High radiation dose possible	All post-mortem cases	Increase in image quality (resolution)
Specific questions for the reconstruction of the incident (e.g. reconstruction of trajectory, age estimation, identification, etc.)	All cases	Adapted scanning protocol necessary, adapted image reconstruction necessary, knowledge of forensic pathology necessary
Importance of lesions on the body surface	Traffic accidents, sharp trauma, ballistic trauma	Application of radiologically visible landmarks
Post-mortem changes	All post-mortem cases (increasing with post-mortem interval)	Knowledge of thanatology necessary

If forensic imaging should be applied in trauma cases, it is also important to know which imaging modality is the most convenient to document and investigate the specific case. For this reason, this book contains also a first part (Chap. 2) giving some basic knowledge about the different forensic imagining techniques. For each technique the main advantages and limitations are summarised in a clearly laid out table, and the main applications and indications are given.

The second part of the book is structured in specific chapters concerning the different types of trauma that are regularly encountered in forensic and legal medicine:

– Blunt trauma
– Sharp trauma
– Ballistic trauma
– Traffic accidents
– Asphyxia
– Thermic trauma
– Explosion

Each chapter is built up using the same schema. First a short introduction including the basic knowledge about the type of trauma is given; then, the most suited imaging methods for its investigation are indicated. Finally it is explained how the trauma type can be recognised, how its consequences should be described and interpreted, and what can be done to correctly reconstruct the medico-legal case. As this book is focused on forensic imaging, it has to be mentioned that it is not meant to replace textbooks for clinical radiology nor for forensic pathology. It shall simply indicate the main aspects of evaluation of trauma in forensic imaging and help the reader to understand what the important issues are in this special field.

References

1. Thomas AMK. Postmortem imaging: development and historical review. In: Grabherr S, Grimm JM, Heinemann A, editors. Atlas of postmortem angiography. Springer; 2016.
2. Dirnhofer R, Jackowski C, Vock P, Potter K, Thali MJ. Virtopsy: minimally invasive, imaging-guided virtual autopsy. Radiographics. 2006;26:1305–33.
3. Egger C, Bize P, Vaucher P, Mosimann P, Schneider B, Dominguez A, Meuli R, Mangin P, Grabherr S. Distribution of artifactual gas on post-mortem multidetector computed tomography (MDCT). Int J Legal Med. 2012;126(1):3–12.
4. Andrews SW. Postmortem changes as documented in postmortem computed tomography scans. Acad Forensic Pathol. 2016;6(1):63–76.
5. Cartocci G, Santurro A, Neri M, Zaccagna F, Catalano C, La Russa R, Turillazzi E, Panebianco V, Frati P, Fineschi V. Post-mortem computed tomography (PMCT) radiological findings and assessment in advanced decomposed bodies. Radiol Med. 2019;124(10):1018–27.
6. de Bakker HM, Roelandt GHJ, Soerdjbalie-Maikoe V, van Rijn RR, de Bakker BS. The value of post-mortem computed tomography of burned victims in a forensic setting. Eur Radiol. 2019;29(4):1912–21.
7. Heinze S, Grunert S, Grabherr S, Labudde D, Arbeitsgemeinschaft Forensische Bildgebung (AGFB) der Deutschen Gesellschaft für Rechtsmedizin (DGRM). Erstellung und Etablierung einer wissensbasierten Fallsammlung für forensische Bildgebung— WiFas. Rechtsmedizin. 2020;30:71–8.

Anastasia Tsaklakidis, Lorenzo Campana,
Gregorz Teresinski, Virginie Magnin,
and Silke Grabherr

2.1 Conventional X-Ray

Anastasia Tsaklakidis

Like visible light, gamma and X-rays are electromagnetic waves. These waves differ in their length and energy—the shorter the wave, the higher its energy. For example, the waves of visible light have a length of 400–780 nm, whereas the way shorter high energetic waves of gamma and X-rays range from 1 pm to 10 nm. Additionally, these high energetic rays, in con-

A. Tsaklakidis (✉)
Institute of Forensic and Traffic Medicine, University Hospital Heidelberg, Heidelberg, Germany
e-mail: Anastasia.Tsaklakidis@med.uni-heidelberg.de

L. Campana · V. Magnin
Unit of Forensic Imaging and Anthropology, University Center of Legal Medicine Lausanne-Geneva, University of Lausanne, University Hospital Vaud, Lausanne, Switzerland
e-mail: lorenzo.campana@chuv.ch;
virginie.magnin@chuv.ch

G. Teresinski
Department of Forensic Medicine, Medical University of Lublin, Lublin, Poland
e-mail: grzegorzteresinski@umlub.pl

S. Grabherr
Geneva University Hospitals and University of Geneva, University Hospital of Vaud, University of Lausanne, University Center of Legal Medicine, Lausanne-Geneva, Geneva, Switzerland
e-mail: silke.grabherr@chuv.ch

trast to others, are able to dissolve an electron from its atom, the so-called ionization. While gamma rays arise out of radioactive decay, X-rays are produced by decelerating fast-moving electrons suddenly.

The X-ray tube is an energy converter, which contains a cathode and an anode and which converts electric energy into electromagnetic radiation. When the cathode, a wire usually made of tungsten, receives energy and is heated up to 2000 °C, an electron cloud or space charge develops around it, and these negatively charged electrons are accelerated. This process at the cathode filaments is called thermionic emission.

After being accelerated the electrons reach the positively charged anode on the other side of the tube, collide, and interact with it. The positively charged anode is either stationary or rotating and usually made of copper, tungsten, or molybdenum and converses the received electron energy into radiation. There are two main ways X-rays are produced at the anode, both by interactions of the decelerated electron with the atom: the characteristic radiation and bremsstrahlung. Characteristic radiation is the consequence of the collision of the cathode's electron with a K-shell electron of the anode. The K-shell electron is ejected from its place, and to stabilize the atom's shells again, this gap is filled up with an electron from an outer shell. This electron from the outer shell emits, when changing its position, its energy as electromagnetic radiation, also called characteristic photon. But more often X-rays are emitted as bremsstrahlung. When the accelerated electrons travel right next to a nucleus at the anode, they get decelerated by the positively charged atomic nucleus immediately. This interaction leads to an emission of the kinetic energy in the form of X-ray photons, more specifically in bremsstrahlung.

When the electrons decelerate at the anode, energy is released in different ways, but mostly as heat and just for a very small amount as X-rays. For example, at 100 kVp (kilovoltage peak), the ratio is just 1% X-rays but 99% heat. In general, the number and energy of X-rays depend on the amount of kVp and also the mAs (milliampere-seconds), which is used in activating the tube. Increasing the mAs increases the number of electrons and consequently of X-rays as well. Increasing the kVp increases the electron energy and consequently the X-ray energy.

The outer shell of the X-ray tube is the tube housing, usually made out of metal, mainly plumb, which avoids an uncontrolled exit of the X-rays outside the tube and allows the exit just at the exit window. In addition, the exit window can be adjusted in its shape and size by a collimator. The X-rays, which exit the tube through the window, are called primary rays, and after being adjusted by the shutter, which is made out of lead lamellas, the X-rays are called usable radiation. Additionally, to visualize the area, which is going to be examined, a lamp is installed, and its beam, which is directed on the patient, corresponds to the settings of the X-ray beam.

The further components inside the housing are in another casing, usually made out of glass, which contains the anode and cathode in an air-free vacuum, so corrosion and oxidation of the unit can be avoided. Usually in medical radiology, the anode is rotating and not stationary, whereas an induction motor rotates the rotor on which the anode is assembled. By rotating the anode heats up less and in addition the anode can be made out of different materials, so its thermic qualities can be improved as well [1].

The tube's generator generates the desired high voltage between 30 and 150 kV.

The X-ray tube is installed in the examination room with a support system. The exit window of the tube is directed toward the patient and the X-ray table. The X-ray table may be stationary, with a floating top or tilting. Furthermore, the X-ray console or control panel as a part of the imaging system is used by the examiner, where the desired parameters and exposure factors can be entered.

The phosphor-containing detector is placed underneath the patient, in computed radiography CR cassettes, and imaging plates are used. These cassettes are positioned either within the Bucky table or on the tabletop and scanned via laser inside the CR reader later on. Their image resolution is determined by the pixel size and the phosphor layer, whereas the higher resolution is reached with thinner layers. In direct radiography the image is directly or indirectly captured and transferred to the computer system directly. The used flat panel detectors can be differentiated in indirect and direct imaging, while indirect detectors convert X-rays first to light, then into the digital output signal, and direct detectors convert the photons without further intermediate steps right away into electricity and the output signal [2]. This process enables real-time applications and may decrease the required exposure and examination time.

The anti-scatter grid is placed between patient and detector. While passing the absorber or the patient, the X-rays and their photons may change their direction (scattering) while interacting with, e.g., free electrons in the patient, and transmit parts of their energy. This is called the Compton effect, which leads to reduced image contrast and clarity. To avoid that effect, an anti-scatter grid, containing lead, can be used to improve the image's quality.

Like in diagnostic radiology in forensic imaging, important information about a crime can be gained by conventional X-rays, whether it is revealing the extent of injuries, detecting metallic and some nonmetallic foreign objects, body packing, or skeletal surveys in cases of child abuse to detect and date fractures. Furthermore, X-rays of the jaw can help to identify a corpse or are part of age estimation like the X-ray of the left hand.

If a corpse has to be examined, radiation doesn't play a role, contrary to ante-mortem imaging, in which of course the ALARA (as low as reasonably achievable) principle has to be obeyed like in diagnostic radiology, when X-ray imaging is used.

2.2   Postmortem Computed Tomography (PMCT)

Anastasia Tsaklakidis

Computed tomography is a technique of cross-sectional imaging using X-rays, which was developed by Sir Godfrey N. Hounsfield in the 1960s and 1970s of the last century and established firmly in diagnostic and forensic radiology since then. A rotating X-ray tube, installed in a circular gantry, produces the fan beam of X-rays. Like in conventional X-ray, the following applies to computed tomography as well: the higher the kV, generated by the generator which produces the high voltage, the higher the energy of the X-ray beam and mainly heat is produced and just a small amount of X-rays. The facing detectors on the opposite side (up to third generation) in the gantry receive the X-ray photons after passing the scanned object and convert the attenuation measurements (especially the photoelectric and Compton effect take part in this process) into an electric signal. Then, this electric signal is converted by the data acquisition system (DAS) into a digital signal which is send to the computer. Afterward this is processed by the computer into multiple tiny cubes, so-called voxels. Out of these voxels, the cross-sectional images, also called slices, are constructed by the computer and can be displayed in 2D or reconstructed into 3D further on. While the 2D imaging is shown in a gray scale of Hounsfield units (HUs) to describe the object's density, 3D reconstructions can show color depending on the computer's software and the used medical image viewer. Values from −1024 HU up to 3071 HU can be saved, when 12-bit images are used. Hounsfield units (HUs) about 0 HU present water, about −100 HU fat, about −1000 HU air, 60–90 HU fresh blood, up to 1000 HU bone, and about 3000 HU metal. The higher the HU's value, the "whiter" the image on the monitor, and the object is described as hyperdense, whereas objects with lower HUs and "blacker" appearance are described as hypodense. Due to the fact that the human eye is able to differentiate only 20–80 gray scales, the images are presented in different windows, for example, bone, soft tissue, and lung window. For the exact value, a software's HU measuring tool can be used.

In a helical scan, the table moves continuously through the gantry while the gantry is rotating and scanning the patient. In fourth-generation CT, just the generator is rotating, while the detectors build in a 360° circle are stationary.

The detector system contains multiple usually solid-state crystal scintillation detectors. The first scanner was a single-slice scanner with one row. Nowadays multi-slice scanners of the third generation with 32, 64, or 128 detector rows are in daily use. For example, in a 128-row multidetector scanner, 128 slices can be scanned with just one rotation. Furthermore, the name of helical scanners is composed of the detector rows: single slice, dual slice, or multi-slice [3].

Besides the known one source computed tomography, dual-source CT scanners are in use as well. These contain, instead of one, two X-ray tubes, which work on different energy levels—one producing low kVp X-rays and another producing high kVp X-rays. The advantage of this technique is the possibility of creating a spectrum of the attenuation inside the scanned object and thus getting a densitometry and spectroanalysis of the examined area for further definition and analysis of the scanned tissue. Bone or foreign bodies, for example, metallic objects, can be differentiated better than in a regular CT scan.

Some helpful terms:

1. Dimensions

    The used three planes in computed tomography are the X-, Y-, and Z-plane. The x-axis corresponds to the horizontal axis, crosswise to the patient table, the y-axis is the slice's vertical axis, and the z-axis as the third dimension corresponds to the orientation of the examination table.

2. Field of view (FOV)

   The scanned area of interest, which should be adapted in its size as small as possible to improve its resolution. In addition, the patient dose decreases as well, when a smaller FOV is chosen, which is only relevant for ante-mortem imaging.

3. Collimation/filtration/automatically adjusted tube current

   Collimators, made out of tungsten or molybdenum, are installed between the X-ray tube and the patient or on the detector side. These are used to adjust and shape the X-ray beam to improve resolution and reduce signal contributions, which are caused by scatter radiation. The size of their opening can be adjusted to the desired slice width and slice thickness. Furthermore, because photons with low energy do not contribute significantly to the relevant detector signal, but increase the patient dose, they can be removed by filtration with, e.g., tin filters as well [4].

   Another optional technique for some scanner is the modulation of the organ exposure. The X-ray exposure of sensitive parts like the breast and thyroid gland can be reduced by reducing the tube current automatically during the scan of the defined area, which should be protected [5].

4. Pitch

   Pitch is defined as table feed (mm) per 360° rotation/number of detector rows x slice collimation (mm). A pitch of 1 is defined if table feed and collimation are identical. The pitch's value can be changed manually. In some scanners when the pitch is increased, the mAs increases automatically as well whereas radiation remains unchanged [5].

5. VRT and MIP

   Volume-rendering technique (VRT) and maximum intensity technique (MIP) are 3D and volume visualization tools in post-processing the generated CT data. MIPs are especially helpful for a detailed vivid visualization of vessels and VRT as a reconstruction tool especially for bones [3].

6. $CTDI_{vol}$ and DLP

   Volume-associated CT dose index, measured in mGy, describes the patient's average local dose, is standardized, and enables the comparison of the examination radiation of different scanners. Furthermore, it shows the influence of adjustable parameters like pitch, mAs, kVp, etc. The abbreviation DLP stands for dose length product, which is a product of $CTDI_{vol}$ and the length of the whole scan and measures the total energy the patient is exposed to. $DLP = CTDI_{vol} \times L$ (mGy × cm). Both values are calculated and displayed in the documentation of every scan [3].

In ante-mortem imaging, the ALARA (as low as reasonably achievable) principle has to be obeyed in every examination which is based on X-rays. In postmortem imaging instead, the exposure of radiation doesn't play a role, so voltage and tube power can be increased to minimize background noise. In postmortem imaging there is no need of restriction of the scanned area to an area of interest, and the whole body should be scanned. For more detailed imaging, especially of small parts, an additional scan with a small field of view (FOV) should be performed. Bigger metallic objects should be removed before scanning to avoid bigger artifacts. If available, a special software for metal artifact reduction should be used as well to increase the expressiveness of the body scan and improve the evaluation, especially if trajectories and projectiles have to be identified after a gunshot. Because of the corpse's rigidity, the position can differ from the usual straight supine position like in ante-mortem imaging. Whether contrast media is used or not, image reconstructions using a bone, lung, and soft tissue window have to be done. To guarantee the possibility of further reconstructions later on or 3D prints and to ensure a detailed evaluation, 1-mm reconstructions of the scan should be saved as well. Often more information and details can be detected if contrast media are used, but many important results can be evaluated native as well—e.g., corticalis blast fractures of burned corpses, localization and morphology of multi-fragmental fractures and in-driven fragments, abnormal gas collections, foreign bodies, or hematomas (especially detectable in fatty tissue) and hemorrhage.

2.3 Postmortem Angiography

Silke Grabherr and Virginie Magnin

Since the very beginning of medical science, the analysis of the vascular system remained a challenge for physicians for two main reasons: firstly, to understand its anatomy, which is full of variants, and secondly to understand its pathology. For this reason, during the seventeenth and eighteenth centuries, pioneers such as Graaf, Ruysch, and Lower started to work on techniques that allowed filling the vascular system in order to render it visible [6]. One of the most famous physicians in this field was Virchow in the nineteenth century [7].

In the beginning, the visualization of the vessels was achieved by injecting substances that would harden after their injection, producing so-called vascular casts once the surrounding tissue was removed. This could be done by using different chemical maceration substances or simply by leaving the tissue to maggots that would clean it up eventually. Injected substances were wax, metals with low melting temperature, later celluloid and celloidin, and finally nylon, neoprene latex, and silicon rubber [8].

With the discovery of X-rays, radio-opaque substances were added to the different injection materials. Except for anatomy studies, the injection of those substances and their nondestructive visualization eventually replaced the use of casting methods. According to the injected liquids, mainly six different groups **of classic methods** could be divided [6]:

- Corpuscular preparations prepared in watery solution
- Corpuscular preparations prepared in gelatin or agar
- Oily liquids
- Hydrosoluble preparations
- Casts
- Miscellaneous

Although modern cross-sectional imaging methods, especially MDCT (multidetector computed tomography), lead to a real revolution in medical imaging, the vascular system remains a "black spot" of the human body. For this reason, methods had to be developed that render visible the lumen of the vessels in order to allow diagnosis of vascular pathologies such as stenosis, occlusions, partial or complete ruptures, and any other pathological or anatomical variations of the vascular system. While in clinical radiology the injection of contrast agent for visualizing the lumen of vessels and contrasting the parenchyma of organs is applied regularly, modern postmortem angiography (PMA) is a technique which is only used in well-equipped centers with a rather long experience in forensic imaging. Even in those centers, PMA is often restricted to specific cases. Latest research also lead to the development of PMA combined with MRI [9]. But those approaches are still in development and do not play a role in the daily routine until now.

Today, different techniques of modern PMA exist which show differences concerning the injection method, the injection site, the injected liquid, and the extent of the perfused vessels [10]. Mainly, whole-body angiographic methods have to be distinguished from targeted angiography methods, which aim to visualize only a part of the vascular system (mostly the coronary arteries) or selected vessels. The most often used **modern methods of PMA** can be divided into five different approaches [11]:

- Postmortem whole-body angiography using aqueous contrast agent (mostly mixed with polyethylene glycol)
- Targeted coronary postmortem computed tomography angiography
- Postmortem computed tomography angiography using cardiopulmonary resuscitation
- Multiphase postmortem computed tomography angiography
- Miscellaneous
- Those techniques find their application in **different postmortem investigations** mainly in:
  - Anatomy (understanding vascular morphology)
  - Clinical pathology (finding pathological changes in the vessels)
  - Forensic pathology (detecting traumatic lesions in the vessels)

In forensic medicine, PMA is mostly used to investigate cases of trauma (blunt trauma, sharp trauma, ballistic trauma) [12], sudden cardiac death [13], or death after medical intervention [14]. Numerous articles show the advantages of the different PMA methods compared to conventional autopsy [15]. It is considered as the method of choice for investigating the vascular system after death, especially if the exact source of bleeding shall be located [16] (Fig. 2.1). It can also lead sampling for histopathology [17]. Thanks to the perfusion of inner organs, it also increases the diagnostic value of postmortem imaging compared to native PMCT, for example,

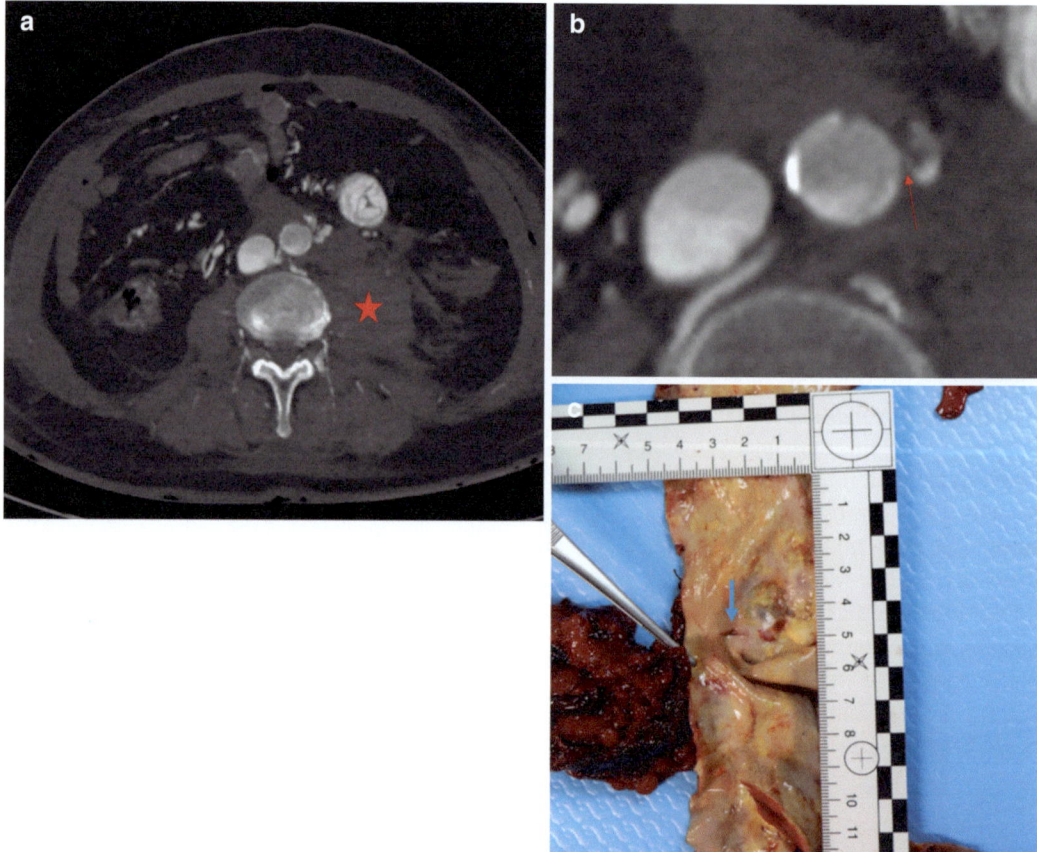

Fig. 2.1 MPMCTA dynamic phase (**a**, **b**), highlighting the exact source of bleeding (red arrow), from an aortic surgical lesion visible on the autopsy section (**c**) (blue arrow). Hemoretroperitoneum (red star)

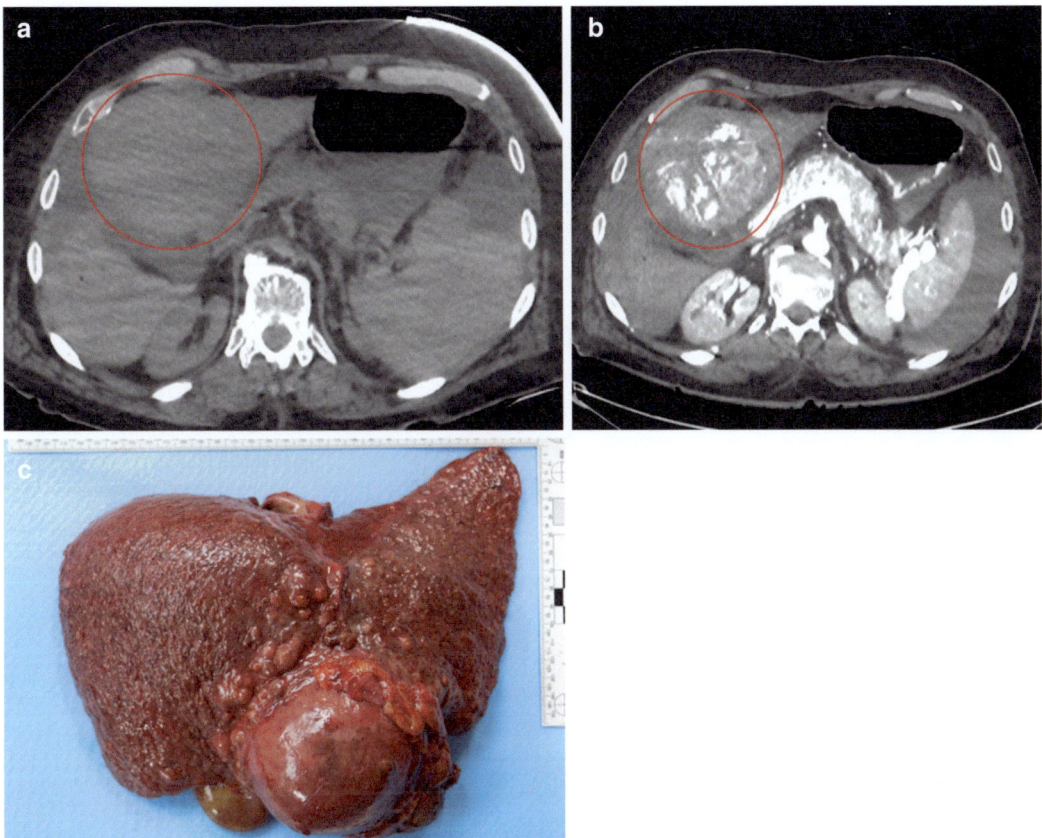

Fig. 2.2 The increase of postmortem diagnostic value after injection of contrast agent. Native CT (**a**), arterial phase (**b**) showing a nodular lesion in the liver paren-chyma (red ellipses) hardly seen on the native CT, well perfused during PMCTA (**b**) and confirmed at autopsy (**c**)

the detection of lesion(s) of plain organs [15, 18] (Fig. 2.2).

No matter which technique is used, it is important to underline that any injection of contrast agent means an important manipulation of the body. Especially in forensic cases, this fact has to be considered and implies a documentation of every step that is done. A standardized protocol, which has been validated via a multicenter study on a huge number of cases, is ideal. However, the only method that fulfills this criterion today is the method of multiphase postmortem computed tomography angiography (MPMCTA) [18] which was developed in the University Center of

Legal Medicine in Lausanne-Geneva and validated by the Technical Working Group of Post-mortem Angiography Methods (TWGPAM) [19] via a multicenter study performed in eight European centers [20].

2.3.1 PMA for Investigating Trauma Cases

For investigating cases of trauma, especially polytrauma, most adequate techniques are whole-body angiography techniques. As mentioned above, the most studied and most often applied

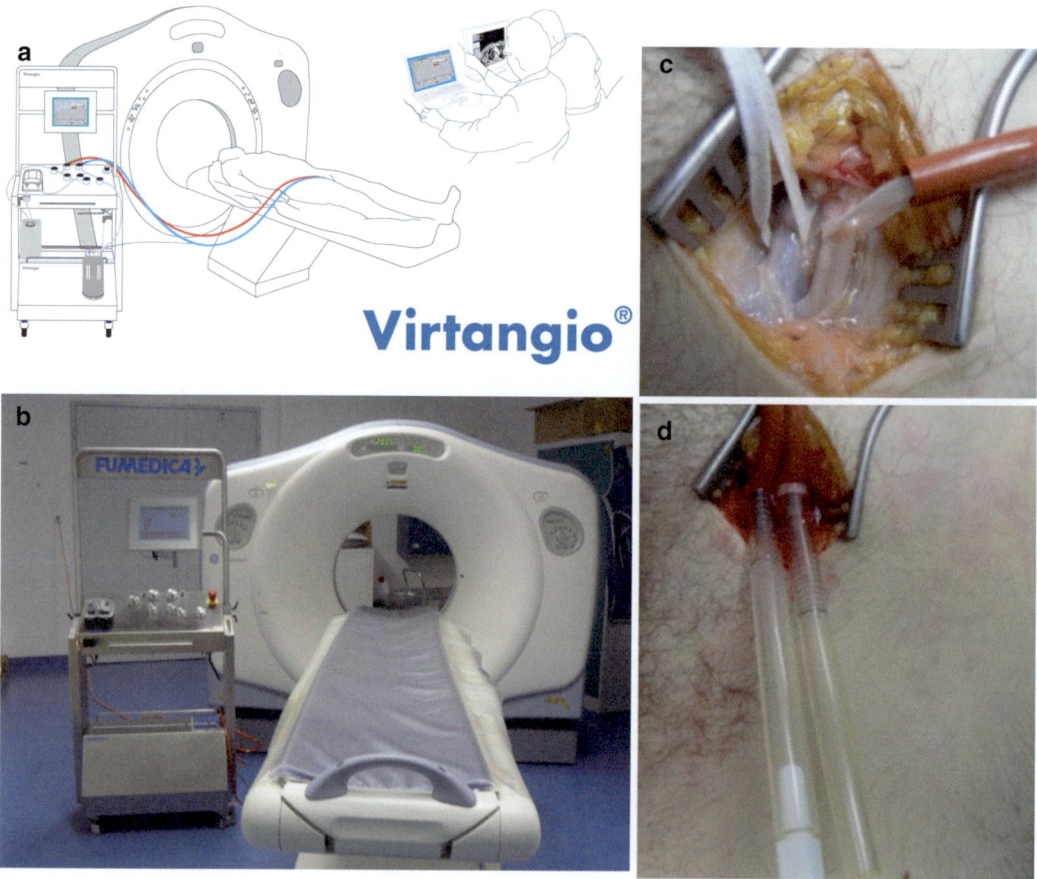

Fig. 2.3 MPMCTA technique: (**a**) Schema as proposed by FUMEDICA. (**b**) Set up using a MDCT scanner and the Virtangio perfusion device, (**c**) femoral artery and vein ready for cannulation, (**d**) cannulas inserted into the femoral artery and vein

Fig. 2.4 MPMCTA standardized protocol for the injection of a mixture of paraffin oil and Angiofil®

MPMCTA Multiphase post mortem CT angiography
Standard protocol

• Parameters:

    • 1200 ml For the arterial phase   in 1 min 30"   (~1/s)
    • 1800 ml For the venous phase   in 2 min 15"   (~13cc/s)
    • 500 ml For the dynamic phase in 2 min 30"   (~3cc/s)

method is MPMCTA (Figs. 2.3 and 2.4). By performing three different phases of angiography after the native MDCT scan prior to any manipulation of the body, it can be applied without any problem on bodies that are the object of forensic investigations. While the native CT scan permits a detailed analysis of the extent of skeletal lesions (Fig. 2.5), the following arterial phase of angiography allows to detect lesions concerning the arteries of the head, thorax, and the abdomen, as well as the upper limbs and one lower limb (the one opposite the injection site or both lower limbs if both have been cannulated). The venous

phase adds information about eventual venous lesions (Fig. 2.6) while the last, so-called dynamic phase, is the one where most information can be gained concerning trajectories of sharp or ballistic trauma (Fig. 2.7).

As mentioned above, it is important to be aware of the advantages and inconveniencies of the PMA method that is applied. According to the injected contrast agent mixture, there can be interferences with additional methods such as histology [21], toxicological analysis [22], etc. Depending on the case, this has to be taken into account, and measures have to be taken accordingly [23] (such as sampling of body fluids for toxicological analysis before the injection of contrast agent, adaptation of the choice of injected contrast agent, etc.). Concerning the most often used mixture of paraffin oil and Angiofil®, it has to be mentioned that injection of this liquid interferes with the detection of fatty embolism. Therefore, two possibilities exist: either performing pulmonary biopsies prior to the injection of the contrast-agent mixture or using water-soluble iodinated contrast medium mixed with polyethylene glycol [24].

In summary, whole-body PMA, especially MPMCTA, is extremely useful for investigating cases of trauma. It permits to:

- Visualize arterial and venous hemorrhages (Fig. 2.6)
- Detect the exact source of bleeding (Fig. 2.1)
- Reconstruct and visualize intracorporeal trajectories (Fig. 2.7)
- Highlight any pre-existing vascular pathology
- Show any pre-existing vascular anomaly (anatomical variation (Fig. 2.8), modified vascular anatomy after surgery (Fig. 2.9), intravascular intervention (Fig. 2.10), etc.)

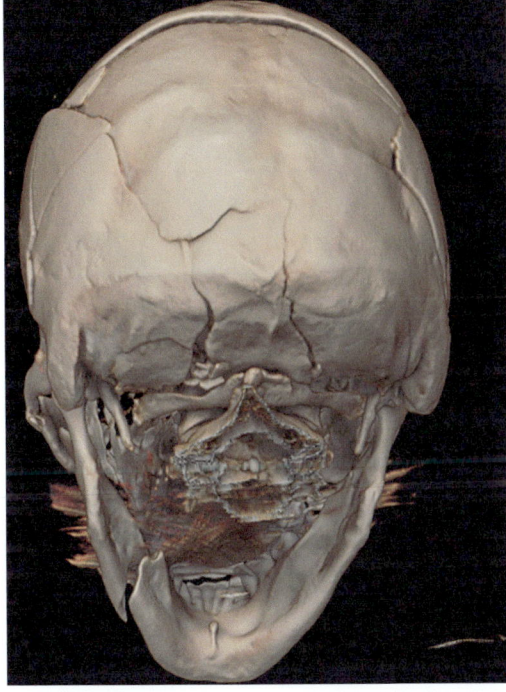

Fig. 2.5 Traumatic lesion of the skull base on a native post mortem CT

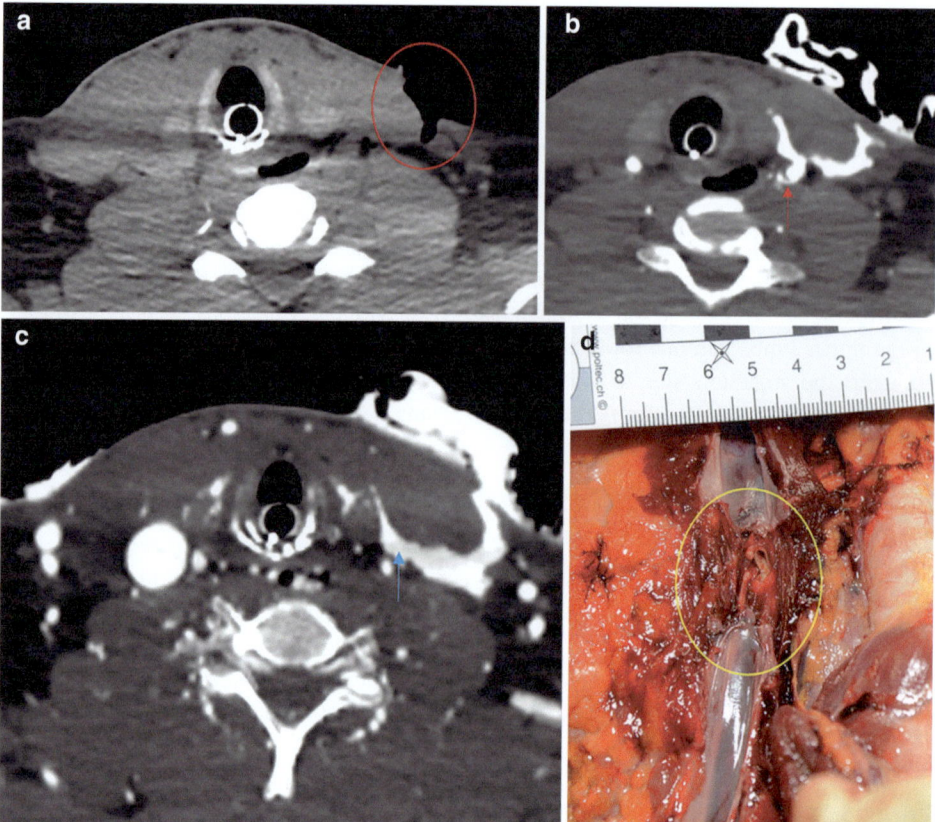

Fig. 2.6 Cervical lesion on native postmortem CT (**a**) red ellipse; arterial phase showing partial lesion to the carotid artery (**b**) red arrow; venous phase showing complete lesion to the jugular vein (**c**) blue arrow and the autopsy finding (**d**) confirming the CT findings (yellow ellipse)

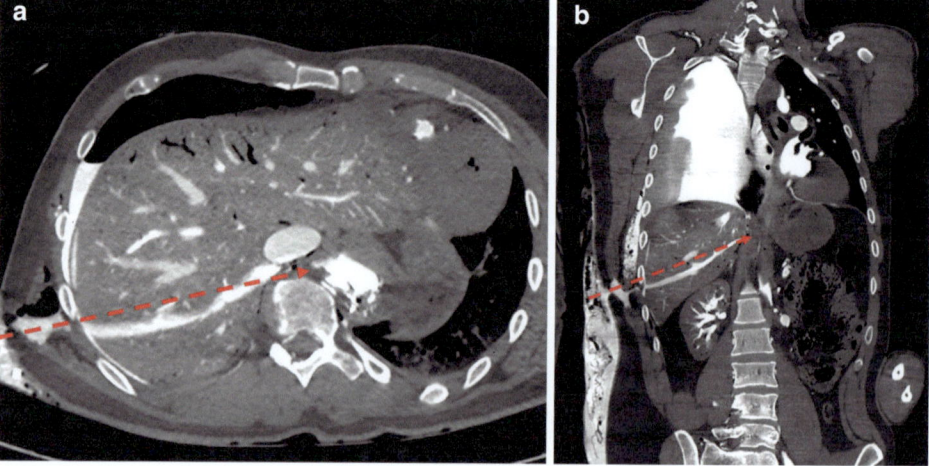

Fig. 2.7 Dynamic phase on axial plane (**a**) and coronal plane (**b**) highlighting the intracorporeal trajectory of a stab wound crossing the liver (red arrows)

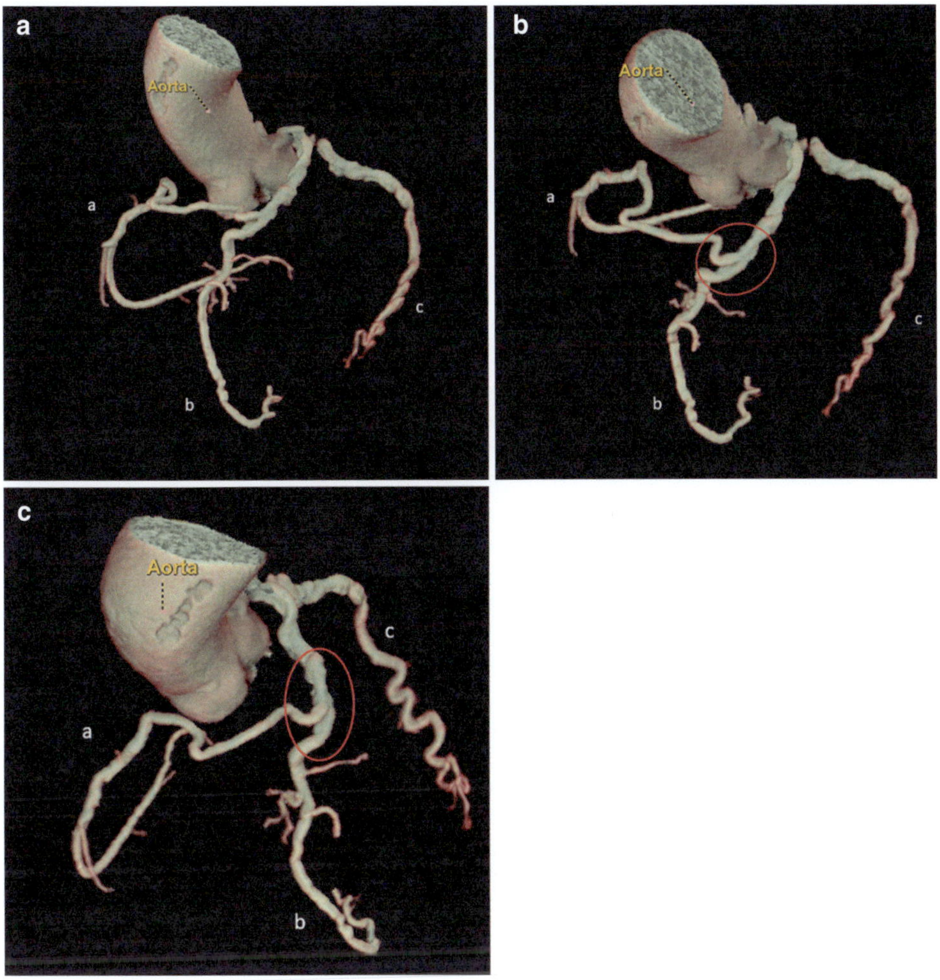

Fig. 2.8 3D reconstruction in arterial phase of the coronary artery vascular system showing anatomical variation of the right coronary artery arising from the left coronary artery (red ellipses). Right coronary artery (**a**), left ascending artery (**b**), and circumflex artery (**c**)

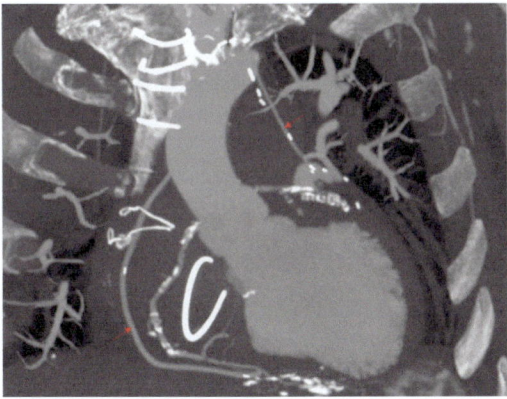

Fig. 2.9 Modification of the arterial system after multiple surgery. Coronal reconstruction MIP, arterial phase, showing different coronary bypass (red arrows)

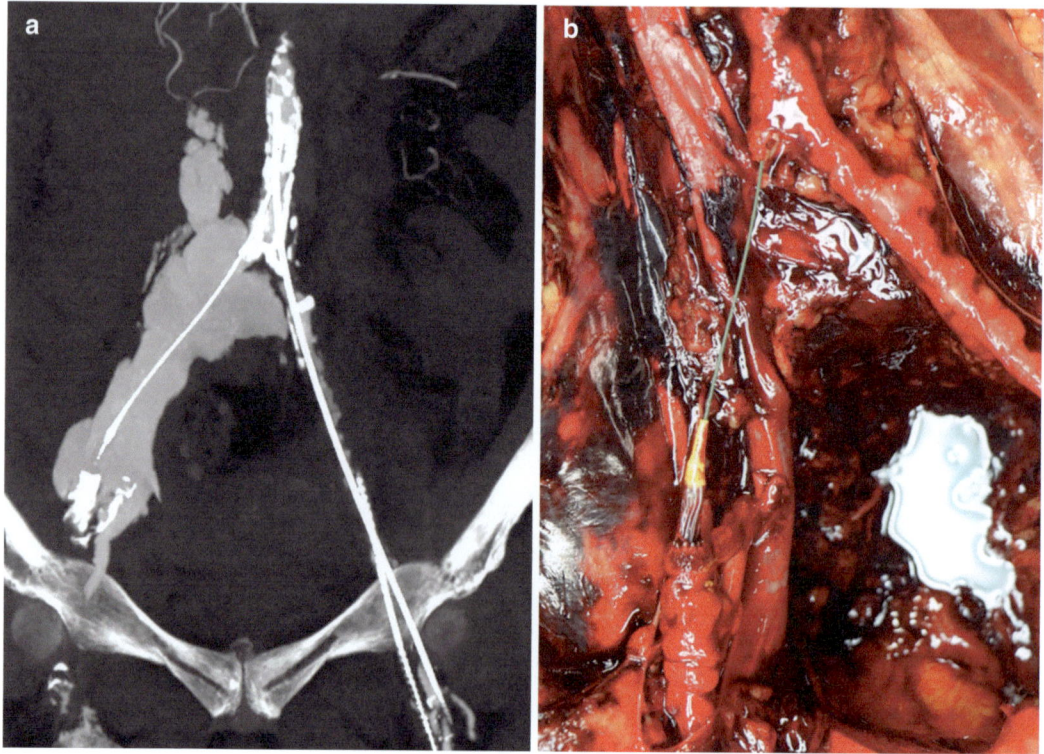

Fig. 2.10 Arterial intervention with intra-arterial catheter introduction in the iliac artery and vascular rupture. Coronal postmortem MPMCTA, arterial phase (**a**) and autopsy finding (**b**)

2.4 Postmortem Magnetic Resonance Imaging (PMMRI)

Anastasia Tsaklakidis

Magnetic resonance imaging is an established technique of cross-sectional imaging based on a strong magnetic field and radio waves, instead of X-ray. Especially alterations of soft tissues including the brain can be displayed with MRI perfectly. Injuries of soft tissue, brain damages; hematomas, e.g., after blunt force trauma; alterations after strangulation; and edema in bones, e.g., in cases of child abuse, can be enhanced and detected with this method. By acquiring 2D or 3D sequences, injuries, fractures, bleedings, or hematomas can be localized correctly and depending on the findings even classified and estimated more precise than by computed tomography in their etiology or age, e.g., if a bleeding or fracture is fresh or chronic.

Generally, the scanner consists of (listed from outside to inside) two tanks, one filled with nitrogen, which cools the liquid helium tank, one with liquid helium to make the coils supraconductive by cooling them near to absolute zero, the supraconductive magnet (so-called cryomagnet), gradient coils, and the radiofrequency (RF) transmitting coil(s) in a circular arrangement around the scanner's bore, in which the sliding patient table is assembled. Besides the integrated body coil and often integrated spine coil, mobile coils can be connected to the device for higher resolution, especially of smaller body parts. These mobile, separate coils are placed directly on the patient and connected to the device with a cable.

The supraconductive magnet produces the homogenous magnetic field ($B0$ field) and is cooled down to -269 °C by the helium, because at this temperature electricity flows without any resistance, so the magnet has to be charged just once to build up its magnetic field, when the scanner is installed or again when the helium is released from its tank. Often MRI scanners with magnets from 1.5 or 3 Tesla (T) are used. The gradient coils are arranged to build up gradients in the x-, y-, and z-axis. The additional magnetic gradients are required to achieve a different magnetic field inside the patient, which is used to localize the received signals in space. The RF coils send and receive the signals to and from the tissue. Often, the mobile coils are receiving and sending coils as well. The mostly used mobile coils are the head coil, a separate body coil, or knee or ankle coil.

Imaging is created by signals of high frequency in different intensity, emitted by the tissue. Basically, after the hydrogen protons of the examined object, which can be seen as small spinning bar magnets, are aligned by the main magnetic field ($B0$), they get deflected by a radiofrequency (RF) magnetic pulse. The frequency, the protons spin in the $B0$ field, is called procession or Larmor frequency. After being deflected protons want to return to their original aligned state. This process is called relaxation. While returning to their original state, different tissues emit different radiofrequencies because of their different content of water. This emission of energy is detectable by the scanner and then turned into an image by the computer. The T2 relaxation (spin-spin relaxation or transverse relaxation) is the expression of the chronological process, the proton needs to dephase while decreasing the magnetization in the transverse plane. T1 relaxation (spin-lattice relaxation time) is called the time the proton needs to finally realign in the main magnetic field ($B0$) again (radiopaedia.org). The relaxation process is described by tissue-specific time constants. T1 relaxation time is 300–2000 ms and T2 relaxation time 30–150 ms [25].

While in computed tomography imaging is described in its density, in MRI the term intensity of a signal is used. Hyperintense means a higher signal and looks "white" on the screen; hypoin-

tense has a lower signal and looks "black" on the screen. The signal's intensity and appearance depend on the tissue's parameters and the used sequence. For example, water appears white in T2 sequences and dark gray in T1 sequences.

Because of the variety of sequences, an in MRI-experienced radiologist should plan the protocol to avoid unnecessary long sequences, time loss, and burden for the patient. Besides the average used sequences in different examinations in ante-mortem imaging, a forensic useful sequence is a coronal T2 TIRM (turbo inversion recovery magnitude)/STIR (short tau inversion recovery) sequence to get the first overview about potential edemas by suppressing the signal of fat. This leads to a clearer signal of fluids and edema, for example, to detect fresh fractures or hematomas after strangulation. Furthermore, like in computed tomography, MRI examinations should always include at least one sequence in which every part of the scanned area, including the cutis, is captured (especially in brain and neck imaging). Furthermore, at least one thin-sliced sequence is helpful to guarantee a complete acquisition without any image gaps, and volume-interpolated 3D GRE sequences are helpful to allow 3D reconstructions. While evaluating the sequences, signal inhomogeneity, especially in the image's margin area, should be registered but not evaluated as a pathological finding mistakenly. Artifacts, you should be aware of, are moving and repetition artifacts in ante-mortem imaging, and in ante- and postmortem imaging folding and susceptibility artifacts.

As already mentioned, in postmortem MR imaging, movement and breathing or pulsation artifacts do not occur, but metallic artifacts, for example, caused by metallic splinters or ferromagnetic bullets, can reduce the examinations' quality like in ante-mortem imaging. Extracorporeal metallic objects should be removed before the scan. Heating effects have to be considered in postmortem imaging for other reasons than in ante-mortem imaging. Often the corpse, which is going to be examined, is cooled down to 4° in advance, which needs adaptions in the sequence programming. While the corpse warms or heats up, changes of the relaxation time occur further. So during the examination and the different used sequences, the tissue heats up and can change its appearance [26]. Gas bubbles in different tissues, bone, or vessels caused by autolysis have to be considered in the analysis of the sequences and should not be mistaken for air bubbles due to an injury or inflammation.

2.5 3D-Surface Documentation

Lorenzo Campana and Gregorz Teresinski

3D-surface documentation as a part of forensic imaging is becoming more and more important in the field of forensic medicine in the last years [27]. At the same time, its methods are developing very fast. They become from time to time faster and easier to apply, and always more forensic institutions apply different 3D documentation methods in their daily work. There are different methods and technics to perform the 3D acquisition of the surface of bodies (e.g., external injuries) or for other objects, and often the combination of various methods is helpful. 3D-surface documentation is useful in the following cases:

- Homicides (firearms, sharp trauma, blunt trauma)
- Traffic accidents:
  - Vehicle vs. pedestrian
  - Vehicle vs. cyclist
  - Vehicle vs. motorcyclist
  - Cyclist vs. pedestrian
  - Cyclist vs. motorcyclist
  - Motorcyclist vs. pedestrian
  - Cyclist vs. cyclist
  - Motorcyclist vs motorcyclist
  - Occupants of accident cars, if the driver has to be determined
  - To visualize the field of view of the driver
- Shaped injuries to be compared with an injury-causing instrument.
- Fractured bones if they have to be reconstructed or compared with an injury-causing instrument.

2.5.1 Methods

The methods of 3D acquisitions vary between expensive high-resolution structured light scanners over laser scanner to the less expensive photogrammetry technique. But every one of these techniques has its advantages and specific targets [28]. For the 3D acquisition of the body, CT scans are additionally used to create 3D models from the interior of the body (mainly the skeleton) and to combine them with the surface scan of the body [29].

2.5.1.1 3D-Surface Scanners
A high-resolution structured light scanner, for example, the ATOS scanner series from the company GOM (Fig. 2.11a), is heavy, time intensive,

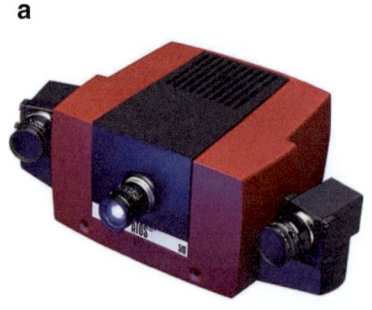
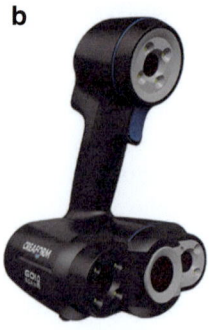
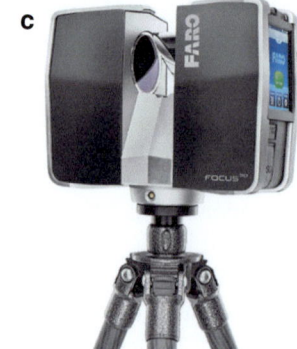

Fig. 2.11 Different types of 3D-surface scanner: (**a**) high-resolution structured light scanner; (**b**) handheld scanner; (**c**) laser scanner

and very sensible for movements. But it is possible to get details in the micromillimeter spectrum concerning the 3D geometry of an object [28, 30]. The scanner is fixed on a heavy stand. Scans are performed statically during some seconds for every view to the object. Several views have to be captured to get almost the whole object. With small objects it can be realized by using a turntable. During the capturing the scanner projects a fringe pattern on the object which is observed by two objectives on the left and on the right side of the projector. Thanks to the deformation of this fringe pattern, the software is able to calculate 3D coordinates for every pixel of the CCD sensor behind the objectives. Thus, every scan can produce millions of 3D points in the space, called point clouds. The software produces a so-called triangle mesh, by connecting the points with wires getting triangles. Every triangle gets a surface which makes the acquisition visible as a surface. This mesh can be exported as STL format, a universal 3D format. The disadvantage of this technology is that no color information is captured. But this can be solved with the fusion method described here under in "Fusion of data coming from different technologies."

Handheld white light scanners [28, 31] are much lighter devices which work similar to the aforementioned type of scanner with a projector and two or three cameras. The difference is that the acquisition procedure is more dynamic. The handheld device can be moved easily around the object during the capturing. It projects a structure like a QR code on the object and takes images from every camera in a high frequency (e.g., 550,000 images per second at the Go!SCAN 50 (Fig. 2.11b) and Go!SCAN 20 from Creaform). This makes the dynamic acquisition possible. At the same time, this is the reason why the accuracy and resolution is limited and lower compared to the static structure light scanner. The big advantages of the handheld scanner are that they are easy to use and fast and many of them have color recording included. Color-textured 3D models are usually exported in OBJ format which supports color information.

Laser scanners (Fig. 2.11c) coming from the surveying field are often used by the police to capture an accident or a crime scene in 3D [32]. It's a device fixed on a tripod, able to turn around its vertical axis and deviating a laser impulse with an oscillating mirror to capture its environment. Most of them use the time-of-flight method by measuring the time a laser impulse takes to come back and thereby calculating the distance. By choosing several different positions for the scanner, gaps of surfaces can be filled which were not visible for the scanner on previous positions. The resolution of such a terrestrial laser scanner is even lower than handheld scanner, but enough to get the environment of an accident or crime scene. The output of a laser scanner is also a point cloud which can be meshed with different software.

2.5.1.2 Photogrammetry

The less expensive way to get true to scale 3D models of the surface is the so-called photogrammetry [28, 33–36], because just a camera (ideally SLR) and a cheap software are needed. It is also a technology coming from the surveying field, which consists of taking photos of an object from different angles by respecting certain rules and camera parameters. In the past, creating 3D models based on this 2D photograph needed a long post-processing time by clicking manually on identical points on every image. Meanwhile high-performance algorithms were developed and implemented in photogrammetry software. After importing all images of a performed photogrammetry, the software will calculate step by step or fully automatically the 3D model of the captured object (Fig. 2.12). The biggest advantage of photogrammetry is the high quality concerning the colors of the 3D models. These are much better and more realistic than the colors acquired from a surface scanner. The accuracy concerning the 3D geometry depends on a lot of factors, for example, the knowledge and experience of the performer, the light circumstances, and if the object or things in the background are moving or not during the phototaking process. But the biggest difference makes

Fig. 2.12 Screenshot from the photogrammetry software. Visible are the positions from where every picture was taken related to the body, and a dense point cloud of the body surface

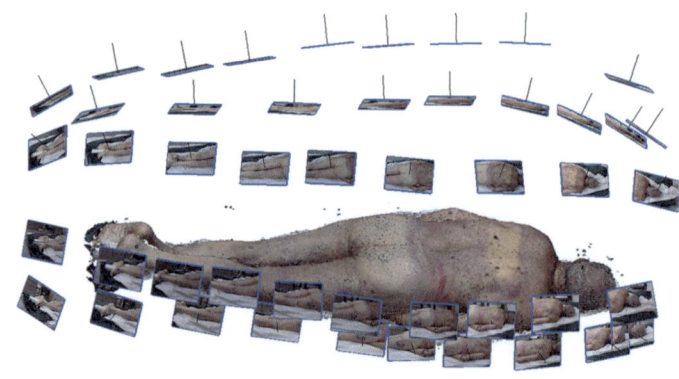

if the photos are taken manually one by one or taken all together with a lot of cameras at the same time with one shot [37–39]. In the latter case, movements between the images can be avoided, which can increase accuracy and bring close attention to detail. The disadvantage of photogrammetry is that there is no control during acquisition. Whereas with surface scanners the captured surfaces are displayed in real time on a screen, the result of the photogrammetry is only visible after the post-processing in the software. This can take some hours, and the object can meanwhile be not available anymore if the 3D reconstruction didn't work, and the 3D acquisition via photogrammetry has to be repeated.

2.5.1.3 Fusion of Data Coming from Different Technologies

Based on MDCT acquisition, relevant parts of the inside of the body can be segmented (often the skeleton) and be exported as well as STL file. This can be very useful with postmortem CT scans, if the acquisition of CT and 3D-surface is performed on the CT table. The body does not change posture and position between the two different acquisitions; this makes a fusion of the different data sets easier and more precise [29, 32, 40, 41]. A segmentation of the skin from the CT data can be used as reference for a best-fit alignment with the surface scan or photogrammetry data (Fig. 2.13). To benefit from every advantage of the two different surface-acquisition methods, it is recommended to perform both. Later the result of both acquisitions can be aligned by common reference points, and the high-quality color of the photogrammetry can be mapped on the high-quality surface of the surface scan.

The treated data of the skin aligned with the models coming from CT data can be placed virtually in the scene, coming from the laser scanning data of the crime or accident scene.

2.5.2 Working in the Virtual Crime or Accident Scene

Unfortunately a 3D model of the body is rigid. It's possible to move the extremities, but it's complicated [29, 42]. To facilitate the procedures, it is better to use a mannequin (called biped in some software) which can be adapted to the real dimensions of the body, with its articulations in the right place, and which can be moved anatomically correct (Fig. 2.14). To use nevertheless the scanned data, the wanted parts of the scan can be cut and linked to the corresponding elements of the mannequin. By moving the elements of the mannequin, the cut parts of the 3D models will follow the movements of mannequin elements (Fig. 2.15) [29, 32, 42].

In the virtual location, created based on the point cloud, coming from the laser scanner (often performed from the police or surveying companies), all other 3D objects like the body surface with its internal 3D models, accident cars and other injury-causing instruments can be repositioned (Fig. 2.16) to perform comparisons

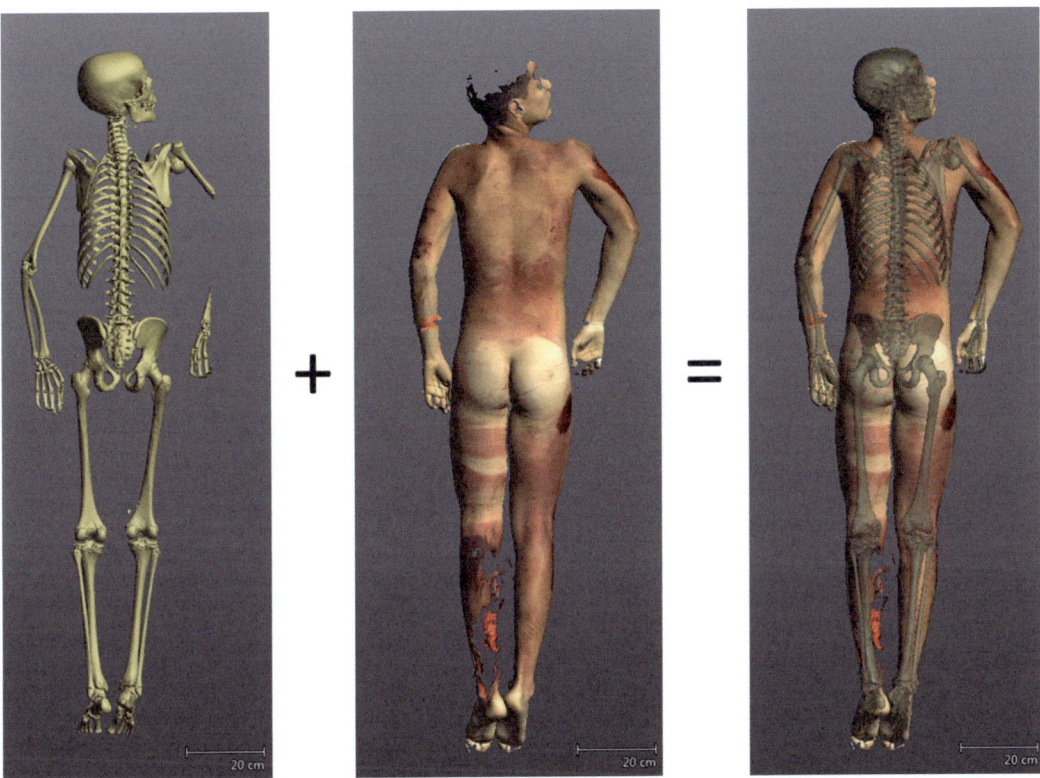

Fig. 2.13 Fusion of 3D models coming from a CT scan (skeleton), with surface scan 3D models (skin)

between object structures and injuries (Fig. 2.17), or measurements on the 3D models or between them can be taken [41]. In cases with shaped fractures, virtual reconstruction is usually achieved with CT scanner and compared with presumed device acquired by SLS (Fig. 2.18).

2.5.3   3D Printing and 3D Identification

Digital substitutes of real physical objects may be archived on electronic storage systems and are possible to be reconstructed physically with 3D printing. The final effect depends on the quality of the 3D model. SLS are characterized by better representation of minor details (better spatial resolution) than CT scans (Table 2.1). SLS should be considered in planned identification of the victim by odonatological studies (Fig. 2.19) due to

typical dental filling artifacts observed in CT. 3D printed models based on CT scans may show layering and loss of minor details—e.g., margins of fractures.

In cases when skeletonized cadaver is revealed, the main use of imaging is related with process of identification:

- Anthropometric analysis (e.g., assessment of body height, age, and body built)
- Identification of previous injuries and effects of treatment (previous fractures, prostheses, etc.)
- Reconstruction of presumed facial appearance of the victim on the base of 3D cranial model

Reconstruction (approximation) of intravital facial appearance of missing person can be achieved by different techniques. The application of modern 3D computer reconstruction (Fig. 2.20)

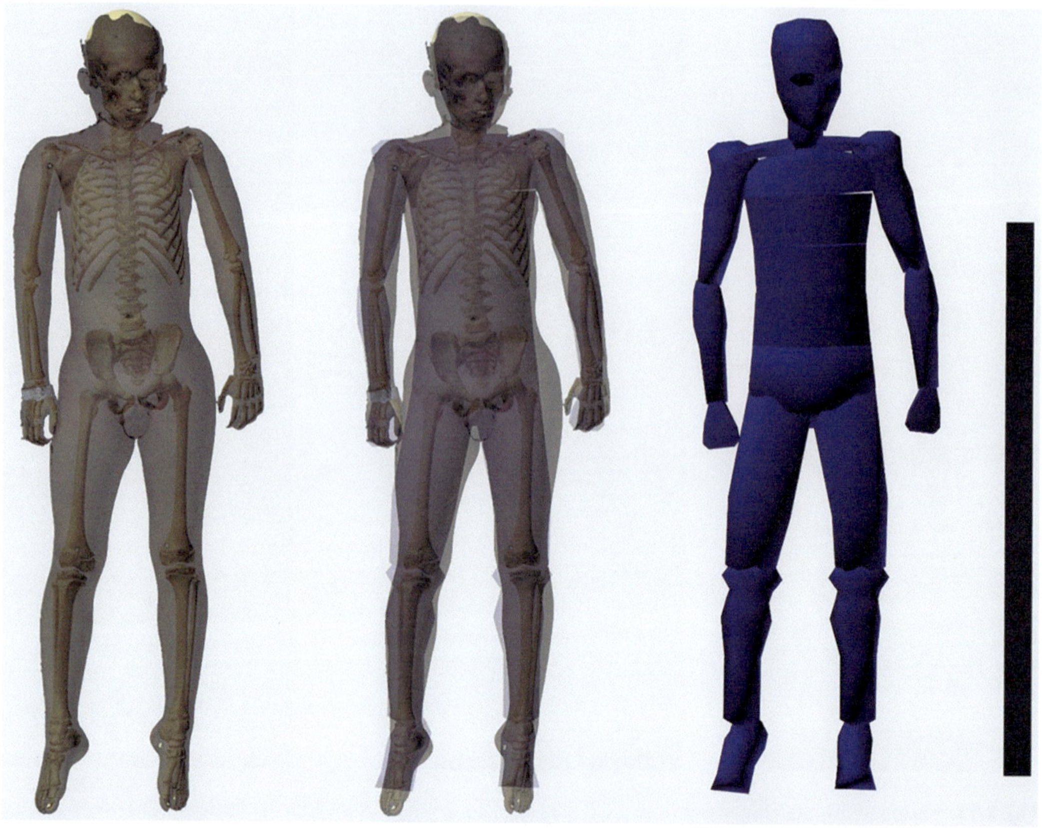

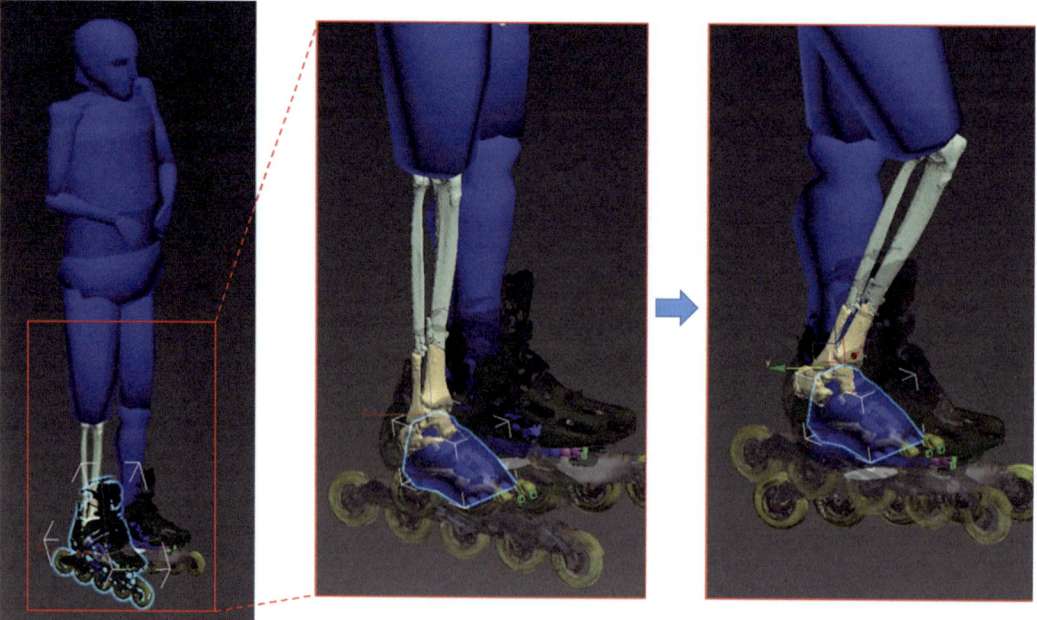

Fig. 2.14 Adaptation of a mannequin, to the real dimensions and proportions of the body

Fig. 2.15 Using parts of the 3D data linked to an element of the mannequin to move them anatomically correct

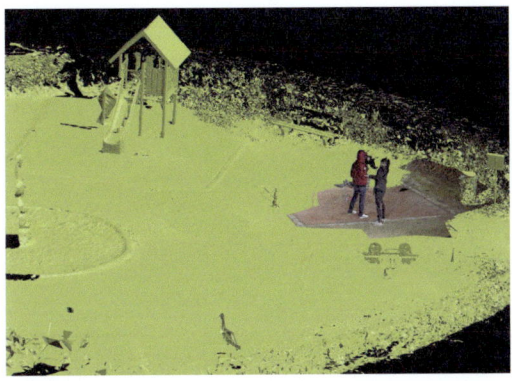

Fig. 2.16 Virtual crime scene and other repositioned elements

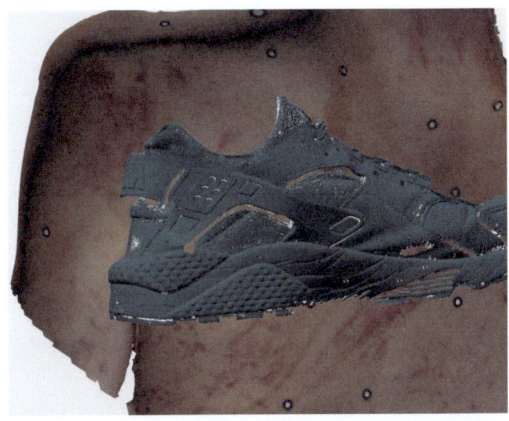

Fig. 2.17 Morphometric comparison between shaped injuries and injury-causing instrument

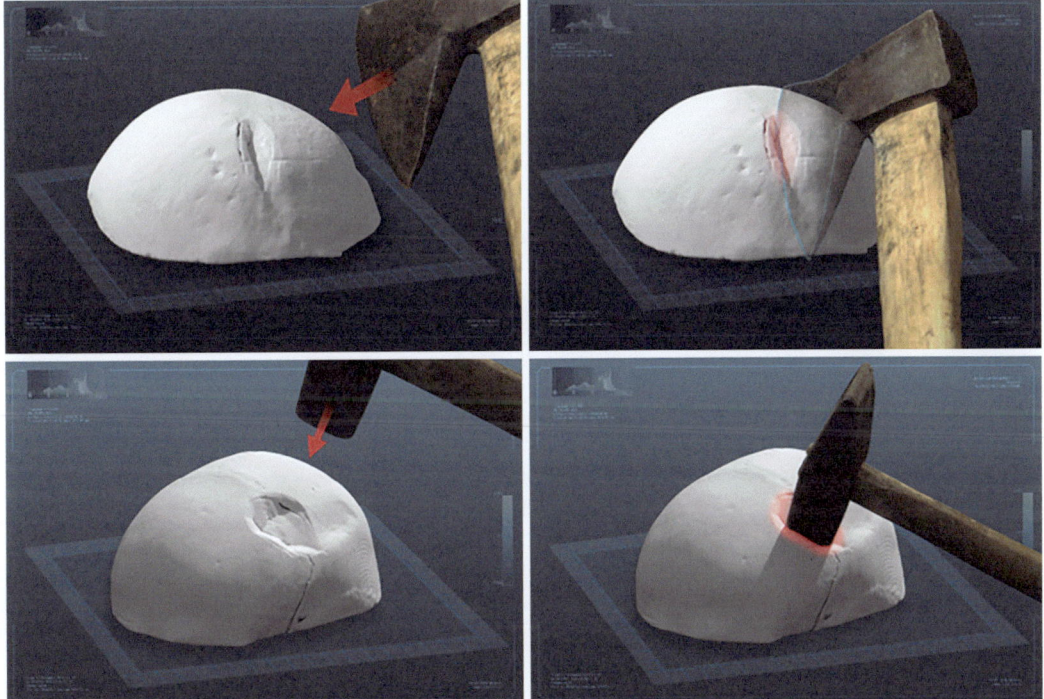

Fig. 2.18 Virtual comparison of cranial vault injuries (3D models based on postmortem CT) with the shape of the presumed device (3D models based on 3D SLS 3D scanning which preserved original textures)

Table 2.1 Weaknesses (o) and strengths (•) of 3D models produced with CT scanning and manual SLS

CT	SLS
o Lower resolution (0.5–1 mm and more) o Artificial smoothing o Clear "layering" o No textures o Significant artifacts from metallic implants	• Better resolution (0.1 mm) • Margins and contours more visible • Homogenous, smooth surfaces • Realistic textures (color and surface) • No effect of metallic foreign bodies
• Better delineation of openings • Structure and channels of diploe	o Worse penetration of recesses o No depiction of diploe

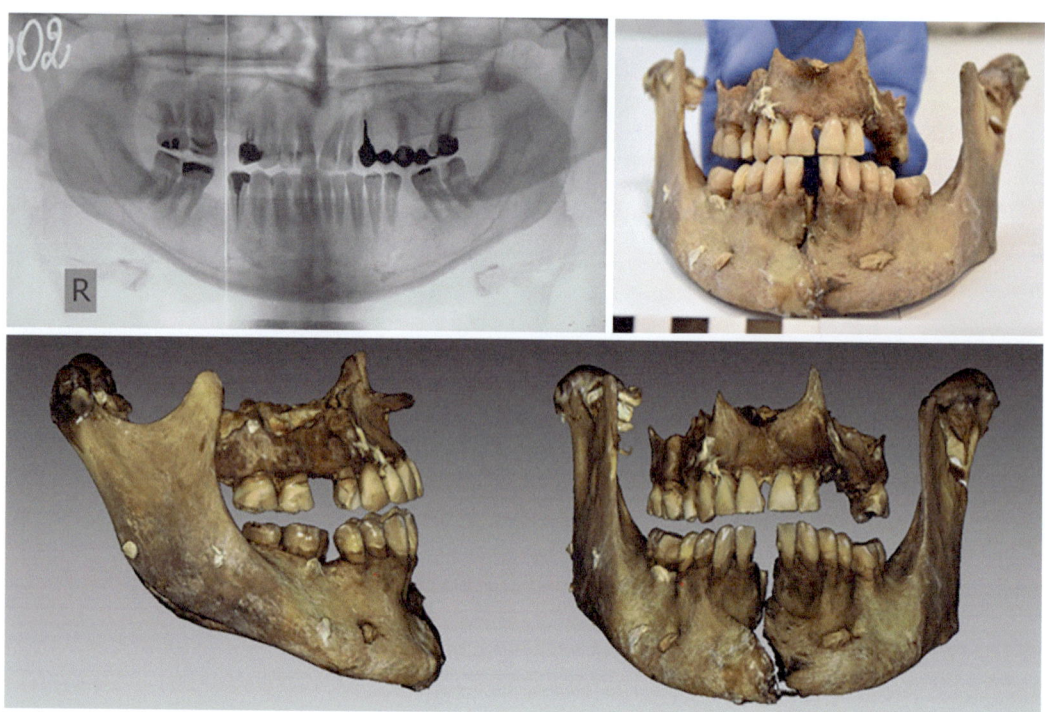

Fig. 2.19 Example of virtual dental reconstruction with SLS scanner (lower part) for identification purposes (on the top intravital panoramic X-ray)

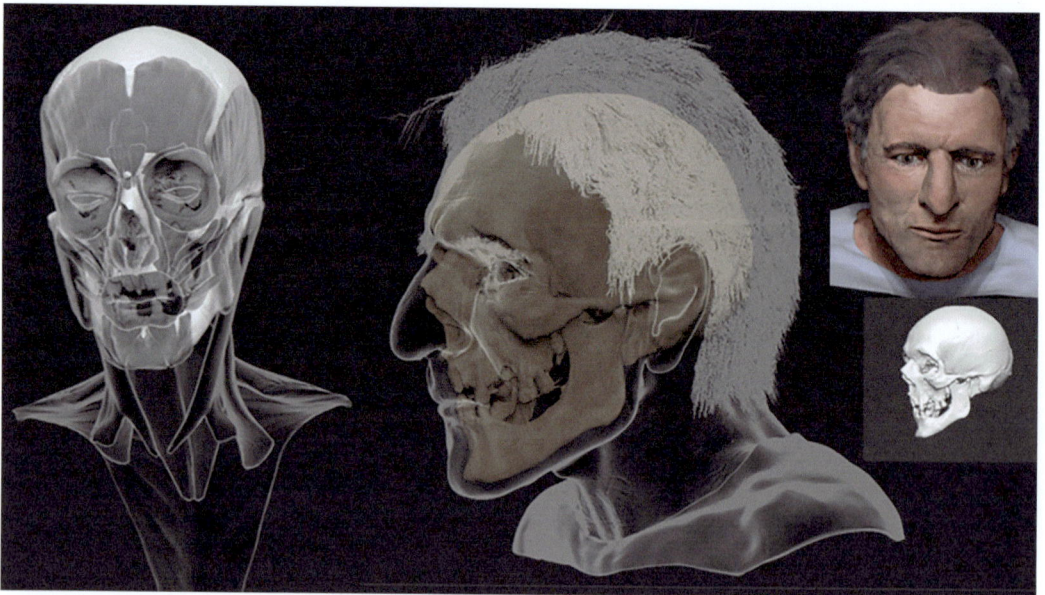

Fig. 2.20 Facial reconstruction by 3D software. (From Forensic Medicine Department, Medical University of Poznań)

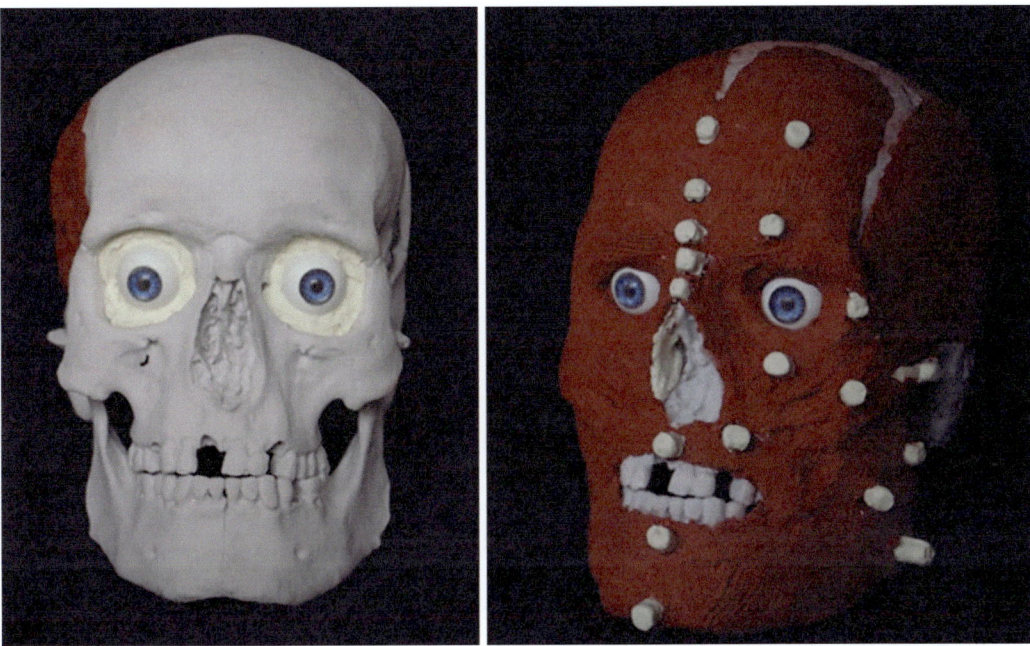

Fig. 2.21 Facial reconstruction by plastic method, using 3D printed skull replica. (From Forensic Medicine Department, Medical University of Poznań)

requires digitization of facial skeleton (preparing 3D model). Traditional artistic method (Gerasimov's plastic facial reconstruction) requires original (macerated) skull; however, its replica might be used (physical backup) produced from 3D model by rapid prototyping—using 3D printer (Fig. 2.21).

In this way 3D documentation becomes an important tool in forensic trauma case, to perform morphometric comparisons or visualize event reconstruction. By looking for matches between an injury and structures of objects (cars, shoe sole, etc.), in 3D and true to scale, injury-causing instruments can be assigned or excluded. Several contacts between a person and a vehicle during the short lap of an accident can be determined. For example, if the persecu-

tor wants to know who the driver of an accident car was, the presumed drivers and the car cabin with the seat on the right position can be scanned. In a second step, the created mannequins of the presumed drivers can be seated in the cabin and checked if pedals, steering wheel, and gear shift are reachable with his extremities (Fig. 2.22). Not to forget the utility in visualizing the trajectory of bullets in shooting cases. And last but not least, 3D documentation has an important role in reassociating fractured bone fragments for better estimation of the sort of trauma or in comparing with probable fracture-causing instruments.

These methods help to understand trauma better for laypersons, and it is an additional helpful element in investigation for the justice system.

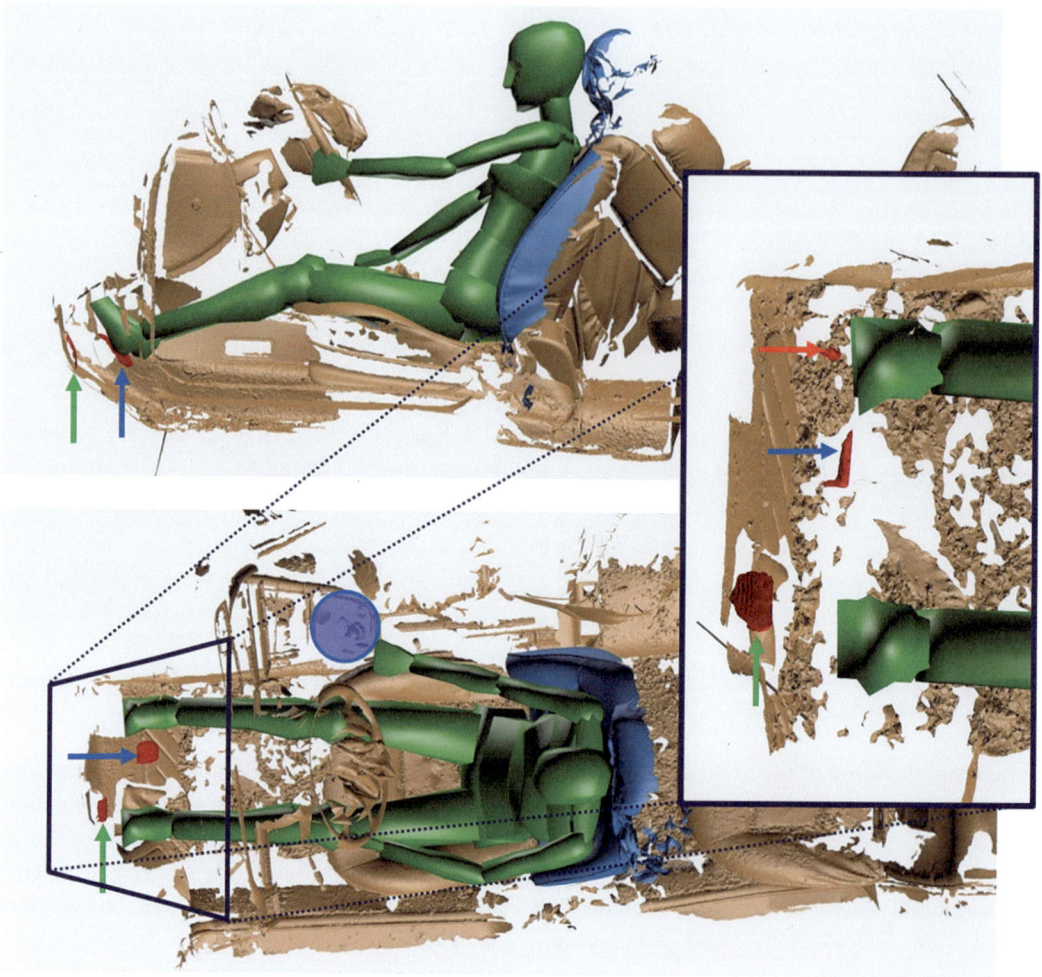

Fig. 2.22 Mannequin sitting in the 3D model of the cabin, to verify who was the driver. It's clearly visible that this presumed drive does not reach the pedals with his feet and also not the gear changer with his right hand

2.6 Ultrasound

Anastasia Tsaklakidis

In contrast to conventional X-ray and computed tomography, this technique uses radiation-free high-frequency sound waves to make different tissues visible by sending ultrasound waves by a transducer in objects and tissues and receiving their echoes. The longer the wave, the lower the frequency—e.g., audible sound waves are located between 20 Hz and 20 kHz. Frequencies above 20 kHz are called ultrasound, and the ultrasound, used in medical examinations, ranges from 1 to 40 MHz [43]. The transducer, which is connected to the ultrasound machine, contains special piezoelectric crystals. These crystals start to vibrate when an electric signal is applied and high-frequency ultrasound is produced. The specialty of these piezoelectric crystals is the fact that they do not just produce ultrasound, but they are able to transform received high-frequency pressure ultrasound waves in an electric signal, as well. The electric signals are sent back to the computer to generate a grayscale (brightness scale) image (B-mode). Because of the different characteristics and densities of the different tissues inside the human body, different echoes are reflected to the crystal element over a 1000 times per second. Depending on the time the ultrasound waves and their echoes have to travel, the distance and depth of tissues and organs to the transducer can be calculated by the machine's computer. Fast-returning signals are assigned to superficial structures, slower-returning signals to deeper structures [43]. The waves' and echo's travel, in other words the speed of sound, depends on the type of tissue. Because of the similar speed through the different tissues inside a human body, ultrasound machines have a saved default speed about 1540 m/s. Just air (330 m/s) and bone (3360 m/s) differ clearly. The saved default speed enables the machine to calculate the position. Deeper structures are shown in the lower part of the image on the computer's screen and superficial structures in the upper image area. But basically, reflection of the echoes is required for this kind of imaging technique, which is achieved by acoustic impedance. When ultrasound waves travel through tissue, echoes are reflected at transition zones of different tissues. The higher the difference, the more echoes are reflected. But if air or bone is hit by the waves, a total reflection is the consequence, and no waves are left to display the deeper structures. The image "behind" the total reflection is "erased" on screen, which is called acoustic shadow. Also because of the pronounced reflection of the ultrasound waves by air, ultrasound gel has to be used to couple and contact the transducer to the skin, to avoid the loss of waves outside the body, and to produce a proper image without shadowing.

The weakening of sound is caused by different mechanisms, e.g., due to:

- Reflection—some waves are reflected to the transducer or in other directions, which means less waves continue travelling toward deeper structures.
- Attenuation—waves are weakened while traveling.
- Scattering—waves are reflected in other directions than the transducer's localization; thus, these get lost for further processing.
- Absorption—waves are absorbed by the tissue and transformed into heat.

Nowadays ultrasound machines are high-resolution real-time machines with different kind of transducers—whether for small or bigger parts or even for interventional diagnostics. For examination areas like the abdomen, musculoskeletal system, neck, or heart, different transducers in different sizes and shapes are used to produce 2D, 3D, or even 4D results. If higher resolution is required, transducers with a higher frequency are needed, usually linear transducers (range between 2 and 24 MHz, often 5 and 10 MHz). If deeper structures are to be presented and more penetration is needed, curved array transducers with lower frequency and lower resolution are used. These curved array transducers (between 1 and 9 MHz) have a bigger aperture and are used in the examinations like abdomen ultrasound. Because of the beam shape, a wider image sector in the deeper regions and a larger field of view can be created. The small configured phased array transducers, which are used especially in cardiac and brain diagnostics, have a range from 1.5 to 4.5 MHz [43]. Their shape with a small aperture allows an easier penetration of regions, where smaller imaging windows due to anatomical features, for example, to examine the heart or lung between the rips, are necessary.

The more echoes return and the higher the impedance change is, the brighter the image gets, for example, fresh blood/hematoma or fat is shown hyper-echoic and "bright" on screen in the grayscale imaging B-mode. On the other hand, anechoic structures, appearing "black" on screen, usually contain fluids like the bladder, a cyst, ascites, or pleural effusion. The M-mode, or motion mode, used, e.g., in cardiac diagnostics, documents and shows movements over time by capturing echoes in one line over a timeline. Doppler is used to visualize moving structures like blood flow. The used colors in color Doppler—usually blue and red—visualize the direction of the movement in the approximate speed, whether the object is moving away or toward the transducer.

Like in ante-mortem imaging, ultrasound can be used in postmortem imaging as well. At the moment it doesn't play a large role in postmortem imaging. But the quick and handy usability makes it attractive for different kinds of diagnostic and forensic questions, though the amount and correctness of findings depend on the examiner's experience. Because of possible decay or gas formations of other origins in the corpse's tissue, the image's quality can be reduced or even lacks important information, so further imaging could still be necessary. In ante-mortem imaging ultrasound imaging is way more in use. In ante-mortem forensic medicine, it can be the easiest and fastest way to rule out injuries and hematomas. Because of the absence of radiation, it is a very attractive and helpful method to examine adults and children at any time, whenever needed.

2.7   Scintigraphy

Anastasia Tsaklakidis

Like X-ray imaging, scintigraphy, also known as gamma scan, uses radiation and ionization. It is an important imaging method in nuclear medicine and is used in the diagnostic and therapeutic field. Gamma rays have the shortest wavelength and the highest frequency of all electromagnetic waves. Generally, in forensic medicine this technique doesn't play a big role, but still, for example, bone scintigraphy can be a helpful tool to detect fractures or to estimate the fracture's age, important in selected cases of child abuse.

Anatomical features are described and documented in details by X-ray, ultrasound, or cross-sectional imaging. But if functional processes have to be evaluated, scintigraphic imaging can be done. This means that it is not a standard technique in postmortem imaging, but in ante-mortem imaging when metabolic processes inside the human body have to be visualized.

Small amounts of radioactive molecules, which are attached to agents, are injected intravenously or inhaled before starting the scan. For example, in a bone scan, phosphates and technetium-99m are used. These attached radio-isotopes accumulate in areas with metabolic activity and emit gamma radiation by radioactive decay. This is captured by a gamma camera and affected areas with higher metabolic activity can

be visualized. In a bone scan, the first scan is usually done a few minutes after injection, whereas the tracer accumulates in the soft tissue periosteal, so inflammation or irritation in this area can be assumed. The second scan after a few hours shows the activity of the bone itself. One single scan lasts up to 40 min, and the patient, lying on the examination table, is scanned by the camera, measuring the emitted gamma rays and radiation and creating a plane image. In addition, a 3D image can be acquired as well to get a more detailed image, so-called SPECT method.

The main components of a gamma camera are the collimator, the scintillator, photomultiplier tubes, and the computer. The collimator, containing lead tubes in a honeycomb shape, absorbs with its lead walls the received nonparallel gamma rays, so that just the parallel rays can be passed on to the scintillator. This step is essential to assign the rays' original direction and anatomical location later on. The scintillator, containing scintillating material like sodium iodide or zinc sulfide, converts gamma photons into outgoing visible photons (scintillations), while the gamma energy is absorbed. Afterward, the photomultiplier tubes receive the visible photons on their cathode, and electrons are released. For a measurable signal, the electrons have to be multiplied by dynodes with an increasing positive potential to generate more and more electrons. These multiplied electrons reach the anode at the tubes end, which converts the multiple electrons into an electric signal. This signal is sent to the computer, and in the end, the computer transfers the electric signal of the photomultiplier tubes into the final image, which is seen on the screen.

2.8   Clinical Forensic Imaging

Anastasia Tsaklakidis

Most of the clinical forensic imaging is done in hospital, directly after the trauma or during the hospitalization and reevaluated by the forensic radiologist later on. This means that the departments of forensic medicine do not have to have their own devices and machines to offer forensic radiology. Authorized monitors should be available to ensure a correct analysis of the transmitted diagnostic data. Because of the diagnostic focus in hospital, cross-sectional imaging, especially computed tomography, is often incompletely calculated for forensic analysis, and superficial parts are not represented completely. For example, subcutaneous hematomas, which often are not important for clinical treatment, can be decisive for the reconstruction of a crime or an accident. Furthermore, to enable reasonable 3D reconstructions or forensic 3D prints, thin-sliced (max. 1 mm thickness) reconstructions of the CT scan should be done in the bone and tissue window and saved.

Sometimes further examinations can be required by the forensic radiologist, for example, sometimes in child abuse imaging should be repeated after a couple of days, because newer fractures can be concealed on the first images and may only be recognizable later on, or a bone scan can be ordered for further information. If a victim was strangulated, a MRI can visualize the soft tissue's injuries, edema, and hematoma, and this can be helpful to reconstruct the probably applied force during strangulation. The process of age estimation includes X-ray of the left hand and the jaw. Furthermore a CT or MRI of the clavicula's medial growth plate can be additionally necessary.

Ultimately the ALARA principle has to be maintained in clinical forensic radiology as well, and further imaging should only be requested, if really needed.

References

1. Loewenhardt B. Bildgebende Diagnostik. Technik Anatomie Pathologie. Dtsch Arztebl. 2006;103(27):A-1896.
2. Bansal GJ. Digital radiography. A comparison with modern conventional imaging. Postgrad Med J. 2006;82(969):425–8.
3. Prokop M, Galanski M, Schaefer-Prokop C. Ganzkörper-Computertomographie: Spiral- und Multislice CT. Georg Thieme Verlag; 2006.
4. Stern C, et al. Pelvic bone CT: can tin-filtered ultra-low-dose CT and virtual radiographs be used as alter-native for standard CT and digital radiographs? Eur Radiol. 2021;31:6793–801.
5. Riemer A. Computertomografie für MTRA/RT. Radiopraxis ed. Georg Thieme Verlag; 2022.
6. Grabherr S, Djonov V, Yen K, Thali MJ, Dirnhofer R. Postmortem angiography: review of former and current methods. AJR. 2007;188:832–8.
7. Virchow R. Einige Bemerkungen über die Zirculationsverhältnisse in den Nieren. Virchows Arch Path Anat. 1857;12:310–25.
8. Schoenmackers J. Technik der postmortalen Angiographie mit Berücksichtigung verwandter Methoden postmortaler Gefäâdarstellung. Ergeb Allg Pathol Anat. 1960;39:53–151.
9. Webb B, Widek T, Scheicher S, Schwark T, Stollberger R. Post-mortem MR angiography: quantitative investigation and intravascular retention of perfusates in ex situ porcine hearts. Int J Legal Med. 2018;132(2):579–87.
10. Grabherr S, Grimm J, Baumann P, Mangin P. Application of contrast media in post-mortem imaging (CT and MRI). Radiol Med. 2015;120(9):824–34.
11. Grabherr S, Grimm JM, Heinemann A. Atlas of postmortem angiography. Springer International; 2016.
12. Woźniak K, Moskała A, Rzepecka-Woźniak E. Imaging for homicide investigations. Radiol Med. 2015;120(9):846–55.
13. Michaud K, Grabherr S, Faouzi M, Grimm J, Doenz F, Mangin P. Pathomorphological and CT-angiographical characteristics of coronary atherosclerotic plaques in cases of sudden cardiac death. Int J Legal Med. 2015;129(5):1067–77.
14. Zerlauth JB, Doenz F, Dominguez A, Palmiere C, Uské A, Meuli R, Grabherr S. Surgical interventions with fatal outcome: utility of multi-phase postmortem CT angiography. Forensic Sci Int. 2013;225(1–3).32–41.
15. Chevallier C, Doenz F, Vaucher P, Palmiere C, Dominguez A, Binaghi S, Mangin P, Grabherr S. Postmortem computed tomography angiography vs. conventional autopsy: advantages and inconveniences of each method. Int J Legal Med. 2013;127:981–9.
16. Palmiere C, Binaghi S, Doenz F, Bize P, Chevallier C, Mangin P, Grabherr S. Detection of hemorrhage source: the diagnostic value of postmortem CT-angiography. Forensic Sci Int. 2012;222(1–3):33–9.
17. Saunders SL, Morgan B, Raj V, Rutty GN. Postmortem computed tomography angiography: past, present and future. Forensic Sci Med Pathol. 2011;7(3):271–7.
18. Grabherr S, Doenz F, Steger B, Dirnhofer R, Dominguez A, Sollberger B, Gygax E, Rizzo E, Chevallier C, Meuli R, Mangin P. Multi-phase postmortem CT-angiography development of a standardized protocol. Int J Legal Med. 2011;125:791–802.
19. Grabherr S, Jotterand M, Grimm J (2016) The technical working group postmortem angiography methods (TWGPAM). In: Grabherr S, Grimm J, Heinemann A. Atlas of postmortem angiography. Springer International Publishing, AG.

20. Grabherr S, Heinemann A, Vogel H, Rutty G, Morgan B, Wozniak K, Dedouit F, Fischer F, Lochner S, Wittig H, Guglielmi G, Eplinius F, Michaud K, Palmiere C, Chevallier C, Mangin P, Grimm JM. Postmortem CT angiography compared with autopsy: a forensic multicenter study. Radiology. 2018;288(1):270–6.

21. Wittig H, Stumm C, Eplinius F, Hecht L. Histology after postmortem angiography. In: Grabherr S, Grimm J, Heinemann A, editors. Atlas of postmortem angiography. Springer International Publishing, AG; 2016.

22. Palmiere C, Grabherr S, Augsburger M. Postmortem computed tomography angiography, contrast medium administration and toxicological analyses in urine. Legal Med (Tokyo). 2015;17(3):157–62.

23. Palmiere C. Complementary analysis after postmortem angiography. In: Grabherr S, Grimm J, Heinemann A, editors. Atlas of postmortem angiography. Springer International Publishing, AG; 2016.

24. Jackowski C, Persson A, Thali MJ. Whole body postmortem angiography with a high viscosity contrast agent solution using poly ethylene glycol as contrast agent dissolver. J Forensic Sci. 2008;53(2):465–8.

25. Debus J. Duale Reihe Radiologie. Stuttgart: Georg Thieme Verlag; 2017.

26. Scheurer E, Boltzmann L (2011) Neuro MRI at the end (necroscopy) forensic/research indications.

27. Grabherr S, Egger C, Vilarino R, Campana L, Jotterand M, Dedouit F. Modern post-mortem imaging: an update on recent developments. Forensic Sci Res. 2017;2(2):52–64.

28. Buck U, Busse K, Campana L, Schyma C. Validation and evaluation of measuring methods for the 3D documentation of external injuries in the field of forensic medicine. Int J Legal Med. 2018;132(2):551–61.

29. Buck U, Naether S, Braun M, et al. Application of 3D documentation and geometric reconstruction methods in traffic accident analysis: with high resolution surface scanning, radiological MSCT/MRI scanning and real data based animation. Forensic Sci Int. 2007;170(1):20–8.

30. Shamata A, Thompson T. Determining the effectiveness of noncontact three-dimensional surface scanning for the assessment of open injuries. J Forensic Sci. 2020;65(2):627–35.

31. Rashaan ZM, Stekelenburg CM, van der Wal MB, et al. Three-dimensional imaging: a novel, valid, and reliable technique for measuring wound surface area. Skin Res Technol. 2016;22(4):443–50.

32. Buck U, Naether S, Rass B, et al. Accident or homicide—virtual crime scene reconstruction using 3D methods. Forensic Sci Int. 2013;225(1–3):75–84.

33. Urbanova P, Hejna P, Jurda M. Testing photogrammetry-based techniques for three-dimensional surface documentation in forensic pathology. Forensic Sci Int. 2015;250:77–86.

34. Villa C. Forensic 3D documentation of skin injuries. Int J Legal Med. 2017;131(3):751–9.

35. Flies MJ, Larsen PK, Lynnerup N, et al. Forensic 3D documentation of skin injuries using photogrammetry: photographs vs video and manual vs automatic measurements. Int J Legal Med. 2019;133(3):963–71.

36. Gitto L, Donato L, Di Luca A, et al. The application of photogrammetry in the autopsy room: a basic, practical workflow. J Forensic Sci. 2020;65(6):2146–54.

37. Sieberth T, Ebert LC, Gentile S, et al. Clinical forensic height measurements on injured people using a multi camera device for 3D documentation. Forensic Sci Med Pathol. 2020;16(4):586–94.

38. Kottner S, Ebert LC, Ampanozi G, et al. VirtoScan—a mobile, low-cost photogrammetry setup for fast post-mortem 3D full-body documentations in X-ray computed tomography and autopsy suites. Forensic Sci Med Pathol. 2017;13(1):34–43.

39. Kottner S, Schaerli S, Furst M, et al. VirtoScan-on-Rails—an automated 3D imaging system for fast post-mortem whole-body surface documentation at autopsy tables. Forensic Sci Med Pathol. 2019;15(2):198–212.

40. Villa C, Flies MJ, Jacobsen C. Forensic 3D documentation of bodies: simple and fast procedure for combining CT scanning with external photogrammetry data. J Forensic Radiol Imaging. 2017;10:47–51.

41. Thali MJ, Braun M, Buck U, et al. VIRTOPSY—scientific documentation, reconstruction and animation in forensic: individual and real 3D data based geometric approach including optical body/object surface and radiological CT/MRI scanning. J Forensic Sci. 2005;50(2):1–15.

42. Villa C, Olsen KB, Hansen SH. Virtual animation of victim-specific 3D models obtained from CT scans for forensic reconstructions: living and dead subjects. Forensic Sci Int. 2017;278(2017):e27–33.

43. Blank W, Mathis G, Osterwalder J. Kursbuch Notfallsonografie. Stuttgart: Georg Thieme Verlag; 2019.

Blunt Trauma

3

Fabrice Dedouit, Fatima-Zohra Mokrane,
Mathilde Ducloyer, Chloé Dorczynski,
Manuelo Turkiewicz, Fréderic Savall,
Hervé Rousseau, and Norbert Telmon

3.1   Introduction

Blunt-force injuries are produced when the body is struck with or strikes a blunt object, or a combination of both [1–7].

Blunt trauma may occur on all anatomical levels:

– Head
– Neck
– Chest
– Abdomen
– Extremities

And also affect all anatomical structures:

– Integuments
– Muscles
– Bone
– Organs
– Vessels, etc.

The lesional panel is consequently large and almost infinite!

Blunt trauma means that the damage to the body can be caused by an impact of a moving blunt object, or by movement of the body against

F. Dedouit (✉)
Medico-Legal Department, CHU Toulouse-Rangueil, Toulouse, France
e-mail: dedouit.f@chu-toulouse.fr

Radiology Department, CHU Toulouse-Rangueil, Toulouse, France

Center for Anthropobiology and Genomics of Toulouse [CAGT, UMR 5288], Toulouse, France

F.-Z. Mokrane
Radiology Department, CHU Toulouse-Rangueil, Toulouse, France

Center for Anthropobiology and Genomics of Toulouse [CAGT, UMR 5288], Toulouse, France
e-mail: mokrane.fz@chu-toulouse.fr

M. Ducloyer
Medico-Legal Department, CHU Nantes, Nantes, France

Radiology Department, CHU Nantes, Nantes, France
e-mail: mathilde.DUCLOYER@chu-nantes.fr

C. Dorczynski · H. Rousseau
Radiology Department, CHU Toulouse-Rangueil, Toulouse, France
e-mail: clarissedubois@orange.fr;
rousseau.h@chu-toulouse.fr

M. Turkiewicz
Medico-Legal Department, CHU Toulouse-Rangueil, Toulouse, France

F. Savall · N. Telmon
Medico-Legal Department, CHU Toulouse-Rangueil, Toulouse, France

Center for Anthropobiology and Genomics of Toulouse [CAGT, UMR 5288], Toulouse, France
e-mail: savall.f@chu-toulouse.fr;
telmon.n@chu-toulouse.fr

S. Grabherr et al. (eds.), *Forensic Imaging of Trauma*, https://doi.org/10.1007/978-3-031-48381-3_3

a hard surface [6, 7]. Both mechanisms produce a transfer of kinetic energy that is high enough to produce an injury. The injury is produced by torsion, compression, scraping, tearing, shearing or crushing.

In general, the greater the force, the smaller the area, or the shorter the duration over which the force is applied, the greater the injury will be. Blunt objects have a relatively large surface. Examples of blunt objects are almost infinite: fists, shoes, pipes, bricks, bats, hammers, roads, cars, trains, airplanes, etc. [1–5, 7].

The severity of the injuries resulting from trauma is a balance between the amount of force, the area over which it is applied, and the duration of the force [2, 8].

In this chapter after a presentation of the general aspects of blunt trauma, including the strike, the authors will detail some particular situations generating blunt trauma: the fall from height, the fall from plain level and some combined trauma. The situations dealing with traffic accidents and ballistic trauma will be treated in specific chapters, but some pictures are presented in this chapter because of a didactic purpose of the presented iconography.

In this chapter the different possibilities of diagnoses and images permitted will be presented:

– In a post-mortem context: with post-mortem radiographies, post-mortem computed tomography (PMCT), post-mortem computed tomography angiography (PMCTA), post-mortem multiphase computed tomography angiography (MPMCTA) and post-mortem magnetic resonance imaging (PMMMR); based on "classical" medico-legal knowledge.
– But also, in a forensic clinical context: with radiographies, computed tomography (CT), and magnetic resonance imaging (MRI). The inclusion of such data in a clinical medicolegal report is an added value and sometimes the main element of the report written by the forensic pathologist.

3.2 Most Suited Imaging Methods in Blunt Trauma

This part describes the most suited imaging methods depending on the anatomical level affected by the trauma.

3.2.1 Blunt Traumas to the Teguments and Muscles

Abrasions can easily be documented with 3D-surface scanner and do normally not have any MSCT visibility [9, 10].

Haemorrhages in the subcutaneous fatty tissue are well documented with PMMR, and appeared in general as hypointense (T1-weighted) or hyperintense (T2-weighted) alterations in signal intensity with a cross-hatched, streaky pattern [11]. The overall sensitivity of MRI for the identification of subcutaneous haematomas in the study by Ross et al. was high (91% specificity; 68% sensitivity) [11].

Superficial haematoma may also reflect the surface texture of the impacting object. For example, in falls from great heights, the texture of the clothing may be visible through patterned superficial haematoma. If the body is struck by a stick, a double "tramline" bruise consisting in two parallel linear haematomas, with an undamaged area between, can be visible. That kind of lesions, like also bitemarks, can easily be documented with 3D-surface scanner [9, 10]. In such cases, the additional use of PMCTA and PMMR is particularly relevant [12, 13].

Skin lacerations can also easily be documented with 3D-surface scanner [9, 14]. Some CT surface reconstructions like the 3D volume-rendering technique (VRT) can also document those lesions. However, some limitations will occur when the body is covered by bloody clothes adherent to the skin and the lesion, or if the PMCT acquisition is performed in decubitus position and in lesions located on the back of the body. In this case, the natural pressure of the weight of the body applying on the CT table may compress the skin and rend some skin laceration invisible. Of course, haemorrhage surrounding the lesion is still more or less visible. In order to eliminate this limit, some authors propose to perform a first PMCT acquisition with a cadaver in decubitus position, and a second one in procubitus [15].

For **parietal muscular haematomas or lacerations**, the use of the PMCT, MPMCTA, PMCTA and PMMR may be particularly relevant [11–13].

3.2.2 Head Injuries

3.2.2.1 Skull Fractures
PMCT is the ideal suited imaging method for those kinds of lesions. Some CT surface reconstructions like the 3D volume-rendering technique (VRT) can document those lesions very plastically [6, 16]. A 3D-surface scanning documentation is also possible on cadavers, after autopsies and bone preparation, or on dry bones [10].

3.2.2.2 Facial Fractures
PMCT is the ideal suited imaging method. Some MPR PMCT reconstructions and 3D CT surface reconstructions like MIP (maximal intensity projection) or VRT can document those lesions.

3.2.2.3 Intracranial Haemorrhages and Cerebral Injuries
Those kinds of lesions can be diagnosed with CT or MRI (in clinical and post-mortem contexts).

3.2.3 Injuries of the Chest

3.2.3.1 Rib Injuries
They can be diagnosed with CT in clinical and post-mortem contexts and to document some ribs' complications as haemothorax, pneumothorax and subcutaneous or mediastinal emphysema. PMCTA and MPMCTA are the ideal suited imaging methods to document also complications of ribs fractures like assessment of the origin of a haemothorax.

3.2.3.2 Lung Injuries
They can be diagnosed with CT in clinical and post-mortem contexts. PMCTA and MPMCTA permit the progressive filling with the contrast agent of the haemopneumatoceles and lung lacerations.

3.2.3.3 Heart Injuries and Pericardium Rupture
As we will see it in the next subchapter, all the injuries like cardiac rupture or injuries of the coronary vessels can be suspected with CT or MRI. However, MPMCTA and PMCTA, which allow vessel opacifications, permit to directly visualise the site of rupture.

3.2.3.4 Aortic Ruptures, Great Vessel, Periaortic Small Vessel Injuries and Diaphragmatic Rupture
Those kinds of lesions can sometimes be diagnosed with CT or MRI, but PMCTA and MPMCTA are the best methods to diagnose such vascular lesions because they permit a direct visualisation of the site of vascular rupture or injury. The source of haemorrhage is easily identified and characterised.

3.2.4 Abdominopelvic Injuries

3.2.4.1 Solid Organs
The parenchymal lesions of the liver, spleen, but also abdominal wall can sometimes be diagnosed with PMCT, but PMMR and PMCTA are the best methods to diagnose such parenchymal lesions. PMCT is limited by the notion of natural spontaneous intertissular contrast, which can be low. It explains why sometimes important ruptures of the liver can be suspected on PMCT due to indirect signs like haemoperitoneum, but the rupture itself is poorly visible.

3.2.4.2 Hollows Organs

Perforation of the stomach and intestine can be suspected based on diffuse or located pneumoperitoneum and intraabdominal gastric contents on PMCT.

3.2.4.3 Abdominal Aortic Ruptures

Those kinds of lesions can sometimes be diagnosed with CT or MRI, but PMCTA and MPMCRTA are the best methods to diagnose such vascular lesions because it permits the direct visualisation of the site of rupture. The source of haemorrhage is easily identified and characterised.

3.2.4.4 Pelvic Fractures

PMCT is the ideal suited imaging method. Some 3D CT surface reconstructions like the VRT can document those lesions as well [6, 16].

3.2.5 Injuries to the Extremities

PMCT is the ideal suited imaging method for these bony lesions. Some 3D CT surface reconstructions like the VRT can also document those lesions [6, 16].

3.2.6 Injuries to the Spine

The most sensitive clinical method for demonstrating a vertebral fracture is the clinical premortem CT [17]. Premortem clinical MRI is sensitive for detection of ligamentous and other soft tissue injuries, which indicate the possibility of a fracture in the adjacent vertebrae. Clinical MRI is accurate for the assessment of the nature and the extent of spinal injuries [18]. Clinical premortem CT and MRI findings are consequently an important part of the assessment by the pathologist of cases of suspected vertebral and spinal injuries that should be checked before the autopsy. Clinical radiographs of the neck, with extension and flexion views, will fail to detect many vertebral fractures.

During the autopsy, the location of haemorrhage in the perivertebral soft tissues or an unexplained bleeding in the prevertebral neck musculature may indicate the possibility of a ligamentous or vertebral injury. These haemorrhages are visible on pre- and post-mortem MRI [11].

3.2.7 Particularities of Chop Wounds

For those kinds of lesions, 3D CT reconstructions are useful in a clinical or a post-mortem context. This may be crucial in clinical forensic medicine because the characteristics of chopping trauma often appear masked or changed by clinical treatment [19]. 3D CT reconstructions will provide additional possibilities for supplementing missing information, such as number and direction of blows as well as sometimes a weapon identification. Furthermore, 3D CT reconstructions facilitate demonstration in court and understanding of the injuries of medical laypeople [19, 20].

3.2.7.1 In Summary

PMCT is essentially indicated for detection and diagnostic of gas bubbles and effusions, fluid effusions and bone trauma in general [14].

MPMCTA and **PMCTA** will allow the detection of the site of vascular injuries or parenchymal injuries. This can be useful for superficial and profound wounds (subcutaneous, muscular or organ injuries) [14, 21].

PMMR allows the detection of parenchymal injuries. This can be useful for superficial and profound wounds (subcutaneous, muscular or organ injuries). It has a high interest for cardiac and neuro-radiological injuries (particularly for the brain and spine) [14].

3D-surface scanner permits documentation of skin lesions, and also of dry bones. The possibilities of image fusion (between different tools like the PMCT and 3D-surface scanner data) make it precious for the understanding of trauma [9, 14].

3.3 The Different Characteristics and Morphologies of Blunt Trauma

Blunt-force injuries occur in many kinds of medico-legal situations and contexts: criminal assaults, physical child abuse, traffic accidents, industrial accidents and falls (which may be of different natures: criminal, accidental or suicidal) [7].

As previously explained, blunt trauma may occur on all anatomical levels and affect all anatomical structures. The different anatomical levels are presented in the text through the different subchapters.

3.3.1 Blunt Traumas to the Teguments and Muscles

Contusions are bruises [2, 3, 5, 6, 8]. They are produced as a result of an impact, where soft tissues and blood vessels underneath or within the skin are torn and produce haemorrhage (Fig. 3.1a–c).

Lacerations are tears of the skin, soft tissues, internal organs or vessels as a result of an impact, overstretching or crushing-type forces [2, 3, 5, 6, 8]. They may be caused by blows from blunt objects (such as a hammer, a rod, a fist, etc.); other lacerations may be produced by impact with vehicles or by falls to the ground. When the force acts on the skin, the subcutaneous tissue is squeezed between the injuring object and the bony platform so that tegument is compressed and crushed until it tears and split sideways.

Lacerations are characterised by abraded, bruised and crushed wound margins. Skin lacerations tend to occur more often over hard surfaces, such as the scalp, knee and elbow. Sometimes foreign material from the causative instrument/surface is visible deep in the wound [2, 3, 5, 6, 8]. The characterisation of the foreign bodies can sometimes be solved by the scanning electron microscopy with energy-dispersive X-ray spectroscopy (SEM EDX) [22].

PMCTA permits a documentation of the source of the superficial bleedings (arterial and/or venous) (Fig. 3.1d) [12].

Some parietal muscular haematomas or lacerations may also be seen (Fig. 3.1e). These lesions may be located in the continuity of penetrating tegumentary lesions or near some bone fractures with sharp ends of the fractured bones, which will perforate adjacent muscular structures. They can also be secondary to localised vascular lesions, secondary to high kinetic trauma or to a crushing mechanism in closed trauma, with sometimes diastatic muscular lesions [23, 24].

3.3.2 Head Injuries

The head is a common target in assaults with blunt objects; other frequent causes of head injuries are traffic accidents, falls from a great height as well as from a standing position [2, 3, 5–8]. The area of impact usually results in injuries of the scalp or the facial skin. Severe and lethal trauma is not necessarily associated with scalp bruise, excoriation or laceration. Classically, an impact site on the vertex suggests that the head has sustained a blow, whereas in falls from a standing position, the scalp injuries are expected under or at the level of the brim of the hat [1, 5, 25–27]. This hat brim line can of course not be used as a single criterion to differentiate accidental falls from blows to the head, and some studies had contradictory results concerning this hat brim line rule [28]. Lefevre indicated that differences in injuries caused by falls from less than 2.5 m high (accidental falls or falls due to sudden death) and homicides showed no statistical differences concerning the hat brim line rule. But they found high percentages of depressed cranial fractures in homicides (37%) and none in either the accidental or sudden death group of falls.

3.3.2.1 Skull Fractures
Skull fractures may involve the cranial vault, the base of the skull and the facial skeleton. There

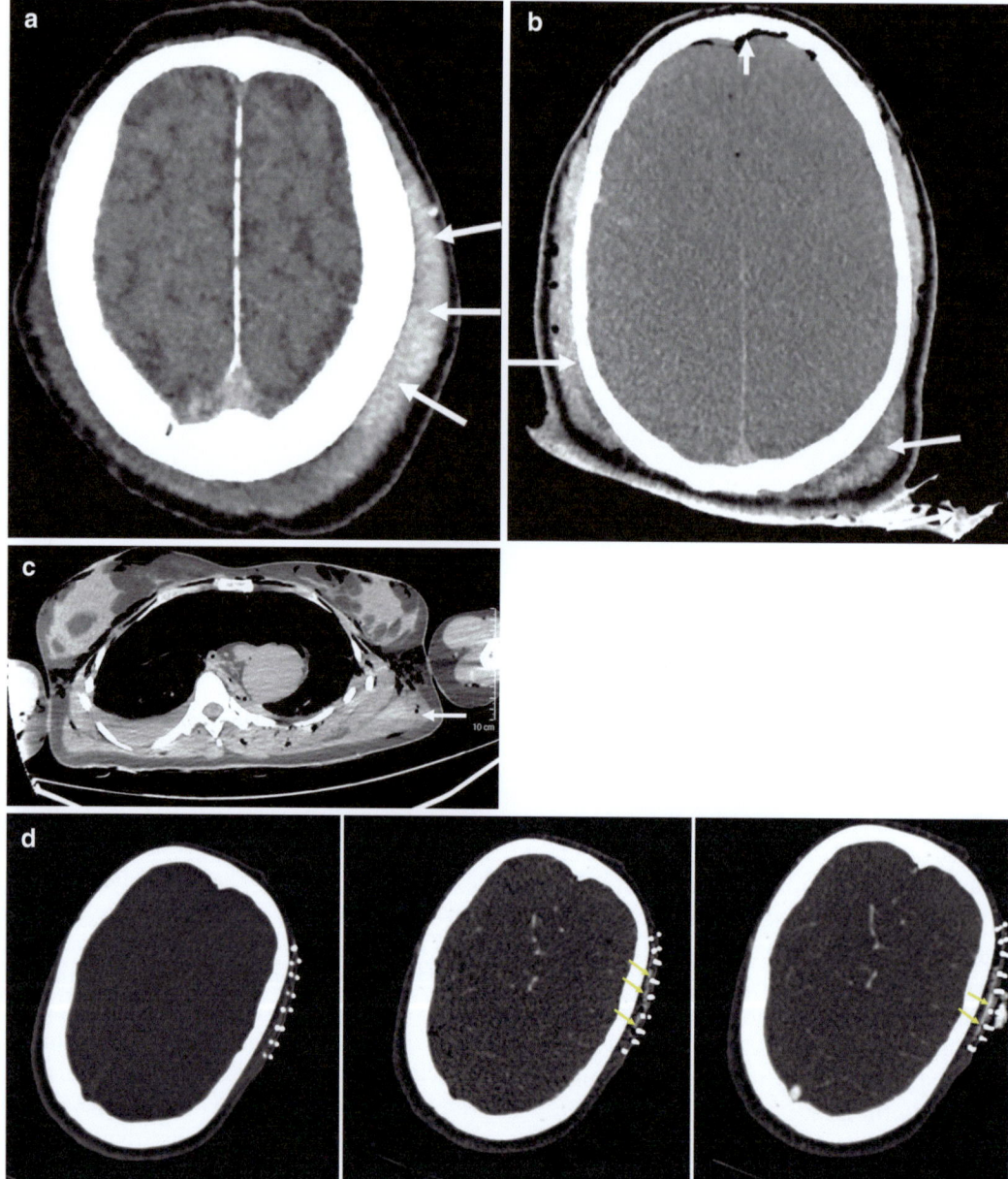

Fig. 3.1 (**a**) PMCT, axial view of the skull, soft tissue filter. Context of a fall in the stairs. Spontaneous hyperdensity of a parietal subcutaneous haematoma (arrows). (**b**) PMCT, axial view of the skull, soft tissue filter. Context of a fight with punching and kicking. Multiple subcutaneous haematomas (arrows) and pneumencephalia (short arrow). (**c**) PMCT, axial view of the chest, soft tissue filter. Context of a fall down the stairs. Large haemorrhagic suffusion into the posterior left thoracic wall (arrow). (**d**) MPMCTA, axial view of the skull, soft tissue filter. Context of fall from great height. Subcutaneous contrast extravasation, located under surgical stitches (yellow arrows). Note the absence of clear lesions in the non-contrast phase. Left image, non-enhanced PMCT;

middle image, MPMCTA, arterial phase; right image, MPMCTA, dynamic phase. (**e**) MPMCTA of the pelvic, soft tissue filter. Context of fall from great height. Severe pelvic fractures with sacroiliac disjunction (white-dotted arrow) associated with a pubic symphysis disjunction (white arrow), and a displaced ischio-pubic branch fracture (yellow circle). Spontaneous haematoma of the anterior abdominal wall (yellow arrow), with severe arterial and venous contrast extravasation both in the anterior abdominal wall (orange arrows) and subperitoneal space (orange-dotted arrows). Superior images: left, PMCT, 3D VRT reconstruction; right, PMCT, axial view. Inferior images: left, MPMCTA, arterial phase; right, MPMCTA, venous phase)

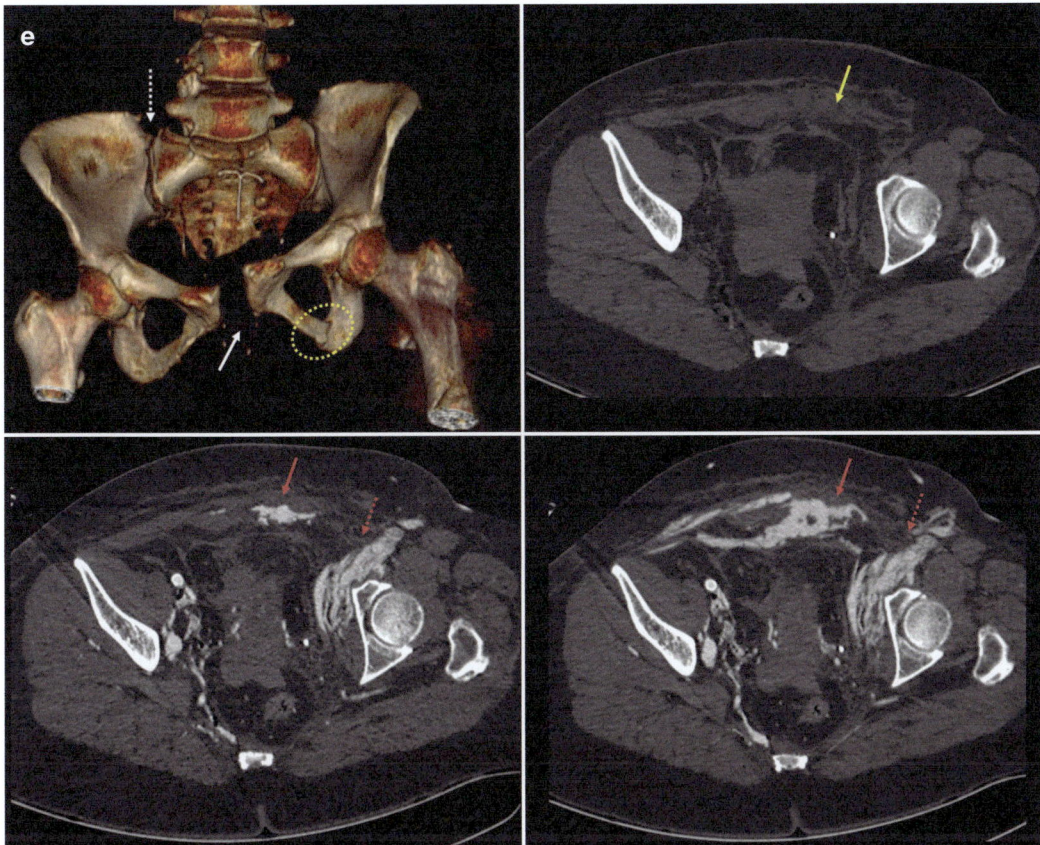

Fig. 3.1 (continued)

are several types of skull fractures that can be distinguished [3, 5, 7, 8]:

- **Single or multiple linear fractures** are caused either by a blow from an object with a broad, flat surface area or by a fall on the head so that the skull is deformed (Fig. 3.2a, b).
- **Spider's web or mosaic pattern**: several fracture lines may radiate outward from a central point of impact where the skull is often depressed and/or shattered to pieces forming a pattern consisting of circular and radiating linear fractures (Fig. 3.2c, d). The sequence of skull injuries may be determined according to Puppe's rule: a fracture does not cross a preexisting fracture line, but terminates when reaching an earlier one [5, 29].
- A hinge **fracture** occurs when a transverse type gaping fracture runs from one side of the cranial base to the other side (Fig. 3.2e) [3, 5, 7, 8].

- **Longitudinal fractures of the base of the skull** frequently occur secondary to a fall on the occiput [3, 5, 7, 8]; in such instances, the linear fractures typically run through the posterior fossa either ending near the foramen magnum or extending to the floor of the middle and anterior fossa.
- **Ring fracture** is located in the posterior fossa and encircles the foramen magnum [3, 5, 7, 8]. It occurs often in a fall from a height onto the victim's feet or buttocks, so that the cervical spine is driven into the skull (Fig. 3.2f).
- **A diastatic fracture** is a fracture that travels through cranial sutures (Fig. 3.2g, h) [3, 5, 7, 8].
- **Depressed fractures and bone impressions** are always located at the point of impact where the head is struck with an object having a relatively small surface area, such as a hammer or a protruding corner of a piece of furniture (Fig. 3.3a–i). The outline of a clean-cut

defect at the outer table may reproduce the shape and the size of a sharp-edged instrument. If a limited force is applied, the depressed fracture can be restricted to the outer or less often the inner table. A depressed fracture from a blow which struck the skullcap at an angle may be concentrically terraced, with lowest fragments lacerating the surface of the brain (Fig. 3.3i). Sometimes the injuring object may be reflected by the shape of the bone injury, giving a particular aspect of the injury which can be patterned as an imprint of the causative object (Fig. 3.3f–i).

- **Pond or ping-pong fracture** is a shallow depressed fracture forming a "pond" (Fig. 3.4). It is more common in pliable bones of infants, for whom a depression can occur without a fracture and is classically compared to the distortion produced by squeezing a table tennis ball.
- **Gutter fracture** is classically defined as a long, narrow, depressed fracture of the skull (Fig. 3.5).
- **Hole fractures**, classically from bullets, but some penetrating objects, may have similar troubling patterns (Fig. 3.6a, b).
- **Comminuted fractures** are classically described as trauma generating three or more fragments (Fig. 3.7a, b). In this case, displacement and some flattening of the skull are encountered.

3.3.2.2 Facial Fractures

There are several types of facial fractures that can be distinguished [3, 5, 7, 8]:

- **Le Fort fractures**

    After an impact on the face, three classical distinct fracture patterns have been described by Le Fort [30]:
    - In Le Fort I fractures: the palate may be separated from the maxilla
    - In Le Fort II fractures: the maxilla may be separated from the face
    - In Le Fort III fractures: the maxilla and parts of the mandibular condyles may be fragmented

    The numerous components seen in Le Fort fractures make it difficult to classify these lesions. Some authors proposed a simplified algorithm [31]:
    - In Le Fort I fractures: the anterolateral margin of the nasal fossa is fractured
    - In Le Fort II fractures: the inferior orbital rim is fractured
    - In Le Fort III fractures: the zygomatic arch is fractured (Figs. 3.3b and 3.8a–c)
    - Le Fort patterns are partially outdated in the first place because Le Fort's experiments used low-velocity trauma; higher-velocity trauma more frequent nowadays results in different midface fracture patterns, although most cases can be

Fig. 3.2 (**a**) PMCT, 3D VRT reconstructions of the skull. Context of a fight with punching and kicking. Left image: right view, showing a left temporo-parietal fracture (short arrow), with multiple facial fractures. Right image: anterior view, showing multiple facial fractures of the fronto-maxillary sutures, nasal bone and both maxillary bones (arrows) with Le Fort II and III fractures. (**b**) Clinical head CT: context of a cranial trauma caused by a kick from a horse. Left image: axial cranial image. Presence of a limited epidural haematoma at the left side (coup) (arrow) and a right temporal intraparenchymal haematoma (contrecoup) (star). Right image, 3D VRT reconstruction; left lateral view, linear left parietal fracture (arrows). This permits to characterise the trauma as a lateral trauma, from the left (coup side) to the right (contrecoup side). (**c**) PMCT, posterior views of 3D VRT reconstructions with circular and radiating fractures. Context of a great height fall. Left image: circular and radiate fractures lines (corresponding to the pattern of spider's web fracture). Right image: circular and radiate fractures lines (corresponding to the pattern of spider's web fracture). (**d**) Clinical head CT: initial context of unconscious victim found on a sidewalk; final context of fall from great height. The CT revealed a spider web fracture at the right parieto-temporal bones. Left image: 3D VRT reconstruction, right lateral view. Right image: 3D VRT reconstruction, superior view. (**e**) PMCT of a cyclist hit by a car. Left image: 3D VRT reconstruction of the skull, posterior view. Parietal linear fractures. Right image: 3D VRT reconstruction of the skull, internal view. Continuity of these fractures within both temporal bones (corresponding to a hinge fracture) with a complete dissociation between the anterior and the posterior fossae of the skull. (**f**) PMCT, axial view of the skull, MIP reconstruction on bone filter. Context of a great height fall. Circular fracture of the occipital bone (corresponding to a ring fracture). (**g**) PMCT, 3D VRT reconstruction of the skull, left view. Context of a pedestrian hit by a car. Diastatic fracture of the left lambdoid suture (arrows). (**h**) PMCT, 3D VRT reconstruction of the skull, superior view. Context great height fall. Diastatic fracture, with an abnormal space of the coronal suture

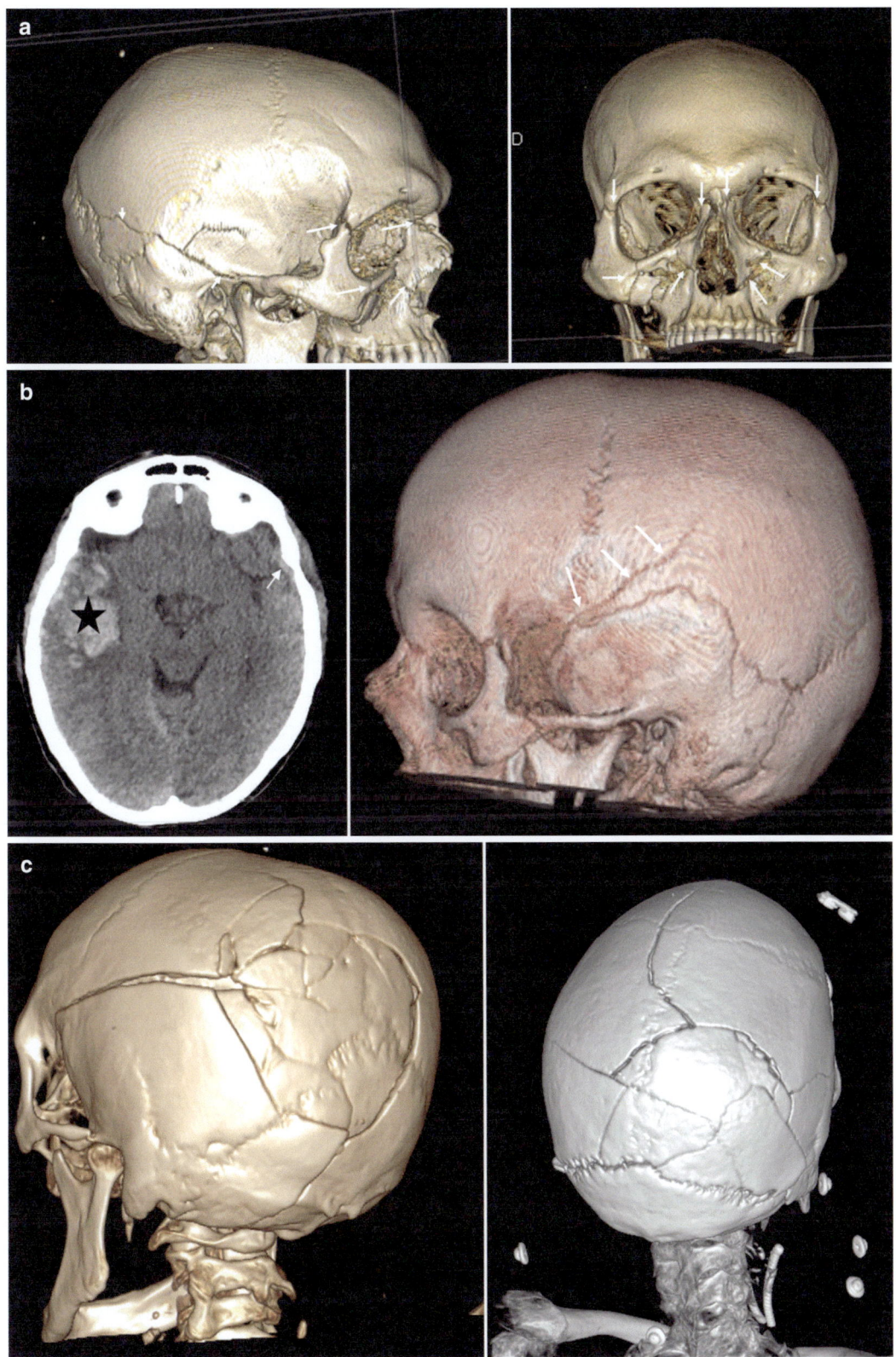

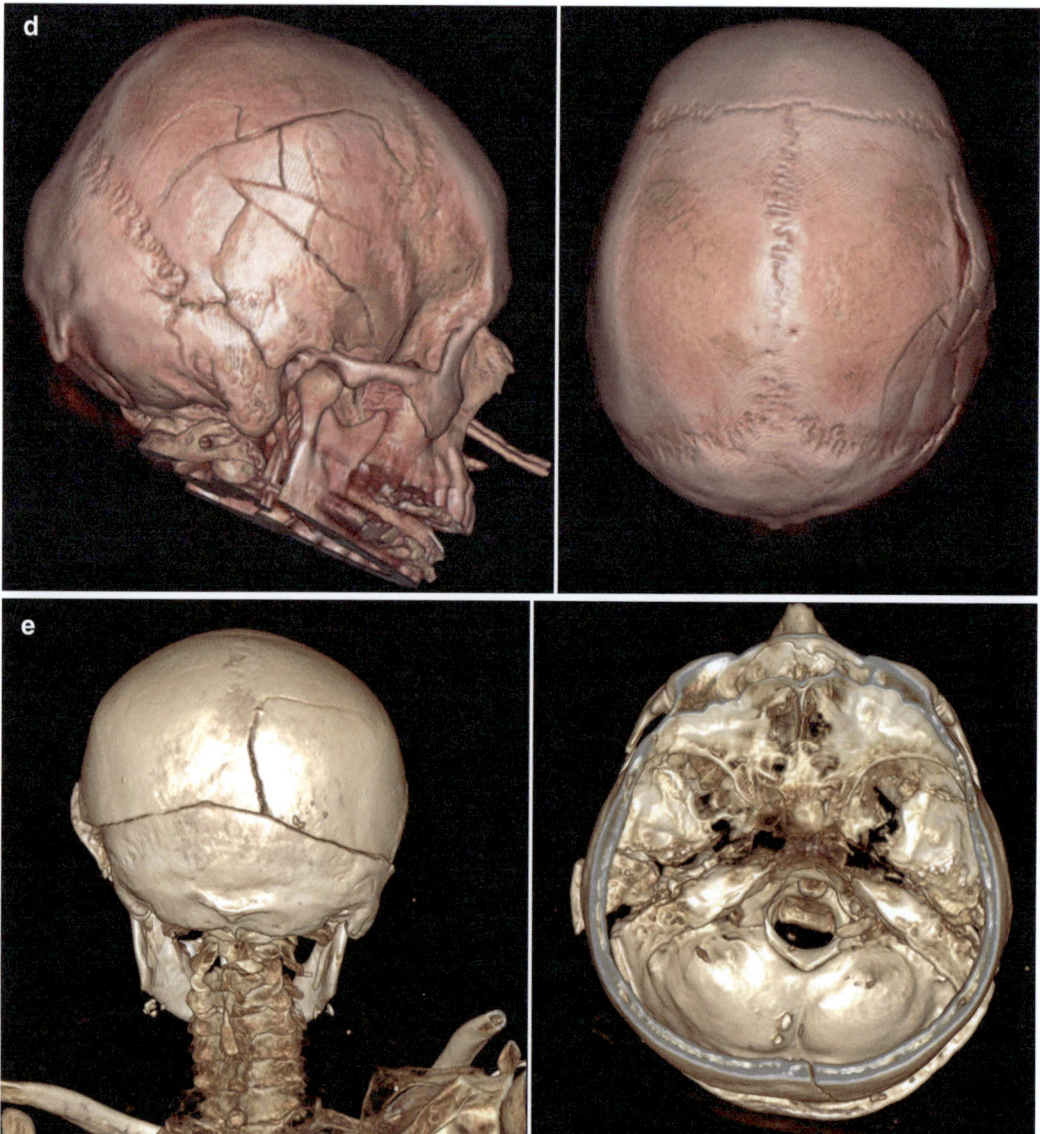

Fig. 3.2 (continued)

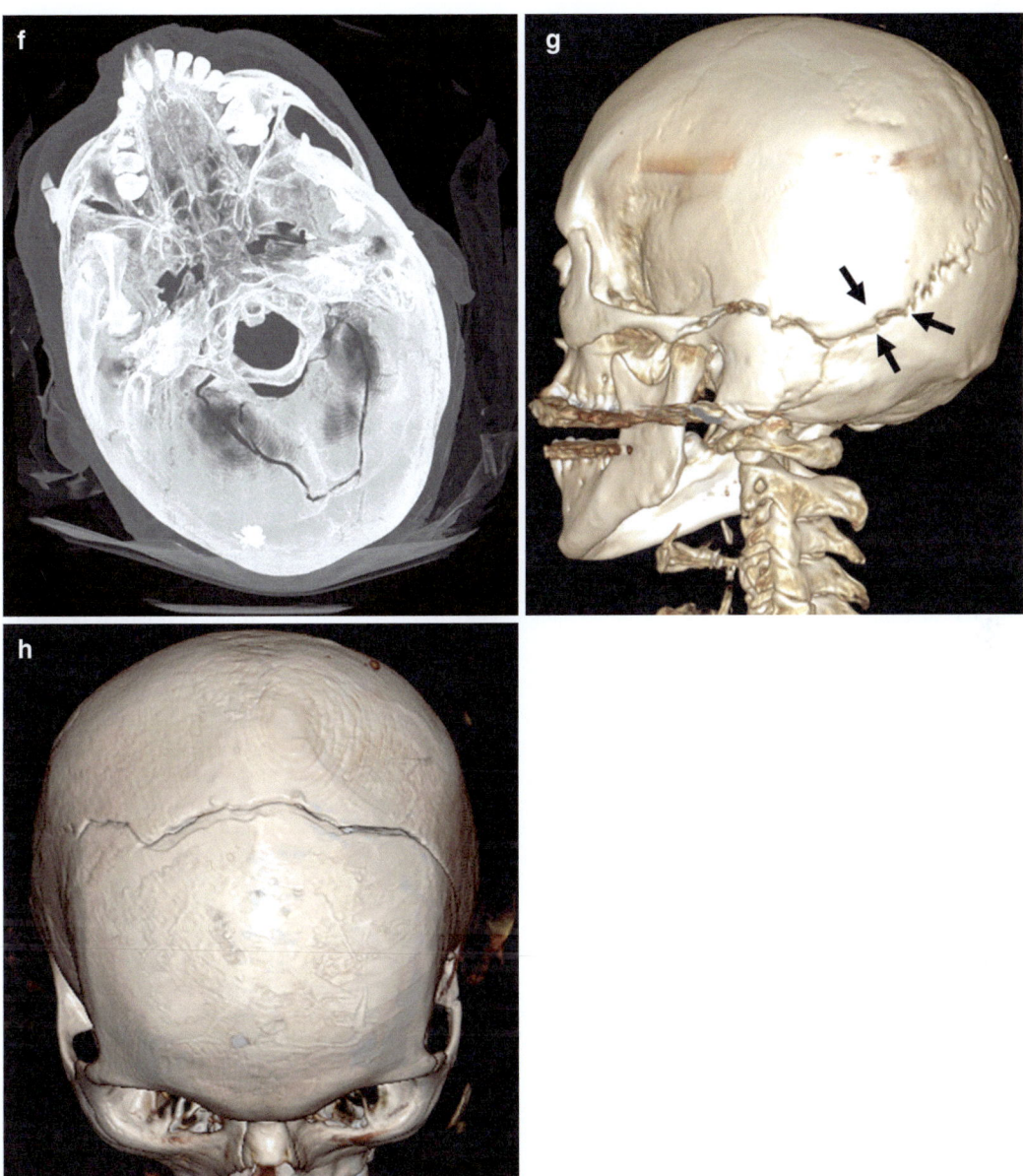

Fig. 3.2 (continued)

described as variants of classical Le Fort fractures [30]. Although pterygoid plate fractures are often described in relation to Le Fort fractures, 37.3% of the patients with pterygoid plate fractures have craniofacial fracture patterns unrelated to Le Fort fractures

– **Frontal sinus fractures**

In fractures of the upper third of the face, the wall of the frontal sinus is usually fractured because this part of the frontal bone is the thinnest (Fig. 3.9a) [30]. These fractures are classified according to:

• Whether the anterior wall, posterior wall or both are involved

• According to the degree of displacement and comminution

– **Blow out fracture** of the orbital wall

This can occur when a sudden blow to the eye pushes the intact globe track into the orbit [4, 30]. The direct traumatic impact on the globe is transmitted to the orbital roof, floor or medial wall, displacing it outward, away from the orbit, while the orbital rim itself remains intact (Fig. 3.9b).

– **Nose fracture**

In low-force impacts, trauma often causes isolated fracture of the nasal bones (Fig. 3.9c). However, because the nasal bones are located close to the ethmoid sinuses and the medial

Fig. 3.3 (**a**) PMCT, 3D VRT reconstruction of the skull, anterior view. Context of a private aircraft accident. Circular and depressed fracture of the right frontal bone due to the impact of a prominent element of the cockpit (arrow). (**b**) PMCT, 3D VRT reconstructions of the skull. Context of a hang-gliding fall. Left image: right view, showing a well-delimited right temporo-parietal depressed fracture (short arrows), with multiple facial fractures (arrows). Right image: anterior view, showing multiple facial fractures of the left fronto-maxillary suture and zygomatic arch, nasal bone and both maxillary bones (arrows) with Le Fort II and III fractures. (**c**) Clinical head CT: context of cranial trauma with a blast ball. Left image: 3D VRT reconstruction, right view, presence of a well-delimitated depressed fracture at the right temporo-parietal bone. Right image: 3D MIP reconstruction, depressed fracture of 8 × 6 cm, with some radiating fractures (at the frontal bone and the mastoid). (**d**) PMCT, context of fight and trauma with a big stone. Well-localised communitive depressed fracture of the left hemi cranium (circles), fracture of the mandible (arrow). Left image: 3D VRT reconstruction, left view. Right image: coronal MPR reconstruction. (**e**) Clinical head CT: context of a cranial trauma with a manhole cover. Presence of a depressed fracture at the vertex, with a coronal long axis (dotted ellipse), and anterior radiating fractures, with a frontal pyramidal-shaped bone fragment (star). Left image: 3D VRT reconstruction, anterior view. Right image: 3D VRT reconstruction, superior view. (**f**) Clinical head CT: context of blunt with the distal extremity of a barrel (hand-gun). The CT revealed a rounded occipital depressed fracture of 2.5 cm in diameter. Left image: 3D VRT reconstruction, posterior view. Right image: 3D coronal MIP reconstruction, coronal plane. (**g**) Clinical head CT: context of a fight with the extremity of a machete handle. 3D VRT reconstruction, superior view: presence of two depressed fractures, one at the left parietal bone, one at the right parietal bone. Left upper inlay: 3D MIP reconstruction, circular-shaped fracture from 20 × 25 mm. Right upper inlay: 3D MIP reconstruction, hemi-circular shaped fracture from 20 × 14 mm. (**h**) Clinical head CT: context of a blunt trauma with an unknown blunt object. Left image: 3D VRT reconstruction, anterior view, presence of a depressed wedge-shaped fracture at the frontal bone. Left superior inlay: 2D MPR sagittal reconstruction, right depressed wedge-shaped fracture. Left inferior inlay: 3D MIP reconstruction, coronal plane, aspect of concentrically terraced fracture. Middle image: axial cranial CT, presence of two depressed fractures, one anterior at the frontal bone; one posterior at the right lambdoid suture. Right image: 3D VRT reconstruction, posterior view, presence a circular fracture of 17 mm in diameter. Right superior inlay: 2D MPR sagittal reconstruction, internal displacement of the bone fragments. Right inferior inlay: 3D MIP reconstruction, circular-shaped fracture of 17 mm in diameter. (**i**) Clinical head CT: context of cranial trauma with an F clamp. Left image: 3D VRT reconstruction, right view, presence of a depressed fracture at the right temporo-frontal bones. Right image: 3D MIP reconstruction, oval depressed fracture of 33 × 48 mm

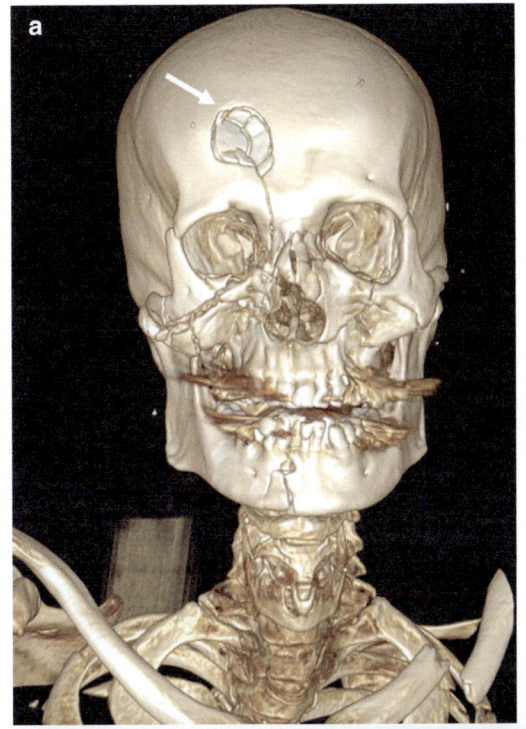

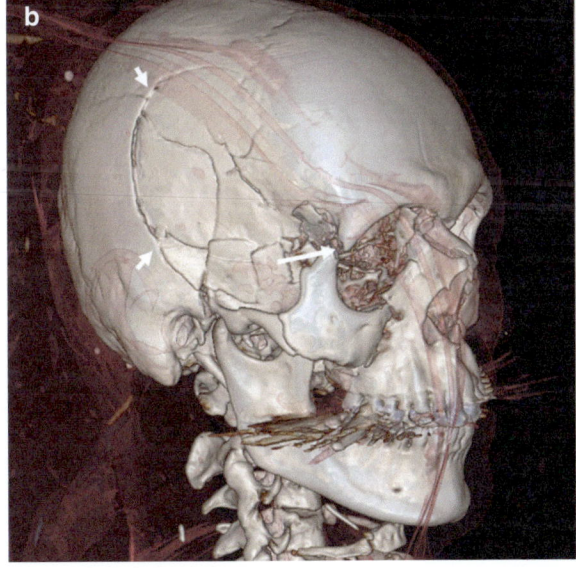

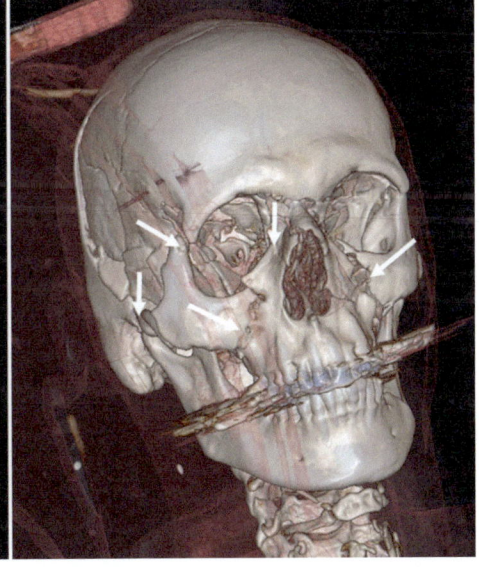

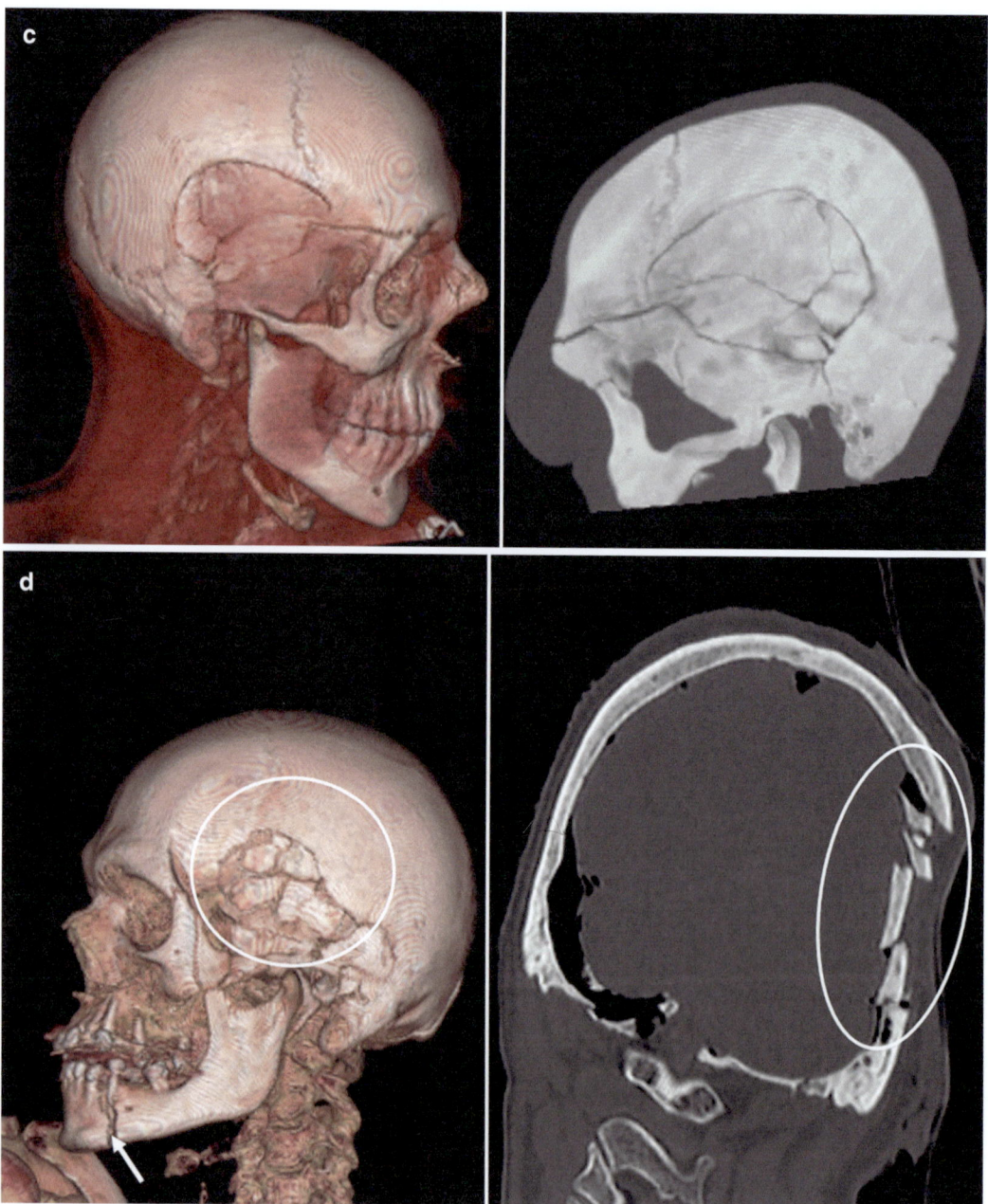

Fig. 3.3 (continued)

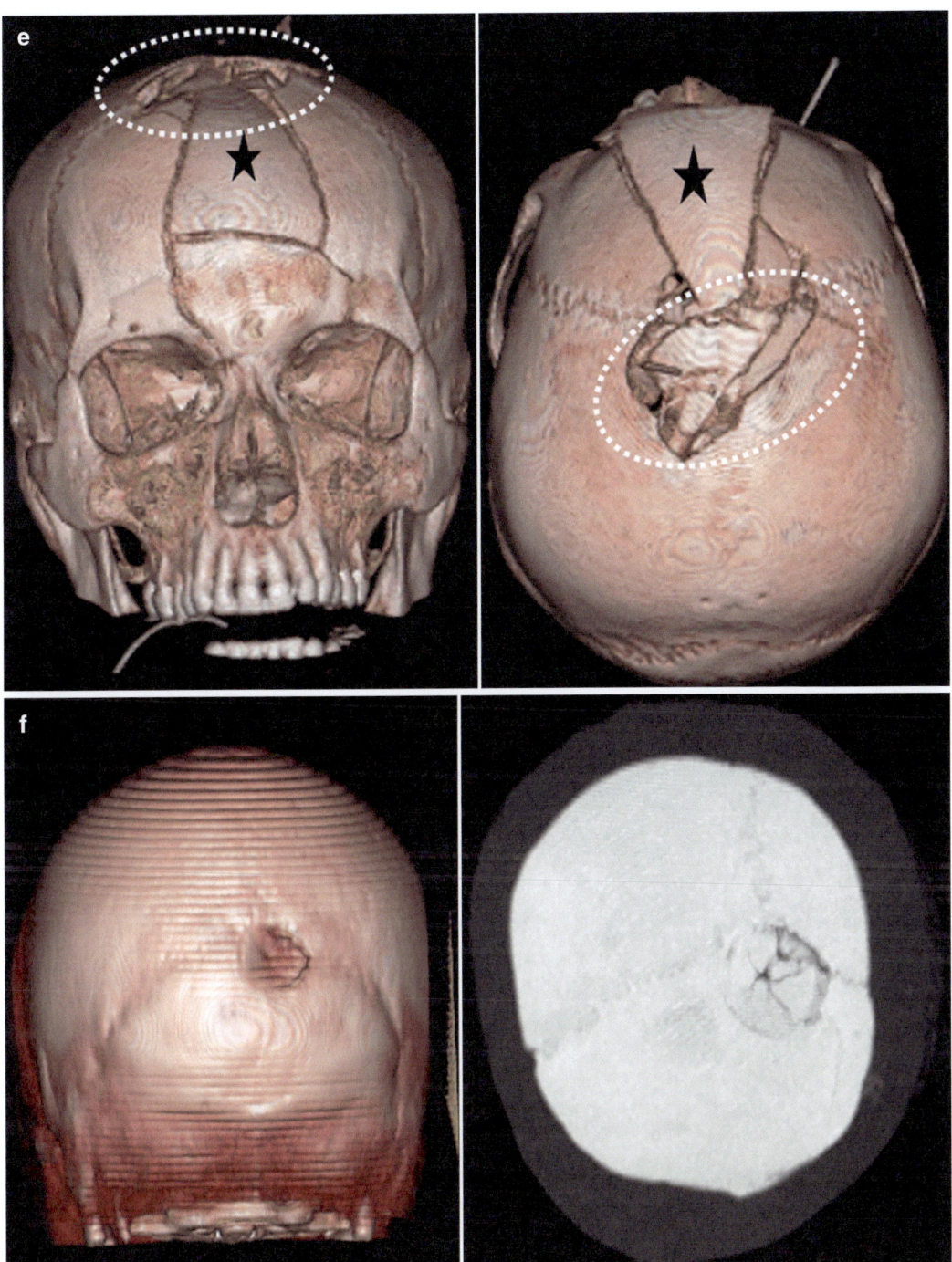

Fig. 3.3 (continued)

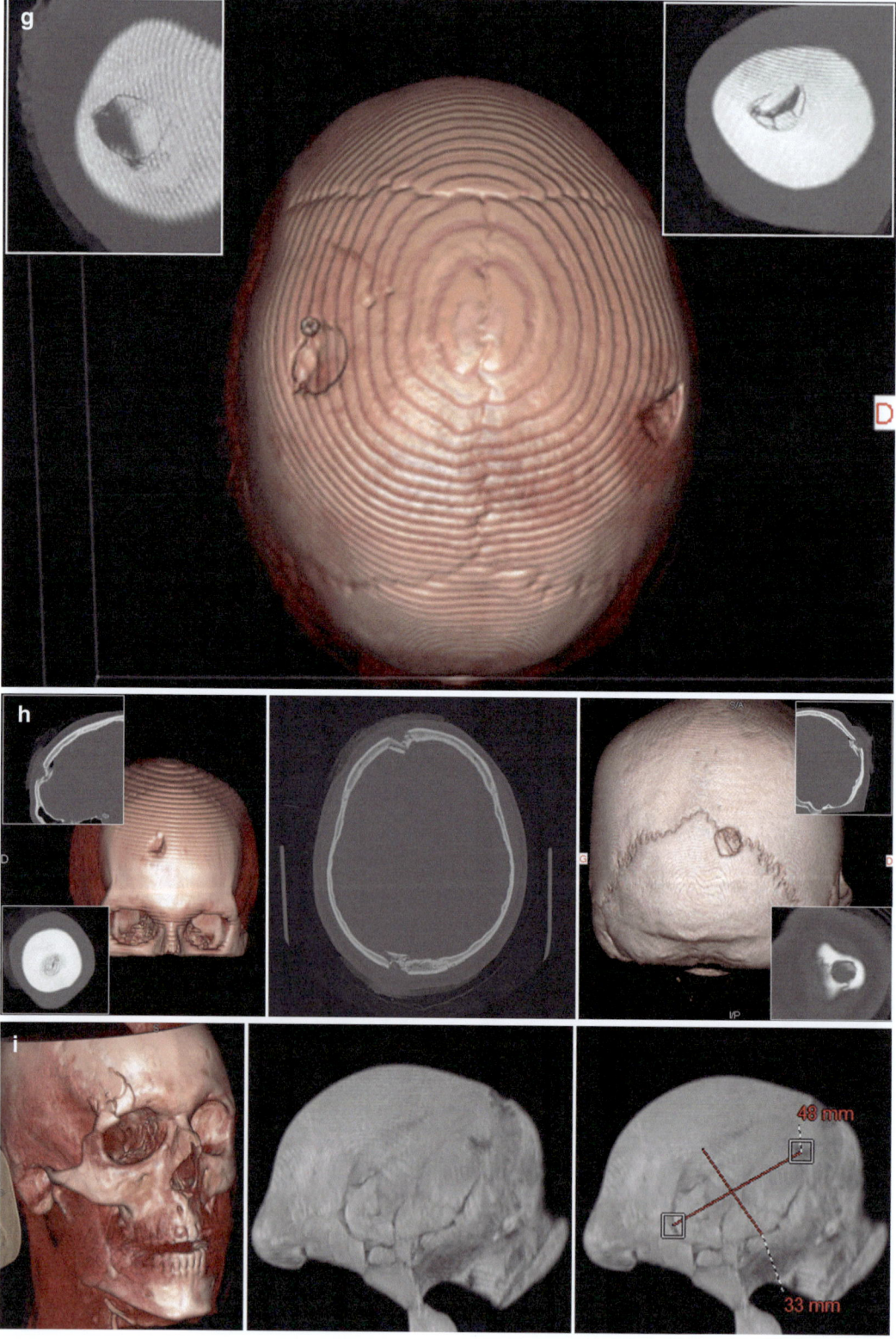

Fig. 3.3 (continued)

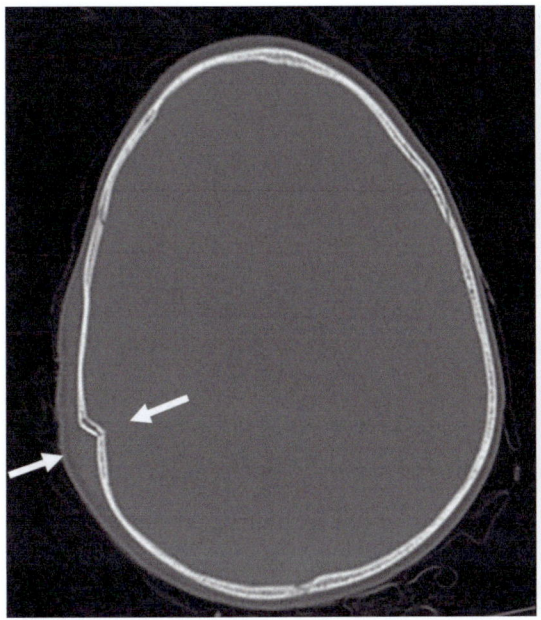
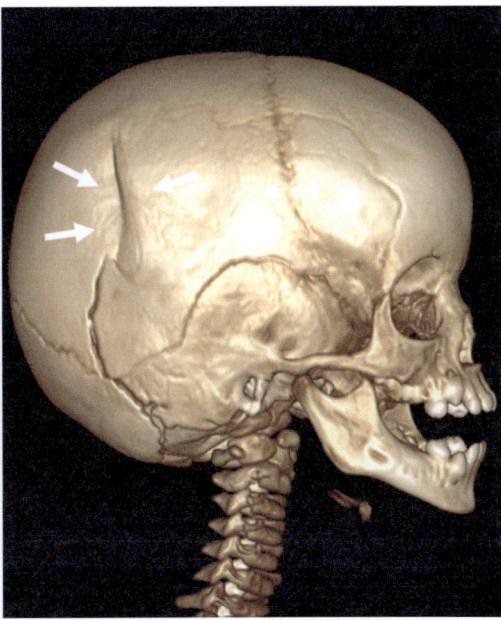

Fig. 3.4 PMCT of a 2-year-old boy hit by a car. Left image: PMCT, axial view of the skull, bone filter. Deformation of the skull (arrows) without rupture of the continuity of the internal and external tables ("ping-pong fracture"). Right image: 3D VRT reconstruction of the skull, right view. Oblong depression (arrows) of the parietal bone at the point of impact

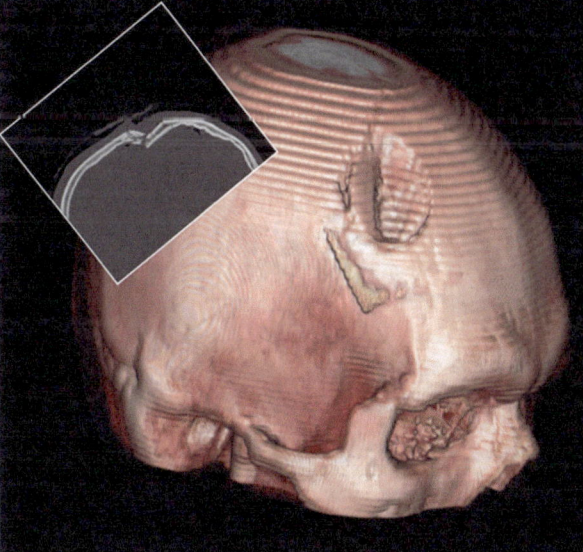
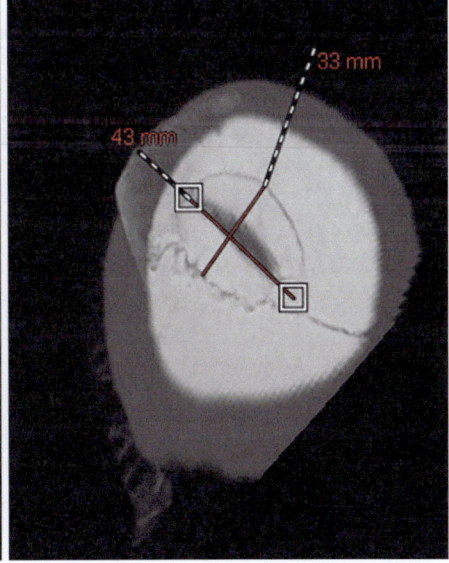

Fig. 3.5 Clinical head CT: initial context of blunt trauma with an unknown object; final context of blunt trauma with a road sign. The CT revealed a right frontal depressed fracture (aspect of a gutter fracture). Left image: 3D VRT reconstruction, anterior and right view. Left upper inlay: oblique reconstruction, short axis of the fracture: visualisation of the "V"-shaped fracture. Right image: 3D MIP reconstruction, oblique coronal plane

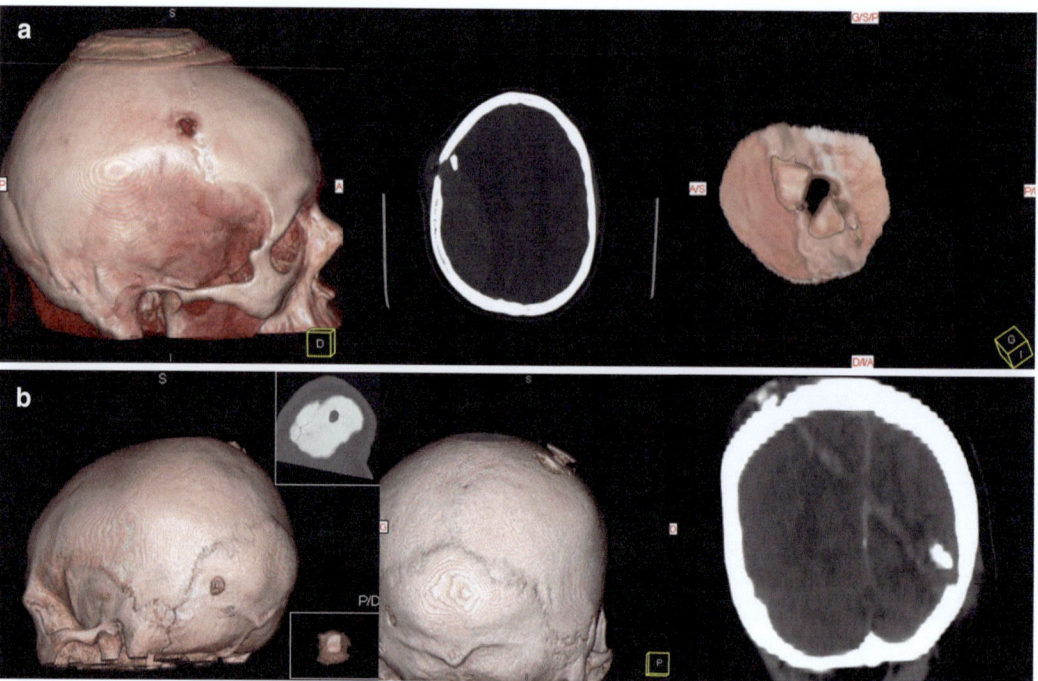

Fig. 3.6 (**a**) Clinical head CT: context of a fight with the extremity of a knife handle. Left image: 3D VRT reconstruction, right view, presence of a bone defect at the right parietal bone. Middle image: axial brain image, epidural haematoma, with one detached intracranial bone fragment. Right image: 3D VRT reconstruction, endocranial view, presence of two triangular-shaped intracranial bone fragments. (**b**) Clinical head CT: Context of fall of a building worker on a long metallic stick. Left image: 3D VRT reconstruction, posterior view, entry hole fracture of 1 cm in diameter at the left part of the occipital bone. Superior inlay: 3D MIP reconstruction, coronal plane; inferior inlay, 3D reconstruction of the detached bone fragment, in intracranial position (which is squared and "mushroom" shaped). Middle image: 3D VRT reconstruction, posterior view, exit hole fracture of 1 cm in diameter, with a subcutaneous detached bone fragment, also with a "mushroom" shape at the right parietal bone. Right image: 3D MIP reconstruction, oblique coronal plane, the haemorrhagic stick path is visible within the cerebral parenchyma, with a direction oriented from left to the right, from down to up, and slightly from the back to the front

orbital walls, high-force impacts can also cause injury to the underlying ethmoid sinuses and orbits [4, 30]. Fracture of the nasal bone is important to know, because bleeding in the nose may provoke a profuse haemorrhage in an unconscious victim, with a passage back through the nasal fossae into the throat, and sometimes cause fatal airway obstruction.

- **Mandible fracture**

    After the nasal bones, the mandible is the most common site of facial fractures (Fig. 3.3e) [30]. When a mandibular fracture results in three or more fragments within the same anatomic region, it is defined as a comminuted fracture. When five or more frag-

ments are present, it is defined as a severely comminuted fracture [4, 30]. A heavy kick or blow to one side of the jaw can cause ipsilateral, bilateral or contralateral fractures.

- **Naso-orbito-ethmoid fractures**

    Injuries combining fractures of the nasal bone, medial orbital wall and frontal process of the maxilla referring to the naso-orbito-ethmoidal complex (Fig. 3.9d, e) [4, 30]. Fractures of the naso-orbito-ethmoidal complex occur when a high-power force impacts the nose anteriorly and is transmitted posteriorly through the ethmoid bone, resulting in severe comminution of both medial maxillary buttresses.

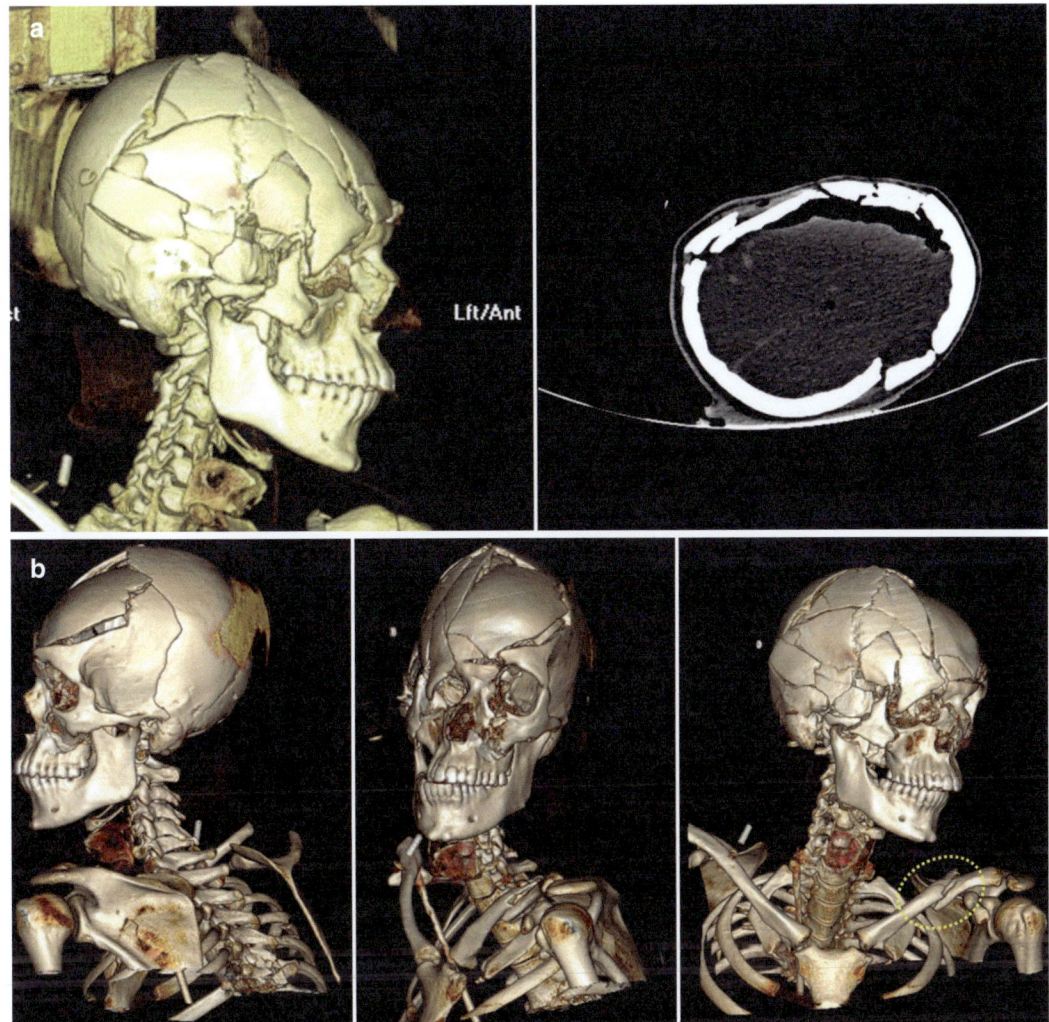

Fig. 3.7 (**a**) PMCT, context of great height fall. Left image, 3D VRT reconstruction, left view, diffuse comminuted fractures. Right image, axial slice: showing the massive flattening in the coronal plane of the skull. (**b**) PMCT, context of great height fall, 3D VRT reconstructions. Multiple skull fractures with massive flattening in the coronal plane of the skull, associated with a left clavicular fracture (yellow-dotted circle). Left image: left view. Middle image: frontal view. Right image: right view

– **Zygomatico-maxillary complex fractures**

A fracture of the zygomatico-maxillary complex results from a direct impact on the malar eminence that causes the underlying zygomatic bone to separate from the calvaria (Fig. 3.9f) [30]. Zygomatico-maxillary complex fractures extend through the four sutures of the zygomatic bone. This fracture is called a tetrapod or quadripod fracture and may extend posteriorly through the sphenozygomatic suture.

3.3.2.3 Intracranial Haemorrhages

– **Epidural (extradural) haematomas** are located between the skull and the underlying dura mater, which is stripped from the bone by

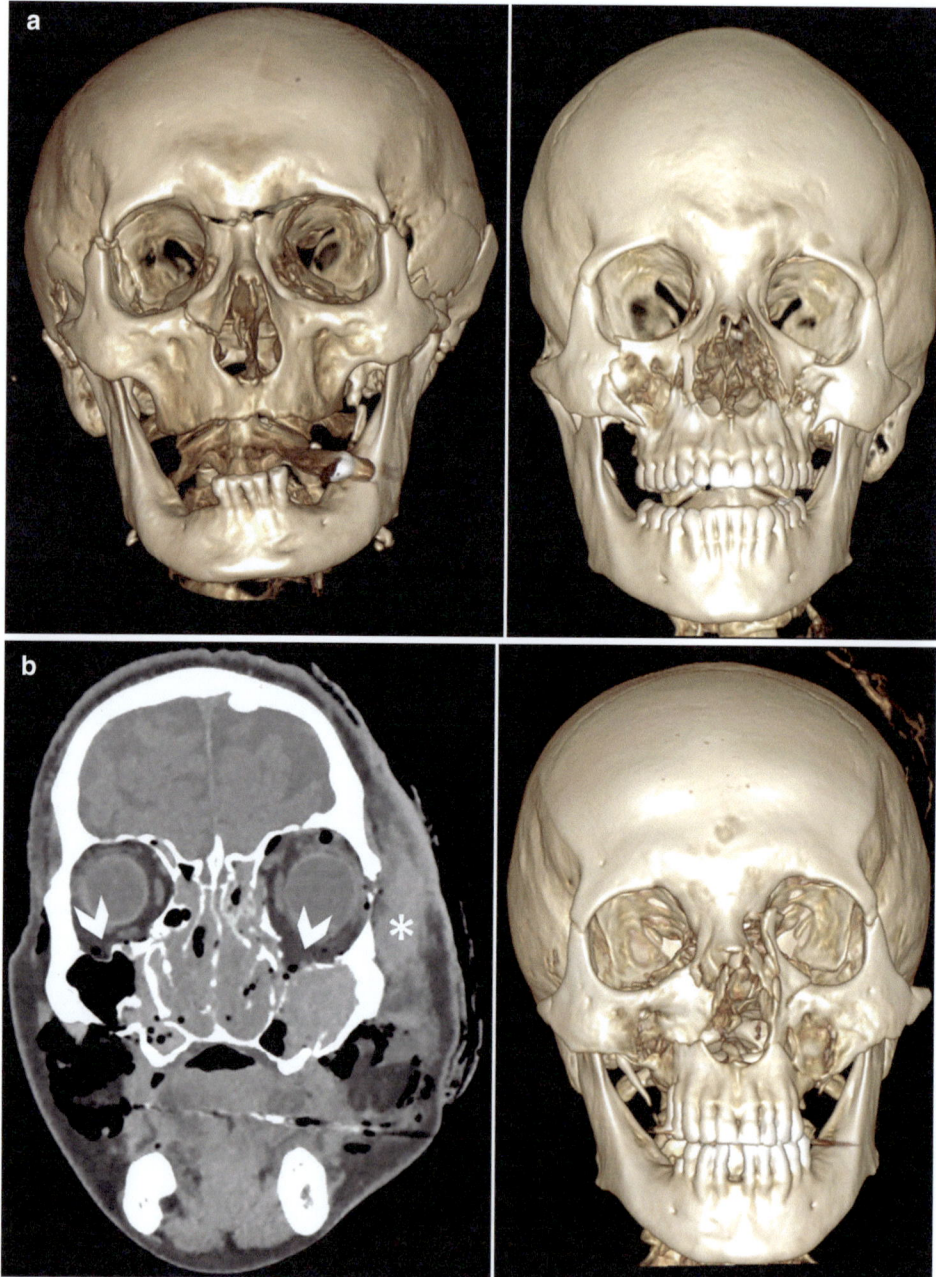

Fig. 3.8 (**a**) PMCT, 3D VRT reconstructions, anterior views. Context of a great height fall. Left image, bilateral Le Fort III fracture: the fractures separate the naso-frontal suture and pass through the medial orbital walls, the zygomatico-frontal sutures and zygomatic arches. Right image, bilateral Le Fort I fracture: fracture of the maxilla (from the dental arches to the base of the nose), with also fractures of both orbital floors. (**b**) Clinical head CT, context of a fall down the stairs. Left image, coronal view of the face in soft tissue filter: fractures of the two maxillary sinuses with subcutaneous emphysema, fracture of the orbital walls (arrowheads); subcutaneous haematoma of the left jaw (asterisk). Right image, 3D VRT reconstruction of the skull, anterior view: bilateral Le Fort I fractures associated with Le Fort III fractures; comminuted fracture of the nasal bone. (**c**) Clinical head CT, context of a fall from standing height. 3D VRT reconstruction of the face, anterior view: bilateral Le Fort I with bilateral fractures of the maxillary bone (arrows)

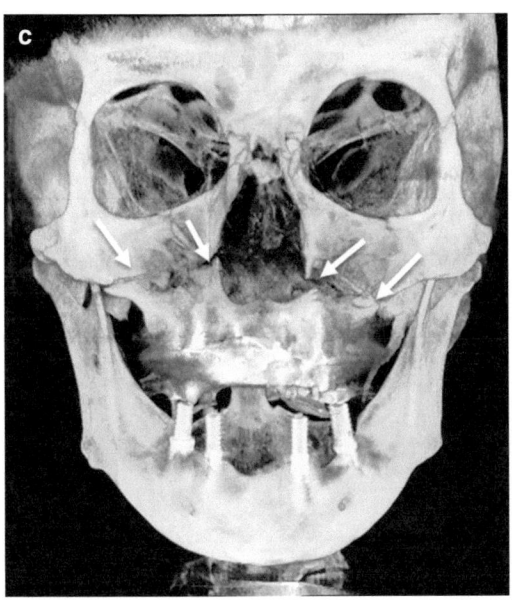

Fig. 3.8 (continued)

bleeding from a vessel. Typically, the haematomas are disc- or lens-shaped (Fig. 3.10a) [1, 5, 6, 32]. In the majority of cases, an extradural haemorrhage is associated with a cranial fracture. The most common locations are the parietal and the temporal regions where branches of the middle meningeal artery are easily lacerated in the course of a transecting fracture line.

– **Subdural haematomas** are intracranial bleedings located beneath the dura mater and above the arachnoid [3, 5–8]. Most often, the bleeding is caused by tearing of overstretched bridging veins that traverse the subdural space between the surface of the cerebral hemisphere and the superior sagittal sinus (Fig. 3.10b). Usually it covers one cerebral hemisphere in a cap-like manner from the parasagittal area via the lateral surface down to the basal fossa, and most often is not associated with skull fractures. An important part of the subdural haematoma is secondary to acceleration or deceleration of the head, for example, in falls with a head impact on a hard surface, and also in traffic accidents.

– Traumatic **subarachnoid bleeding** may result from damage to the cerebral cortex from penetrating injuries or from a vessel laceration within the subarachnoid space (Fig. 3.10c, d) [3, 5–8]. A haemorrhage around the brainstem may arise from laceration of an artery belonging to the circle of Willis or from basilar or cerebral arteries.

– In some skull trauma cases with significant pneumencephalia, the PMCTA can reveal vascular ruptures (arterial or venous) with quite complete pericerebral filling with the contrast agent [6] (Fig. 3.10e).

3.3.2.4 Cerebral Injuries

– **Contusions** are traumatic lesions of the brain that are frequently seen in the cortex and sometimes extending into the underlying white matter (Figs. 3.2b and 3.10f) [1, 5, 6, 32]. The cortical lesions are often covered with subarachnoid bleeding. The word laceration implies severe anatomical destruction. Most cerebral contusions occur in brain regions that are directly opposite the point of impact. This contrecoup is classically due to a fall on the occiput, when the moving head is suddenly decelerated with preferential localisation at the poles and under the surface of the frontal and temporal lobes. The coup contusion arises at the area of impact. Severe coup and contrecoup lesions are not necessarily associated with skull fractures.

– **Diffuse axonal injury** (DAI) is a consequence of shear and tensile strains from sudden acceleration and deceleration or rotational movements of the head [1, 32].

– **Cerebral oedema** is a frequent finding. The enlarged volume of the oedematous brain results in a displacement of cerebral tissue downwards through the midbrain opening, resulting in grooving of the unci and/or hippocampal herniation.

– **Herniation** with concomitant compression of the brainstem may be followed by secondary

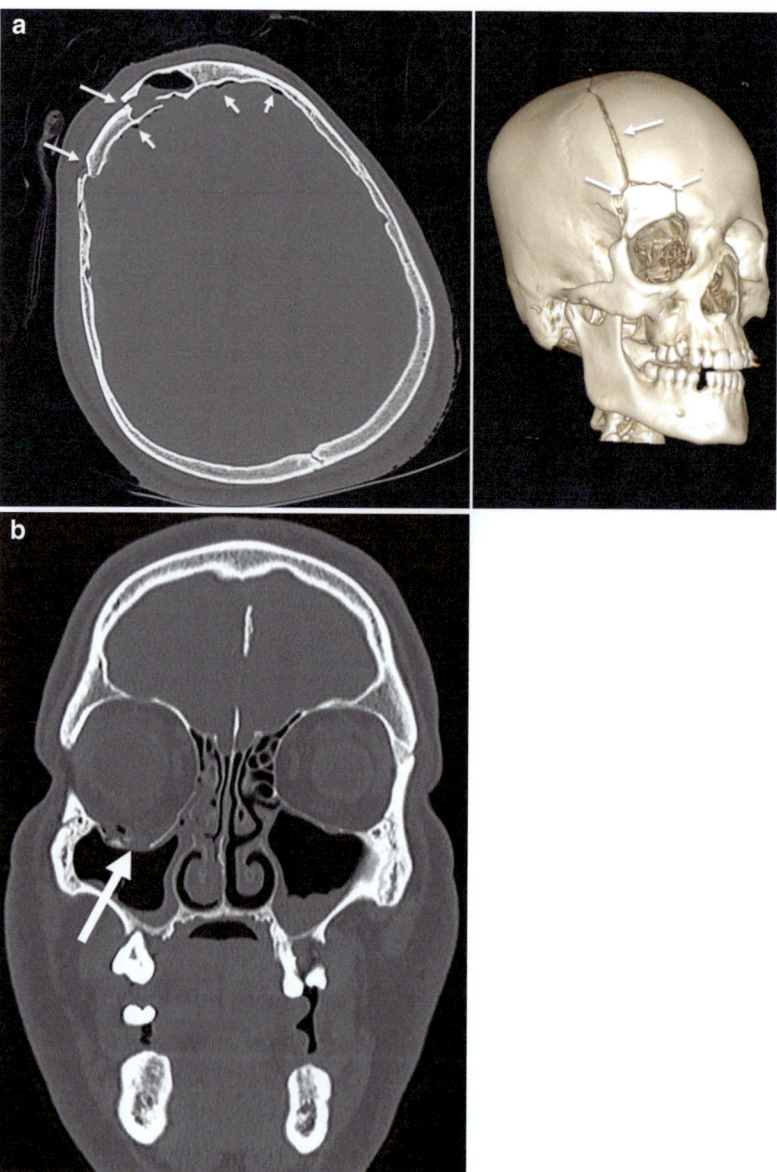

Fig. 3.9 (**a**) PMCT, context of a fall from great height. Fracture of the frontal bone with a depressed fracture with a right linear frontal fracture (arrows) with a fracture of the right frontal sinus, generating gas bubbles in the extra-dural space (short arrows). Left image: axial view, bone filter. Right image: 3D VRT reconstruction, anterior view. (**b**) PMCT, coronal view, bone filter. Context of a punch in the face. Fracture of the right orbital wall (arrow) without incarceration of the orbital fat or the ocular muscles. (**c**) Clinical head CT, axial images, bone filter. Context of fight with punching and kicking. Left image: displaced fracture of the nasal bones (circle). Right image: displaced nasal septal fracture (arrow). (**d**) PMCT, 3D VRT reconstruction of the skull, anterior view. Context of a facial trauma after a brawl. Comminuted fracture of the

left maxilla, with depression of the anterior wall of the maxillary sinus, associated with a complex fracture of the zygomatic arch. (**e**) PMCT, 3D VRT reconstruction. Context of a great height fall. Comminuted fracture of the maxilla, with depression and displacement of the maxillary sinus, associated with a complex fracture of the left zygomatic arch, the mandible and the different walls of the orbits. Note the multiple skull fractures associated with massive facial fractures. Left and middle images: anterior view. Right image: left-side view. (**f**) PMCT, 3D VRT reconstruction of the skull, anterior view. Context of fight with punching and kicking. Comminuted fracture of the left maxilla, with a depression of the anterior wall of the maxillary bone, associated with a fracture of the zygomatic arch, the fronto-maxillary suture and the nasal bone

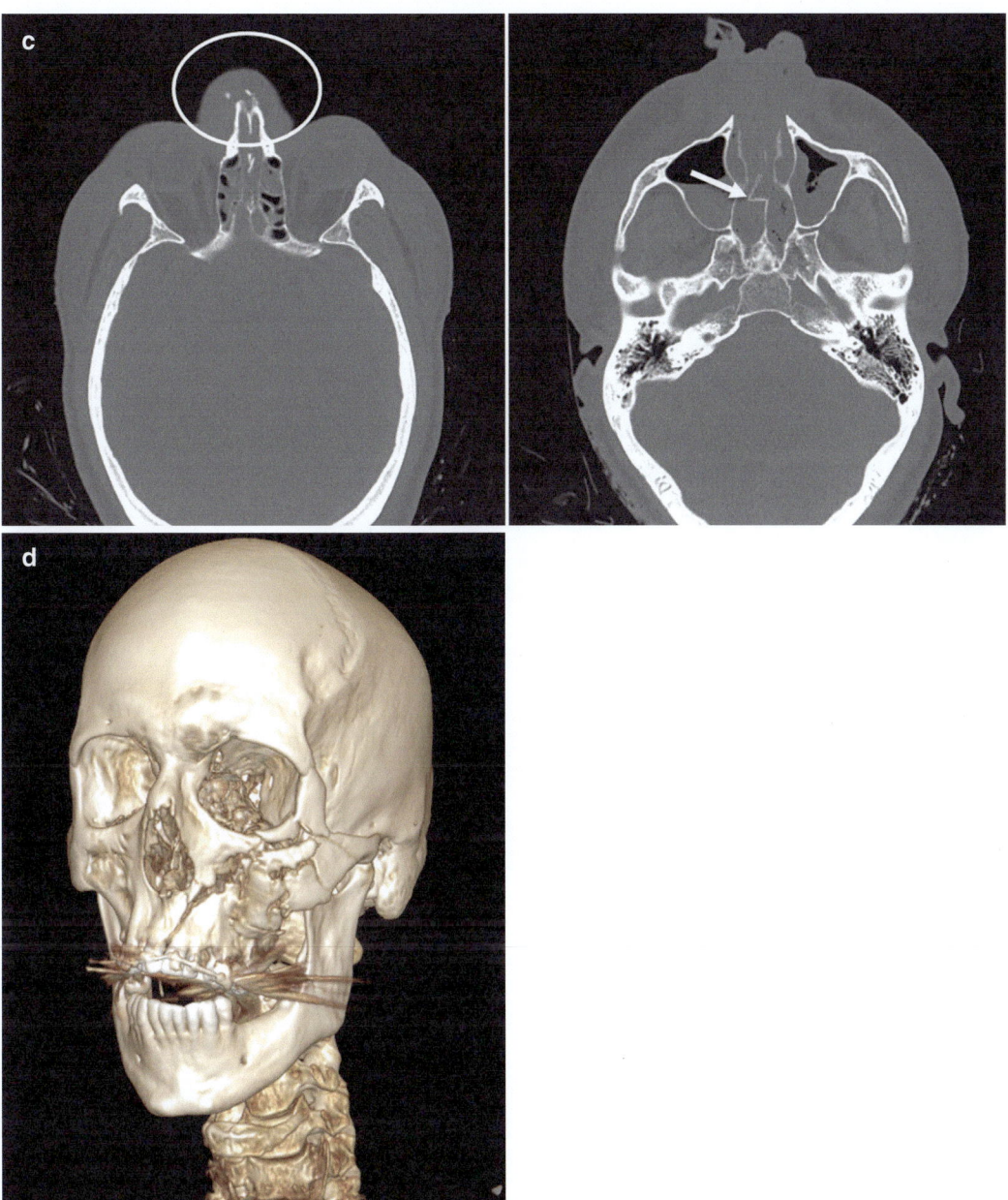

Fig. 3.9 (continued)

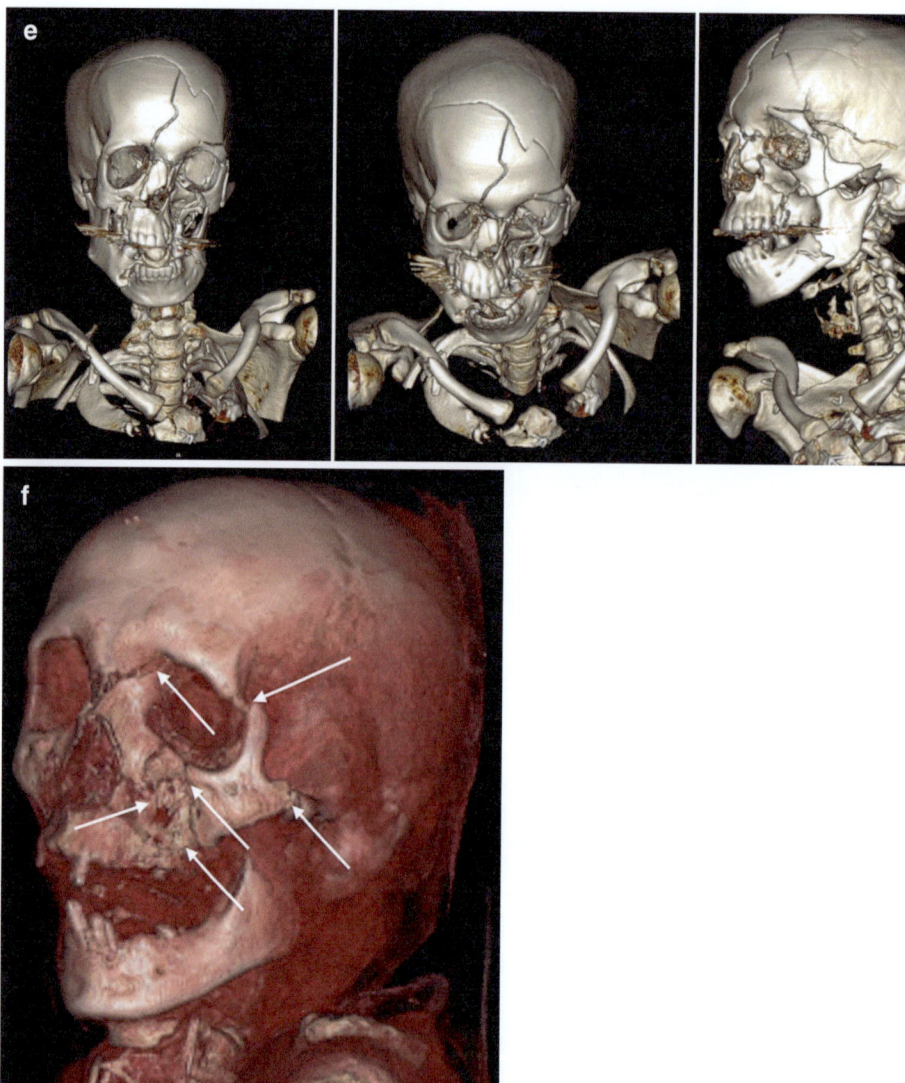

Fig. 3.9 (continued)

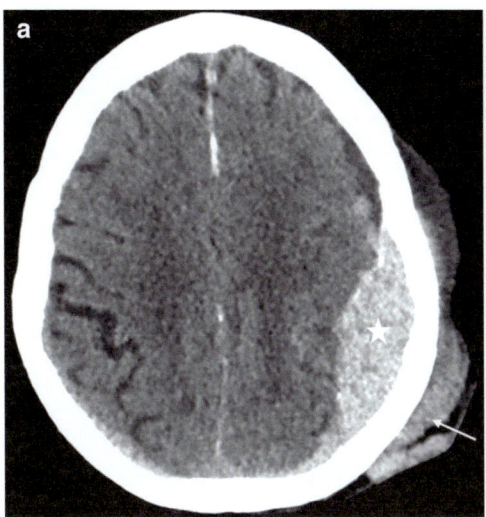 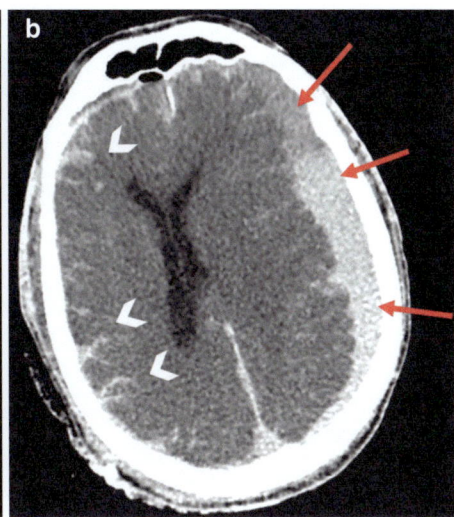

Fig. 3.10 (**a**) PMCT, axial view of the brain, soft tissue filter. Context of a 90-year-old woman, who fall from standing height. Acute left epidural haematoma (star) associated with a parietal fracture (not shown) and left parietal subcutaneous haematoma of the scalp (arrow). (**b**) PMCT, axial view of the brain, soft tissue filter. Context of a 70-year-old pedestrian hit by a car. Acute subdural haematoma (red arrows), with deviation and compression of the lateral ventricles, associated with diffuse subarachnoid bleeding in the sulcus (white arrowheads) and parenchymal oedema. (**c**) PMCT, axial view of the skull, soft tissue filter. Context of a fight with punching and kicking. Multiple subcutaneous haematoma (arrows), subarachnoid haemorrhage (short arrow) and massive pneumencephalia (star). (**d**) PMCT, axial view of the brain, soft tissue filter. Context of a fall from great height. Subarachnoid bleeding filling the lateral fissures and the interpeduncular cistern; diffuse brain oedema with disappearance of the cerebral sulci. (**e**) MPMCTA, axial view of the skull, soft tissue filter. Context of fall from great height. Severe head trauma associated with severe skull fractures (yellow-dotted circles) and contrast agent extravasation. Intraventricular haemorrhage (yellow arrow) and intraparenchymal haematoma and laceration (yellow arrowhead). Note the severe pneumencephalia (yellow star) totally filled with contrast agent at the dynamic phase (yellow star), confirming the severe vascular injuries. Left image: non-enhanced PMCT. Right image: MPMCTA, dynamic phase. (**f**) PMCT, axial view of the skull, soft tissue filter. Context of a fight with punching and kicking. Left image: intraventricular haemorrhage located in the occipital horns of the lateral ventricles (stars), subarachnoid haemorrhage (arrows) and a subtle single gas bubble of pneumencephalia (discontinuous arrow). Right image: subcutaneous right frontal haematoma (stars), massive right intraparenchymal temporal haemorrhage (arrows) in a sequellar hypodensity (medical history of a stroke) (short arrows) and pneumencephalia (discontinuous arrow) (**g**) MPMCTA, axial view of the skull, soft tissue filter. Context of fall from great height. Important head trauma associating severe skull fractures (yellow dotted circles), with contrast extravasation. Intraventricular hemorrhage (yellow arrow) and intraparenchymal hematoma and laceration (yellow arrowhead). Note the important contrast extravasation in the subcutaneous space (orange arrowhead) and the contrast extravasation inside the fourth ventricle (orange arrow) confirming thus the important vascular injuries. Note the important pneumencephalia (white star) totally filled with contrast at dynamic phase, confirming thus the important vascular injuries (orange star).

- Left image: non enhanced PMCT.
- Middle image: MPMCTA, arterial phase.
- Right image: MPMCTA, dynamic phase.

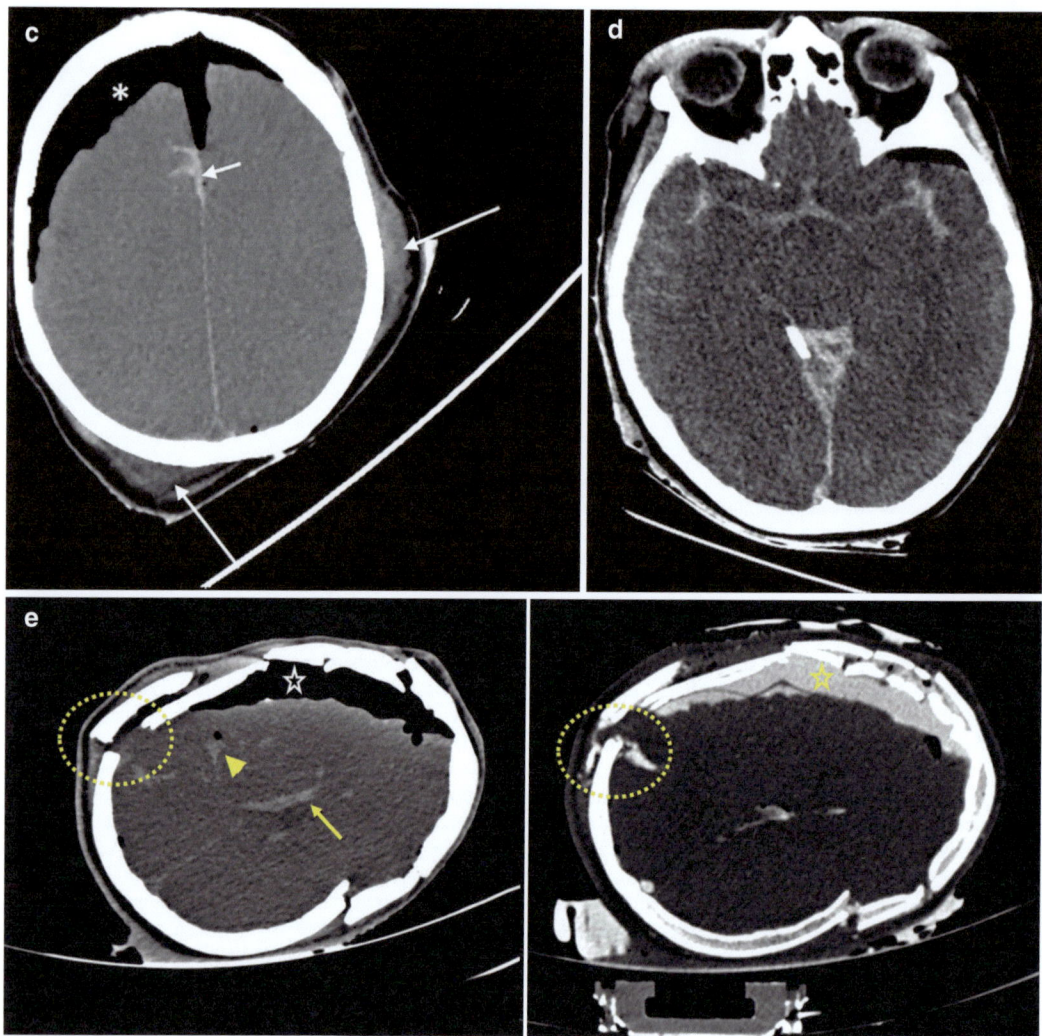

Fig. 3.10 (continued)

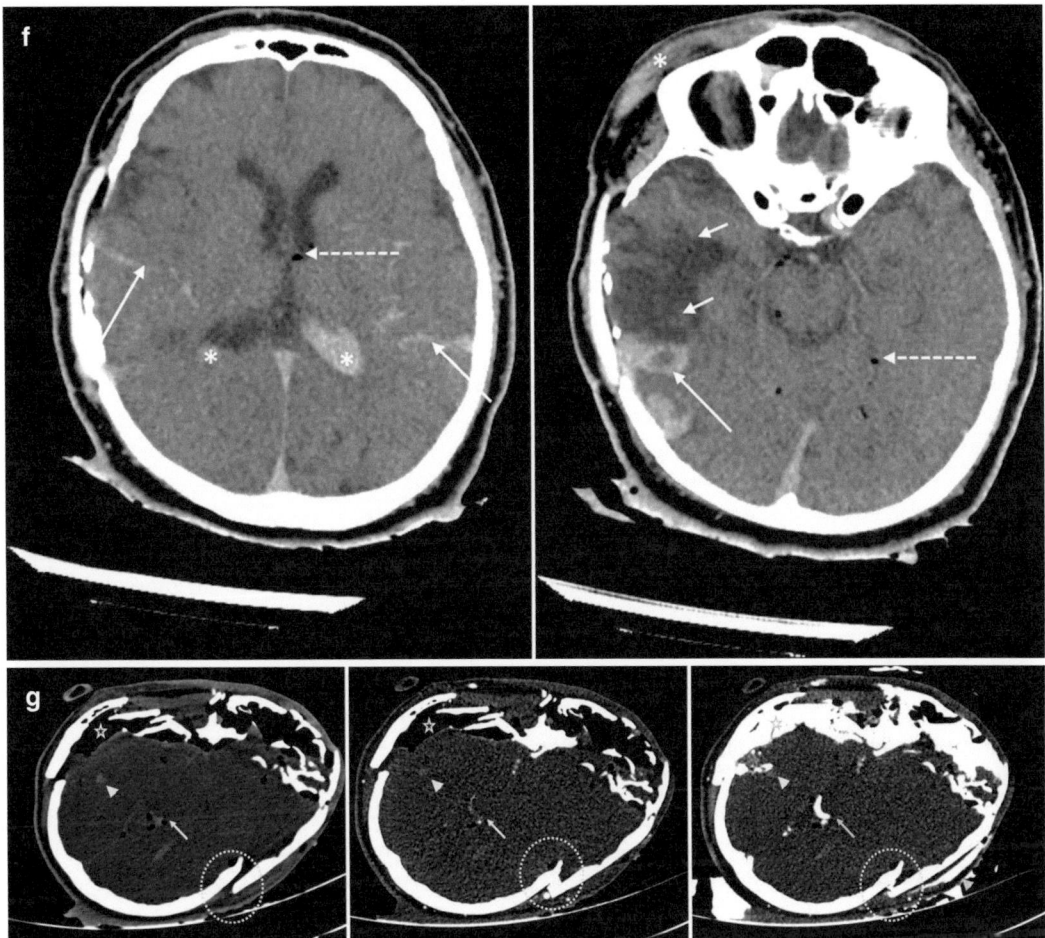

Fig. 3.10 (continued)

haemorrhages and finally lethal dysfunction of the vital centres. Expansion of the subtentorial brain leads to herniation of the cerebellar tonsils [1, 6, 32].

3.3.3 Injuries of the Chest

3.3.3.1 Rib Injuries

These are caused either by direct localised force, producing fractures in the contact area, or—more frequently—indirectly due to compression of the chest [1, 5, 6, 24, 33, 34]. The fracture sites depend on the site of compression (Fig. 3.11a, b):

– Anterior force generates sternal and anterolateral rib fractures.
– Posterior force generates posterior rib fractures.
– Lateral force generates posterior rib fractures and costochondral disruption.

Different complications of rib fractures are possible:

– **Flail chest** corresponds to contiguous fractures, involving at least three ribs and having two fracture sites along each of the affected ribs, creating a loose segment that moves paradoxically with respiration (Fig. 3.11a) [6, 34].
– **Haemothorax** is, for example, possible when sharp ends of fractured ribs induce a laceration of the pleura of the lung (Fig. 3.11c–e). Haemothorax can also be caused by heart or great vessel trauma. Injuries of intercostal vessels are another source of this kind of bleeding (Fig. 3.11f) [18, 35]. Internal mammary artery or vein lacerations are rare, and often associated with clavicle or rib fractures [6, 24, 36, 37]. Sudden deceleration can avulse the internal mammary artery from its origin at the subclavian artery and cause haemothorax or mediastinal haematoma.
– **Pneumothorax** is caused by a leak in the visceral pleura that permits air entry into the pleural cavity [6, 24, 38]. A valve-like leakage of the pleura may induce a tension pneumo-

thorax, caused by an increasing pressure of trapped air in the pleural cavity, following a complete collapse of the affected lung and a shift of the mediastinum to the opposite side (Fig. 3.11g–i) [3, 5–8].
– **Subcutaneous and mediastinal emphysema** may derive from injuries of the trachea, bronchi, the thoracic wall or the lungs by air entering within the adjacent soft tissues (Fig. 3.11d) [1, 6, 24, 32, 39].

3.3.3.2 Lung Injuries

– **Contusion** is very common and is caused by an impact of the chest with consecutive inward bending of the thoracic cage (Fig. 3.11h, i) [6, 24, 40]. Rib fractures are not necessarily associated with lung contusions, especially when the thoracic cage is highly pliable, as in children. It is defined either as a subpleural suffusion or as an intrapulmonary haemorrhage.
– A concussive wave from a chest impact overexpands and tears alveoli. Alveolar septae are disrupted when a concussive wave encounters a liquid-gas interface. **Pneumatoceles** or **haemopneumatoceles** may also be seen in these cases (Fig. 3.11h–j). In some cases, pneumatoceles on native CT are completely filled by the contrast agent during the following PMCTA.
– **A laceration** is secondary to compressive or crushing forces, generating pulmonary tissue to burst or tear, or secondary to inward intrapulmonary displacement of a fractured rib [6, 24, 40]. Tears from rib fractures typically involve the pleural surface, and lacerations which are caused by other mechanisms occur typically at the hilum.
– **The trachea and major bronchi** are rarely injured [6, 24, 39]. The trachea within 2 cm of the carina and right mainstem bronchus are common sites of injury.

3.3.3.3 Heart Injuries

Blunt trauma of the heart is caused directly by precordial impact, with or without lacerating rib and sternal fractures, and indirectly by increased intracardiac pressure from compression and deceleration [6, 24, 33]. Different kinds of lesions are possible:

- **Concussion, contusion and myocardial rupture** are possible [41]. In most cases, the mechanism is due to the force applied on the anterior chest, which compresses or crushes the heart between the sternum and the vertebral column (Fig. 3.12a).
- **Lacerations** of the heart are most often seen in the relatively thin right ventricle or in the atria or the atrial appendage [6, 24, 41]. The anterior surface of the heart underlying the chest wall is composed of the right ventricle (55%), the left ventricle (20%), the right atrium (10%), the ascending aorta, the pulmonary artery (10%) and the vena cava (5%). The frequency of cardiac rupture is the same. Septal ruptures are uncommon.

- The risk of **cardiac rupture** is high during the diastole when the heart chambers are filled with blood and easily burst when suddenly compressed [6, 24, 41]. Heart rupture induces death by either massive blood loss and haemorrhagic shock (pleural cavity filling through a pericardial sac rupture) or cardiac tamponade (Fig. 3.12b) [7].
- **Injuries of the coronary arteries** are uncommon. A dissection, thrombosis, laceration and/or rupture may occur (Fig. 3.12c) [6, 42].

3.3.3.4 Pericardial Injuries

Pericardial laceration is frequently associated with penetration in chest-wall fractures [6, 24, 43]. Cardiac rupture and great vessel trauma may be associated. Laceration is observed on the diaphragmatic, superior, mediastinal or lateral parts of the parietal pericardium [43, 44]. However, the left side is most commonly affected. Lateral

Fig. 3.11 (**a**) PMCT of a car passenger who died in a road traffic accident. Multiple and bilateral fractures of the anterior part of the ribs (arrows) producing a flail chest panel. Left image: 3D VRT reconstruction, anterior view. Right image: axial view in bone filter of the chest. (**b**) PMCT, 3D VRT reconstruction, left view. Context of a fall from great height. Multiple rib fractures and associating lesions of the posterior arches (yellow-dotted circle) anterior arches (white-dotted circle) and a displaced rib fracture of the ninth (orange-dotted circle). (**c**) PMCT, axial view of the chest, pulmonary filter. Context of a fall from great height. Right haemothorax (arrows), right pneumothorax with significant deviation of the mediastina to the left (arrowhead) and subcutaneous emphysema illustrating a tension pneumothorax. (**d**) MPMCTA, axial view of the chest, soft tissue filter. Context of a fall from great height. Haemothorax progressively filled with contrast agent at the venous phase (orange stars). Note the better visualisation of the lung parenchyma at the venous phase (white star). Left image: MPMCTA, arterial phase. Right image: MPMCTA, venous phase. (**e**) MPMCTA, axial view of the chest, soft tissue filter. Context of fall from great height. Intercostal arterial bleeding (orange arrows) responsible for the haemothorax, with progressive contrast agent filling at venous phase (yellow-dotted circle). Left image: Displaced rib fractures (yellow arrow and yellow-dotted circle) responsible of haemothorax (white stars) progressively filled with contrast (yellow stars). Fracture of the middle arch of the fifth left rib responsible of subcutaneous contrast extravasation (yellow arrowhead) and subcutaneous emphysema (orange arrows). PMCT. Middle image: MPMCTA, arterial phase. Right

image: MPMCTA, dynamic phase. (**f**) MPMCTA, axial view of the chest, soft tissue filter. Context of a fall from great height. Intercostal arterial bleeding (orange arrows) responsible of the haemothorax (white star), with progressive contrast filling at venous phase (yellow-dotted circle). Left image: MPMCTA, arterial phase. Right image: MPMCTA, venous phase. (**g**) PMCT, context of hanggliding fall. Left image, coronal MPR: right pneumothorax with significant deviation of the mediastinum to the left. Right image, axial slice of the chest, lung filter: right pneumothorax with significant deviation of the mediastinum to the left. Presence of gas within the cardiac cavities (stars), due to a massive gas embolism. (**h**) PMCT, axial view of the chest in lung filter. Context of a fall from great height. Left image: pneumatoceles (arrows) of the posterior part of the left lung; one of the pneumatoceles is partly filled with blood, with a gas-fluid level (arrowhead). Left pneumothorax. Right image: ground-glass opacities of the anterior part of both lungs (arrows) due to lung's contusions. (**i**) PMCT, axial view of the chest in lung filter. Context of a fall from great height. Left image: bilateral pneumothoraxes (arrows), pneumopericardium (star) and presence of gas within the great thoracic vessels and right cardiac cavities, due to a massive gas embolism. Right image: diffuse ground-glass opacities corresponding to lung contusions and crazy paving aspect due to intra-alveolar haemorrhage. (**j**) MPMCTA, axial view of the chest, soft tissue filter. Context of a fall from great height. Visualisation of two pneumatoceles (black arrows), progressively filled with contrast agent (orange arrowheads). Left image: non-enhanced PMCT. Right image: MPMCTA, dynamic phase

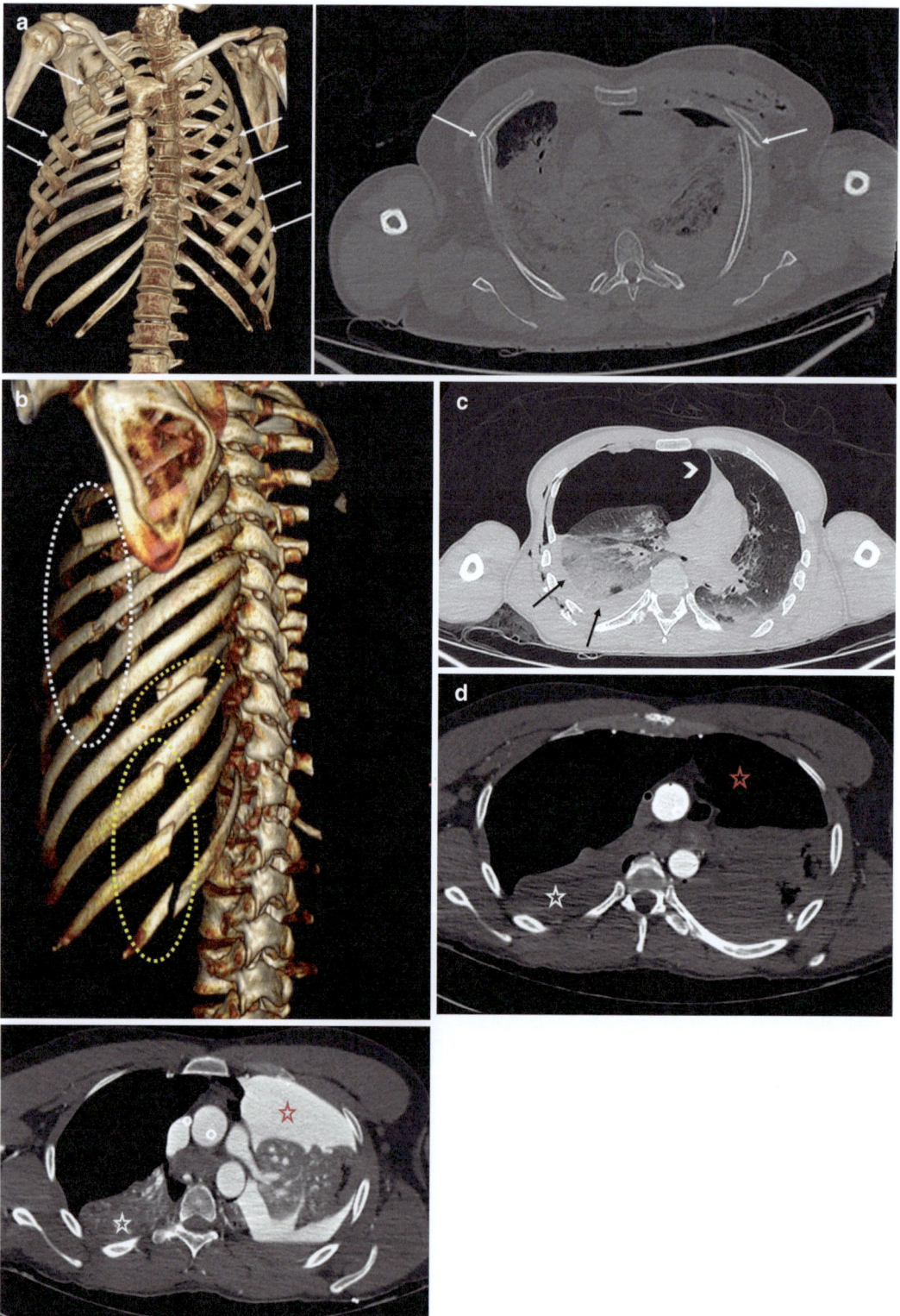

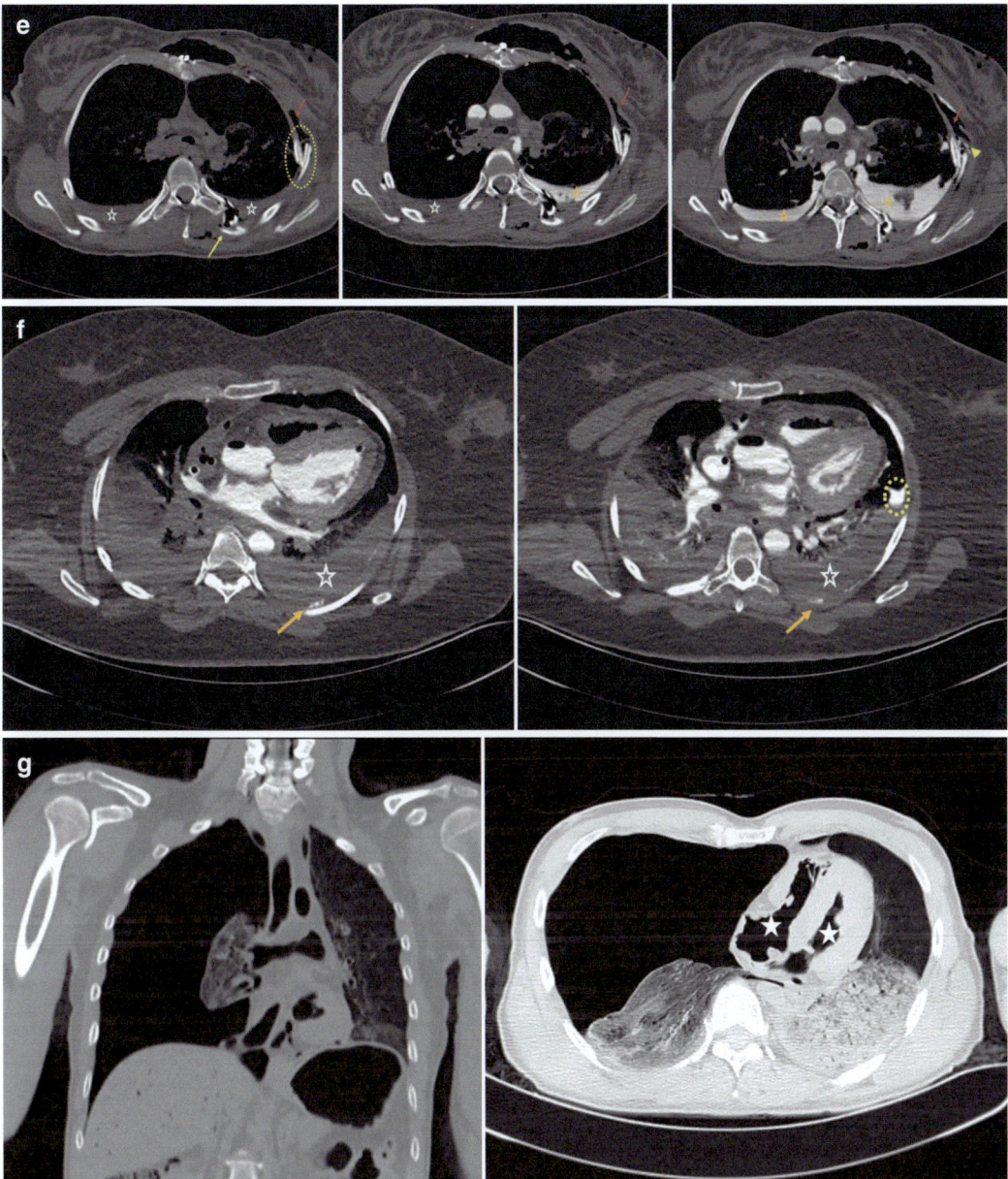

Fig. 3.11 (continued)

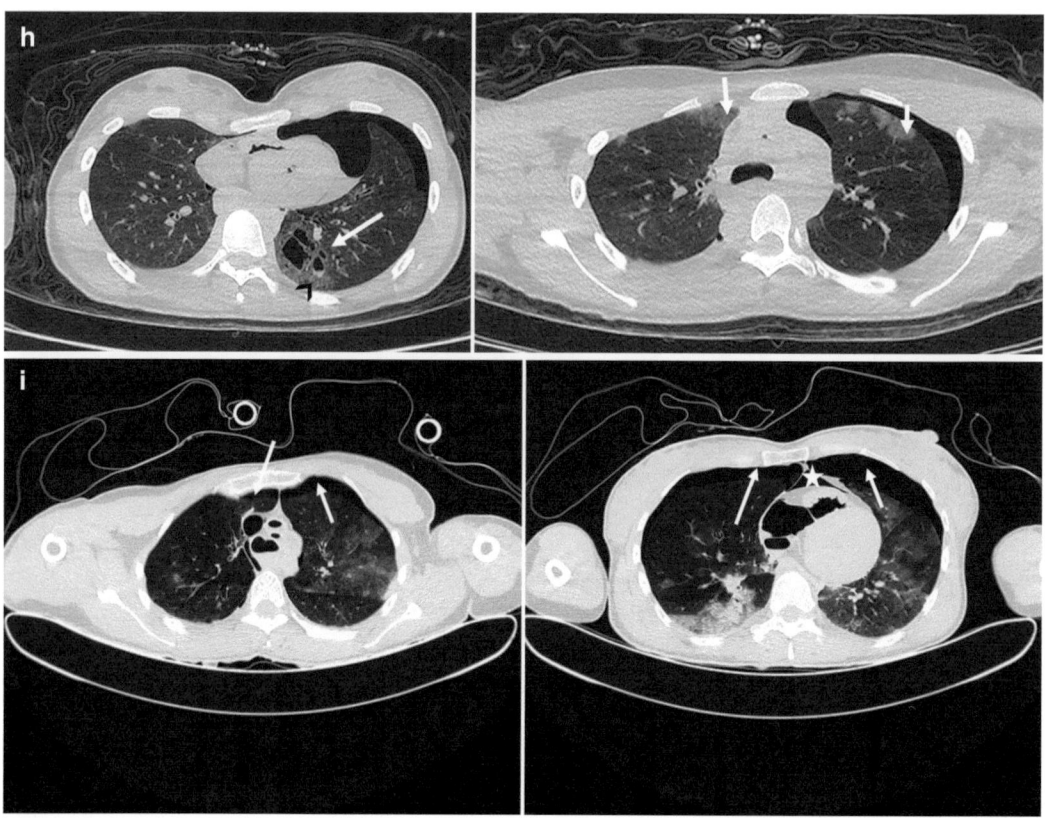

Fig. 3.11 (continued)

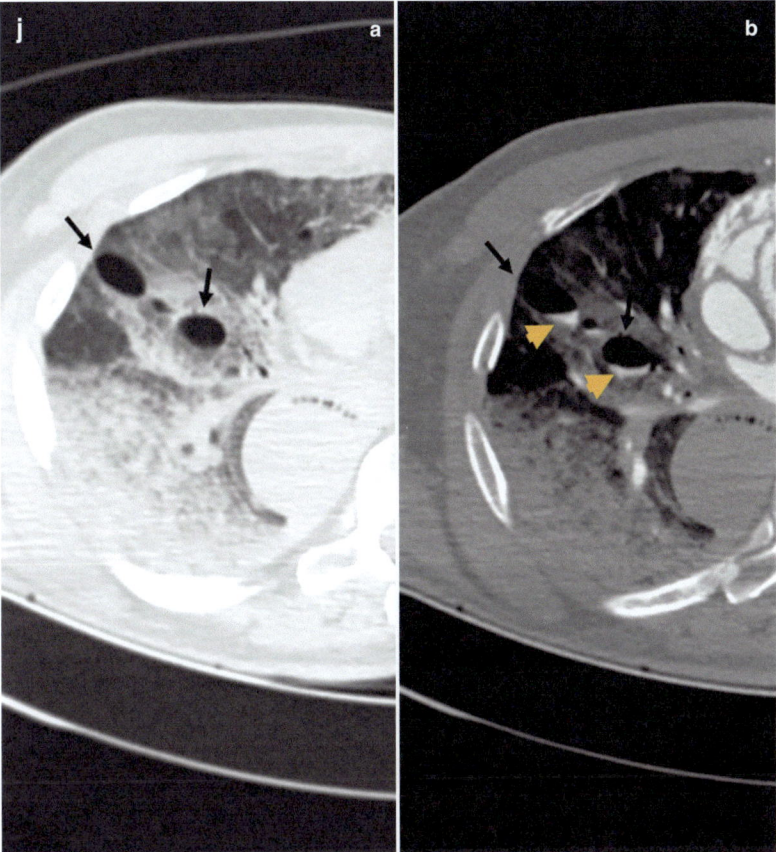

Fig. 3.11 (continued)

Fig. 3.12 (**a**) PMCT, coronal view of the chest, soft tissue filter. Context of a child who deceased after a fall of a piece of furniture on her chest. Rupture of the great vessels and cardiac luxation through the diaphragm (arrowheads). Right haemothorax. (**b**) PMCT, coronal view of the chest, soft tissue filter. Context of a fall from great height. Voluminous bleeding (arrowheads) around the heart in the pericardium leading to death by cardiac tamponade. (**c**) MPMCTA, soft tissue filter, arterial phase. Context of a fall from great height. Right coronary artery rupture (yellow arrowheads) responsible of contrast agent extravasation into the pericardial space (white stars). Left image: axial view of the chest. Right image: coronal oblique view of the chest. (**d**) MPMCTA, axial view of the chest, soft tissue filter, venous phase. Context of a fall from great height. Pericardial rupture clearly identified after contrast agent injection (yellow arrowhead) associated with progressive contrast agent filling of the pericardial space (white star). Note the contrast agent extravasation into intercostal soft tissues, due to rib fractures (yellow arrow). (**e**) PMCT of a man who deceased after a large tree branch fell on his chest. Left image, coronal view, soft tissue filter: laceration and rupture of the right ventricle (arrow). Right image, axial view of the chest in lung filter: severe pneumomediastinum, pneumopericardium and left pneumothorax due to the rupture of the tracheal carina (not shown)

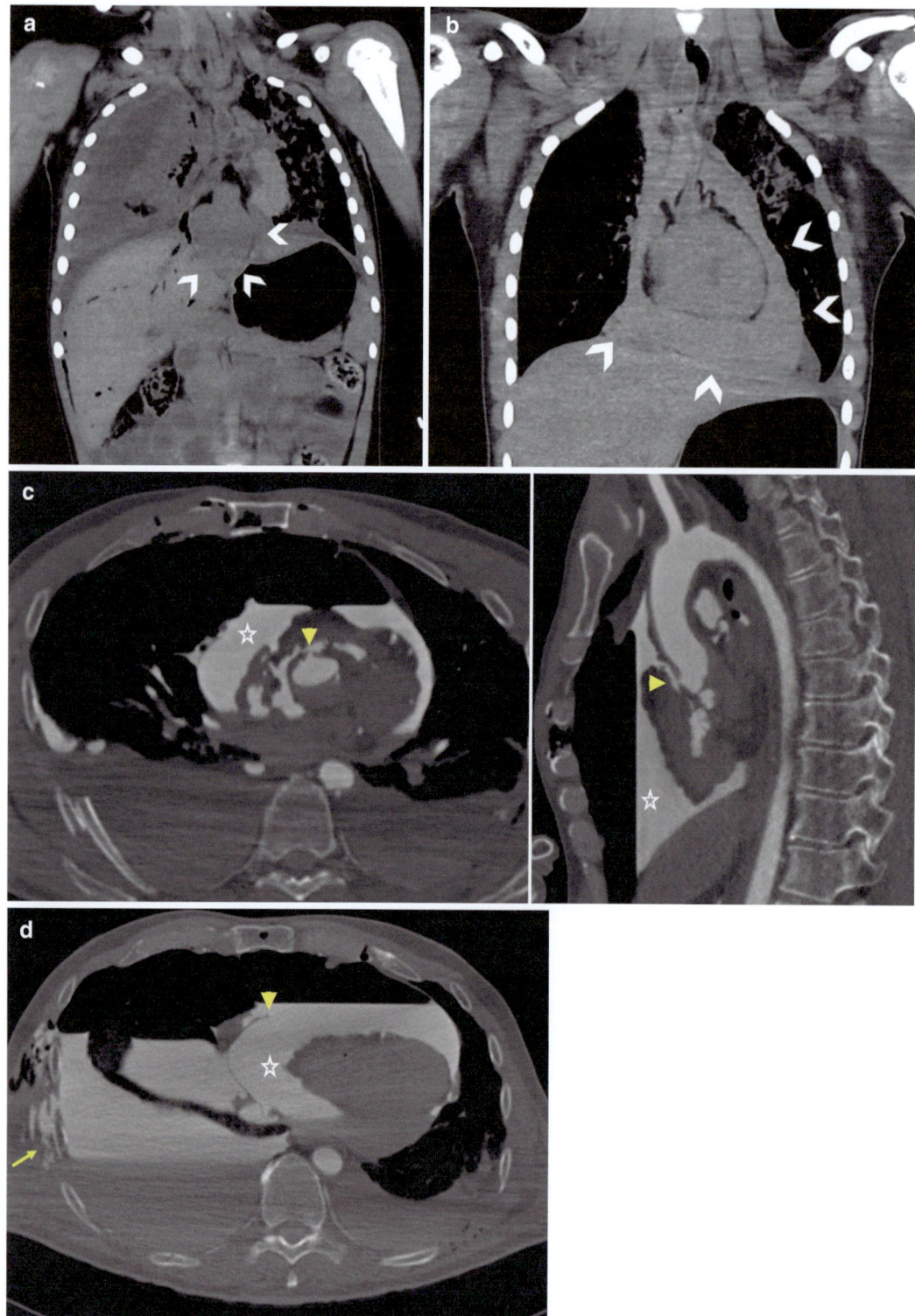

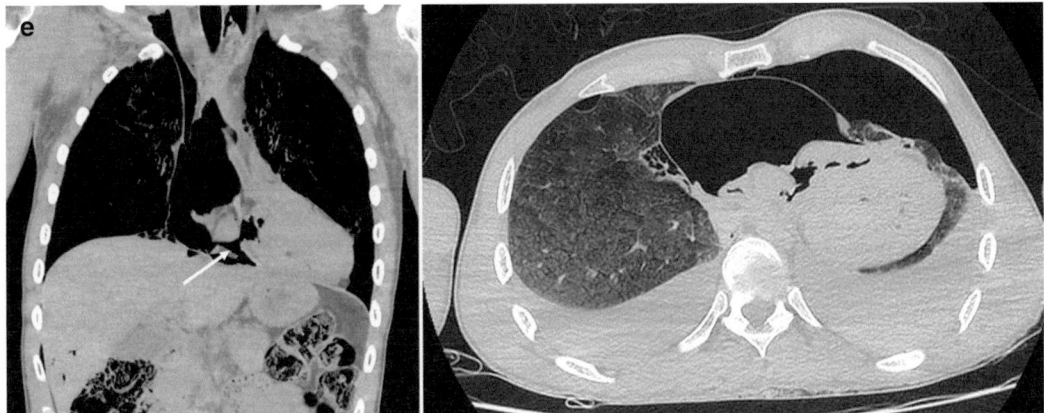

Fig. 3.12 (continued)

pleuro-pericardial tears are usually vertical. Pericardial tears preclude cardiac tamponade and may provoke haemothorax, haemoperitoneum and haemomediastinum (Fig. 3.12d, e).

3.3.3.5 Aortic Ruptures

These typically occur in traffic accidents or falls from height in the context of sudden deceleration that is sometimes associated with compression or shearing mechanisms [6, 24, 45, 46] (Fig. 3.13a, b).

Traction forces tear the aorta transversally at two possible sites [24]:

– The isthmus (the area of the descending thoracic aorta below the left subclavian artery ostium) is the most commonly injured site. It is a fixation point at the junction between the mobile aorta and the descending thoracic segment, which is bound to the spinal column. It is an inherently weak part of the aorta because of the ligamentum arteriosum, the scarred remnant of the foetal ductus arteriosus. The isthmic laceration is a cause of left site haemothorax.
– The ascending aorta, immediately above the cups of the aortic valve.
– Other locations are rare and often associated with vertebral fractures or affect the descending thoracic aorta at the diaphragmatic opening, the aortic arch [6, 24].

Aortic lesions may be complex with the occurrence of multiple aortic lacerations. A laceration may also be complete or partial.

3.3.3.6 Great Vessel Injuries

– Tears and dissections of the major aortic arch vessels secondary to blunt trauma are rare. Stretching or rotational stress from neck hypertension may play a role in this type of injury. The subclavian artery is well protected by the clavicle and the first rib [6, 24, 47]. Fractures of these bones and the presence of a haemothorax raise the possibility of a subclavian vessel tear (Fig. 3.13a).
– Intrathoracic veins may also be injured [6, 24]:

• Isolated ruptures of the main pulmonary artery, its major branches or a pulmonary vein are rare [48].
• Laceration of the superior or inferior vena cava is uncommon (Fig. 3.14a, b) [49].
• Tearing of the azygos vein is uncommon, provoking haemothorax or haemomediastinum [6, 24]. A midthoracic spine fracture can directly tear the vein, but in most cases, the laceration occurs either close to the superior vena cava/azygos vein junction or along the azygos vein arch. Shearing from deceleration is a proposed mechanism [50].

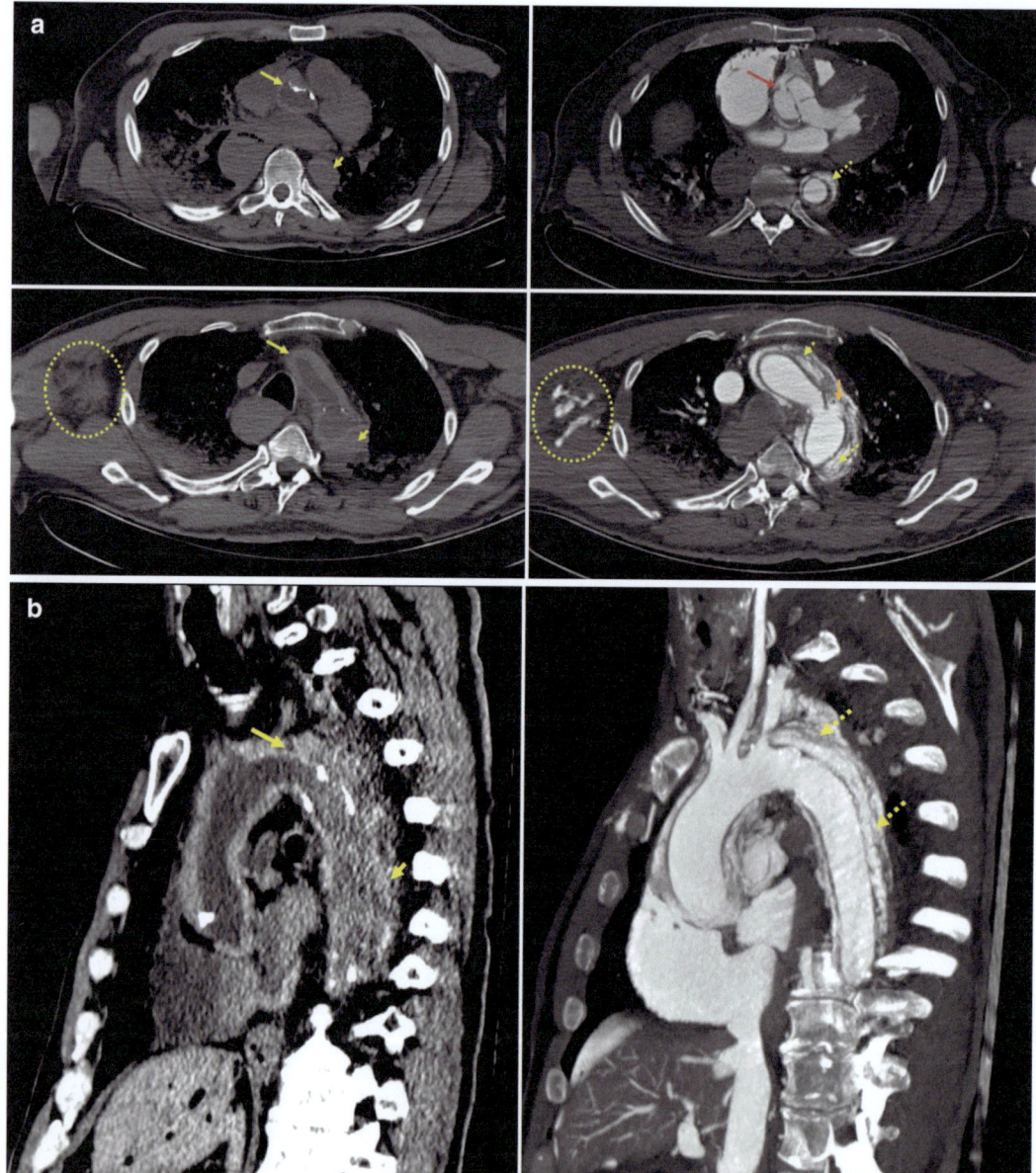

Fig. 3.13 (**a**) MPMCTA, axial view of the chest, soft tissue filter. Context of a fall from great height. Double aortic dissection (ascending aorta and aortic arch; orange arrows) illustrated contrast agent injection. These ruptures are responsible for spontaneous periaortic haematoma (yellow arrows) progressing with contrast agent after injection (yellow-dotted arrows). Note the bleeding caused by axillar vascular injuries with contrast agent extravasation in the axillary space (yellow-dotted circles). Superior image, left, PMCT; right, MPMCTA, arterial phase. Inferior image, left, PMCT; right, MPMCTA, arterial phase. (**b**) MPMCTA, sagittal oblique view of the chest, soft tissue filter. Context of a fall from great height. Aortic arch dissection (orange arrows) illustrated by contrast agent injection. These ruptures are responsible of spontaneous periaortic haematoma (yellow arrows) progressively filled with contrast agent after the injection (yellow-dotted arrows). Left image: PMCTA. Right image: MPMCTA, phase

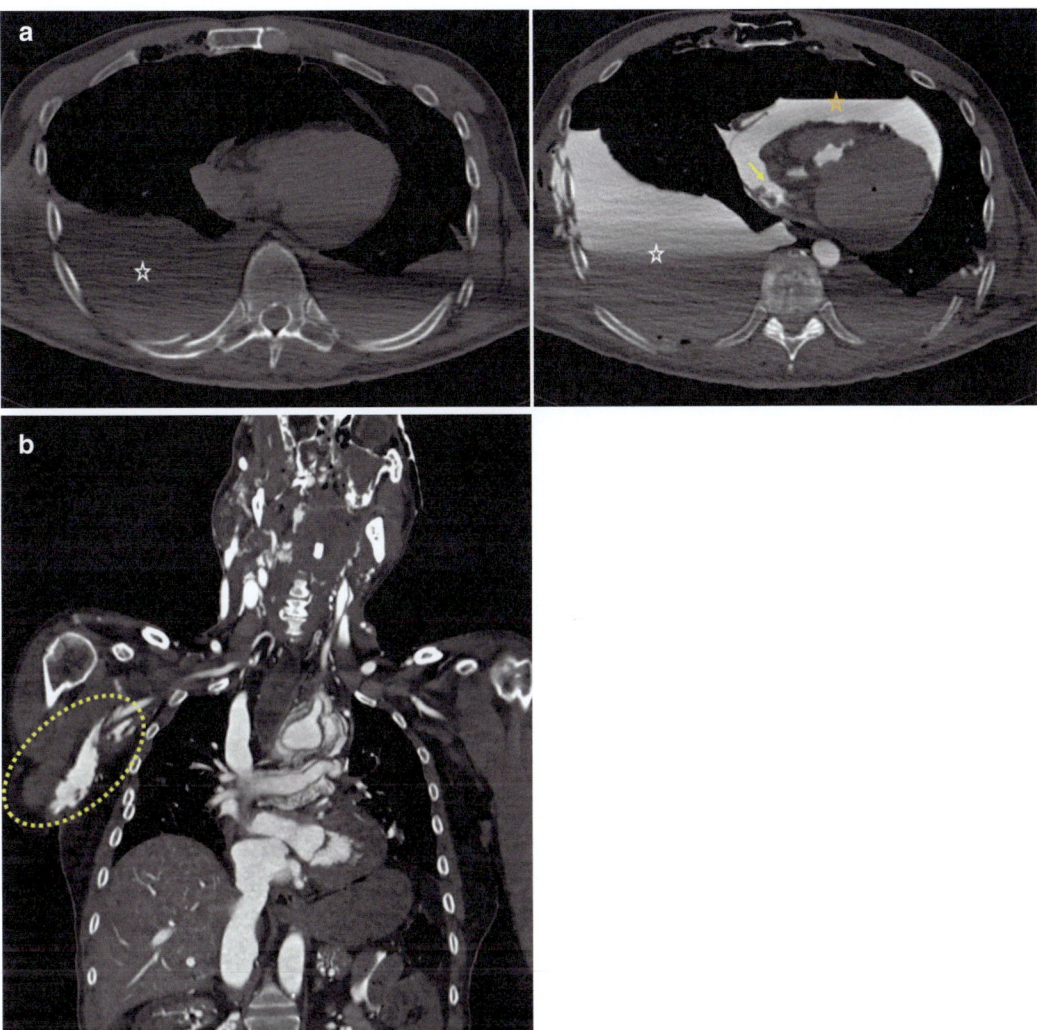

Fig. 3.14 (**a**) MPMCTA, axial view of the chest, soft tissue filter. Context of a fall from great height. Severe inferior vena cava laceration (yellow arrow) responsible for the contrast agent extravasation in the pericardium (orange star). Note the right pleural effusion progressively filled with contrast agent (white stars). Left image: non-enhanced PMCT. Right image: MPMCTA, dynamic phase. (**b**) MPMCTA, coronal reconstruction of the chest, soft tissue filter. Context of a fall from great height. Contrast extravasation in the axillary space related to axillar vascular injuries (yellow-dotted circle)

3.3.3.7 Periaortic Small Vessel Injuries

Tears, dissections and ruptures of small arterial vessels that directly branch from the aorta, secondary to blunt trauma, are rare. Retroperitoneal bleeding in lumbar arteries is rare and mostly related to trauma involving a large amount of kinetic energy with associated lesions of the pelvis and/or the vertebral column (Fig. 3.20h) [6, 24, 51].

MPMCTA may allow to understand the source of a haemothorax due to a laceration of the intercostal arteries in some cases (Fig. 3.11f).

3.3.3.8 Diaphragm Injuries

The incidence of diaphragm laceration caused by blunt trauma is 2% [6, 18, 24, 52]. Rarely isolated, they are usually associated with other severe injuries. There is a left-side predominance, which is explained by the fact that the right side is protected by the liver (Figs. 3.12a and 3.15a, b). Bilateral tears are uncommon [24].

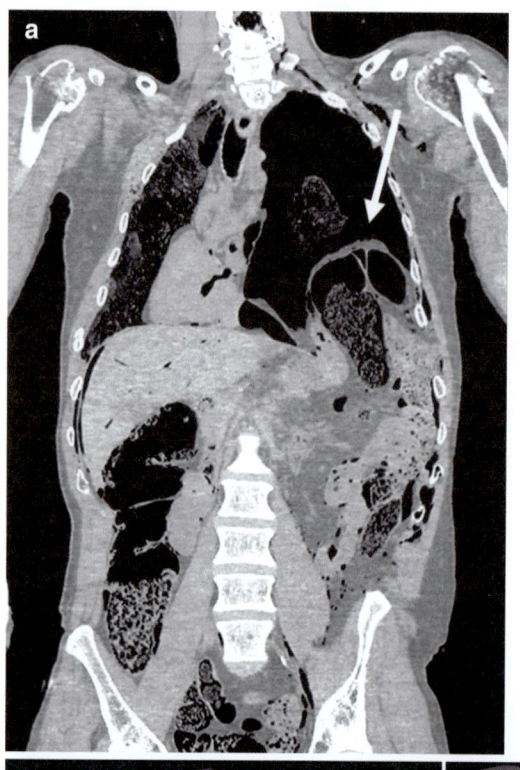

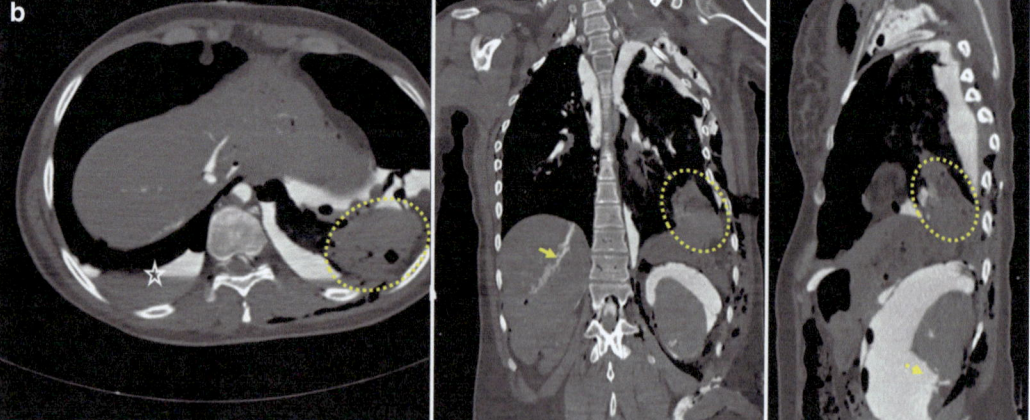

Fig. 3.15 (**a**) PMCT, coronal view of the chest and the abdomen, soft tissue filter. Context of a crash of a private aircraft. Diaphragmatic rupture (arrow) with herniation of the abdominal content (colon) in the left part of the thorax. Please note the bilateral humeral fractures. (**b**) MPMCTA of the chest, arterial phase, soft tissue filter. Context of a fall from great height. Severe thoracic injuries demonstrated by pleural effusions and pleural contrast agent extravasations (white star) associated with diaphragmatic rupture with intra thoracic spleen (yellow-dotted circles). Note the absence of splenic enhancement, related to severe splenic vascular injuries. Severe other organ lesion, as hepatic (yellow arrow) and kidney (yellow-dotted arrow) injuries. Left image, axial view; middle image, coronal view; right image, sagittal view

3.3.4 Abdominopelvic Injuries

3.3.4.1 Solid Organs

The most vulnerable anatomical structures are the liver, spleen and the mesentery [6, 24] (Figs. 3.16a–g and 3.17) [6, 24, 53]. Traffic accident is the most common cause of these injuries. Solid organ injuries such as laceration produce internal bleeding into the peritoneal cavity. The lacerations are classified as transcapsular (lesion of the capsule and the parenchyma) or subcapsular:

– The **liver** is frequently injured in the posterior-superior area of the right lateral lobe [6, 24, 53]. When the phenomenon of compression occurs, it creates a bursting injury. Other patterns of injuries are possible, including linear capsular laceration, haematoma under an intact capsule and intraparenchymal tearing (Fig. 3.16a, b).
– **Spleen** injuries are frequently associated with severe trauma and other severe lesions (Fig. 3.16c, d) [6, 24, 53, 54].
– The **kidneys** are rarely a source of severe bleeding because of their retroperitoneal location (Fig. 3.16e) [6, 24, 55]. Dissection of the aorta and major branches (e.g. renal artery) has been described, and arterial and venous bleeding from renal vessels secondary to a laceration is possible. Renal cortical tears may also induce retroperitoneal haemorrhage.

3.3.4.2 Hollow Organs
– The **stomach and intestine** are less susceptible to blunt trauma, unless they are filled with food or fluid [6, 18, 56]. Sometimes a squeezing of the organs between the abdominal wall and the vertebral column is possible. The stomach is usually associated with trauma of the adjacent solid organs and the chest wall. A stomach rupture may involve any portion, but most commonly the anterior wall is injured, followed by the greater curve, lesser curve and posterior wall (Fig. 3.16f).
– The **bladder** can also rupture (Fig. 3.16g). When empty, the rupture side is mostly extra-peritoneal (with pelvic fractures); when urine filled, the rupture side lies typically intraperitoneal [5–7, 24]. Associated urinary bladder tears and lacerations of the major pelvic vessels are possible.

3.3.4.3 Abdominal Aortic Laceration
Rupture of the abdominal aorta is rare because it lies in a protected retroperitoneal location and is attached to the spine [6, 24, 57]. However, a fractured vertebra can directly injure the aorta. Deceleration forces acting on points of major arterial attachments (e.g. the inferior mesentery artery) and the iliac bifurcation can initiate tearing (Fig. 3.17). In practice, dissection may also occur in any segment of the aorta.

3.3.4.4 Pelvic Fractures
Pelvic fractures may induce intense haemorrhage as a result of torn iliac or obturator vessels, and are the most frequent source of traumatic retroperitoneal haemorrhage (Fig. 3.18a–c) [6, 24, 55].

3.3.5 Injuries to the Extremities (Fig. 3.19a–e)

These injuries include skin, subcutaneous fat tissue, muscular, bone and articular injuries. Extensive crushing of the soft tissues, formation of blood-filled cavities, communitive fractures and severance of large vessels are frequent in victims of automobile-pedestrian accidents [5–7]. Injuries provoke internal bleeding (for closed injuries), external bleeding (with traumatic amputation, severe avulsion wounds and compound fractures) and pulmonary and systemic fat embolisms [5, 7, 24].

In assaults of any kind, the natural reaction of the victims is to protect themselves [4]. Defence wounds are usually noted in those cases where the assault occurred at close range [58]. The limbs used for protection can be injured, and these defence injuries may be of considerable medico-legal significance, as they indicate that the victim was conscious, at least partly mobile and not taken completely by surprise [4].

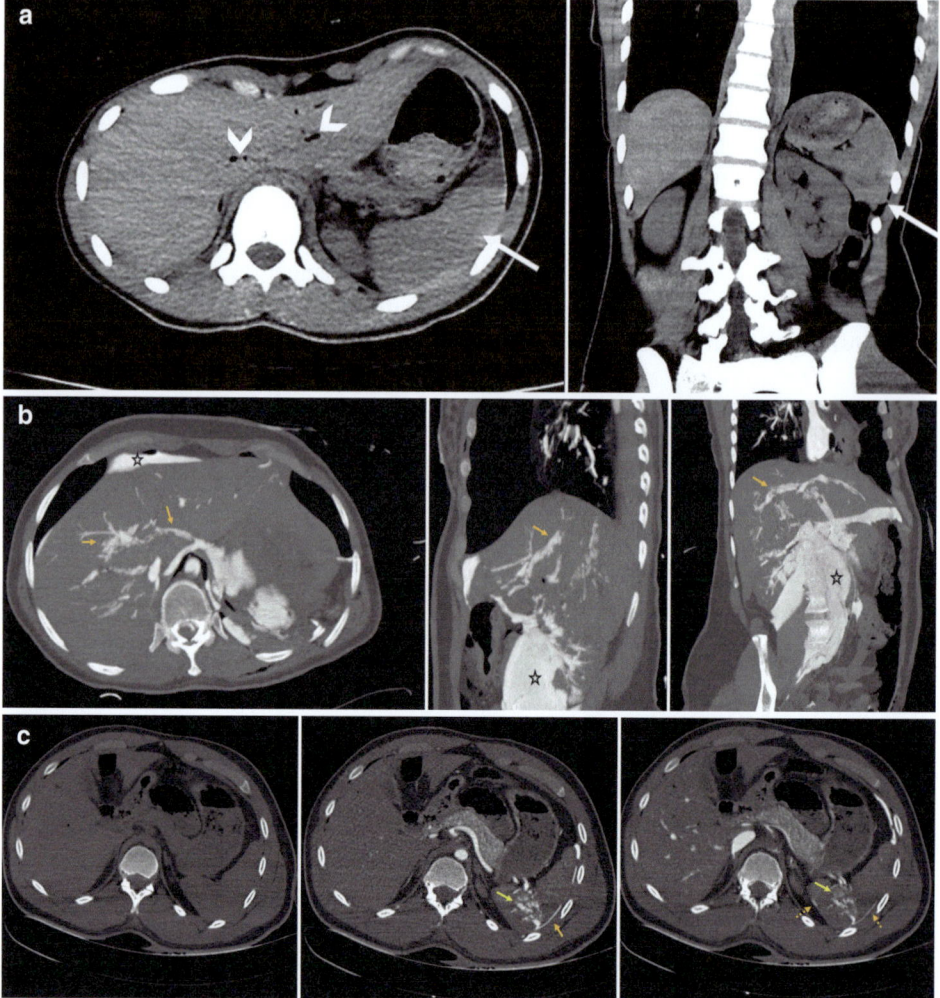

Fig. 3.16 (**a**) PMCT. Context of a fall from great height. Haemoperitoneum around the spleen (arrow), as an indirect sign of spleen rupture. Bubbles of gas within the liver (arrowheads) due to liver ruptures. Left image, axial abdominal slice; right image, coronal MPR reconstruction, soft tissue filter. (**b**) MPMCTA of the abdomen, venous phase, soft tissue filter. Context of a fall from great height. Contrast agent extravasation in the hepatic parenchyma (orange arrows), associated with intra- and retroperitoneal contrast agent extravasation (black star). Left image, axial view; middle image, sagittal view; right image, coronal view, MIP reconstruction. (**c**) MPMCTA of the abdomen, axial view, soft tissue filter. Context of a fall from great height. Contrast agent extravasation in the splenic parenchyma both at arterial and venous phases (yellow arrows), related to severe traumatic splenic injuries, and associated with peri-splenic peritoneal contrast agent extravasation (orange-dotted arrows). Note the absence of obvious splenic lesions during the non-contrast phase. Left image, PMCT; middle image, MPMCTA, arterial phase; right image, MPMCTA, sagittal phase. (**d**) PMCT, sagittal reconstruction, view of the abdomen, soft tissue filter. Context of a fall from great height. Contrast agent extravasation in the splenic parenchyma showing several paren-chymal lacerations (orange arrows), and an intra splenic haematoma (yellow arrow). (**e**) MPMCTA of the abdomen, venous phase, soft tissue filter. Context of a fall from great height. Severe kidney ruptures (yellow arrow) associated with retroperitoneal perirenal contrast agent extravasation (white stars). Note the absence of obvious splenic lesions during the non-contrast phase, and the absence of renal enhancement during the venous phase. Left image, PMCT, axial view; middle image, MPMCTA, axial view; right image, MPMCTA, coronal view. (**f**) PMCT, axial view, abdomen, context of a fall from great height. Visualisation of subcutaneous gaseous infiltrations (short arrow) and a massive pneumoperitoneum (long arrow) due to intestine perforation. (**g**) MPMCTA of the pelvic, sagittal views, soft tissue filter. Context of a fall from great height. Spontaneous haematoma of the anterior abdominal wall (orange arrow). After contrast agent injection, severe arterial and venous contrast agent extravasation both in the anterior abdominal wall (yellow arrows) and the pre-vesical space (yellow -dotted arrow). Note the contrast agent filling of the bladder (yellow-dotted circle), related to severe posttraumatic vesical injuries. Left image, PMCT; middle image, MPMCTA, arterial phase; right image, MPMCTA, venous phase

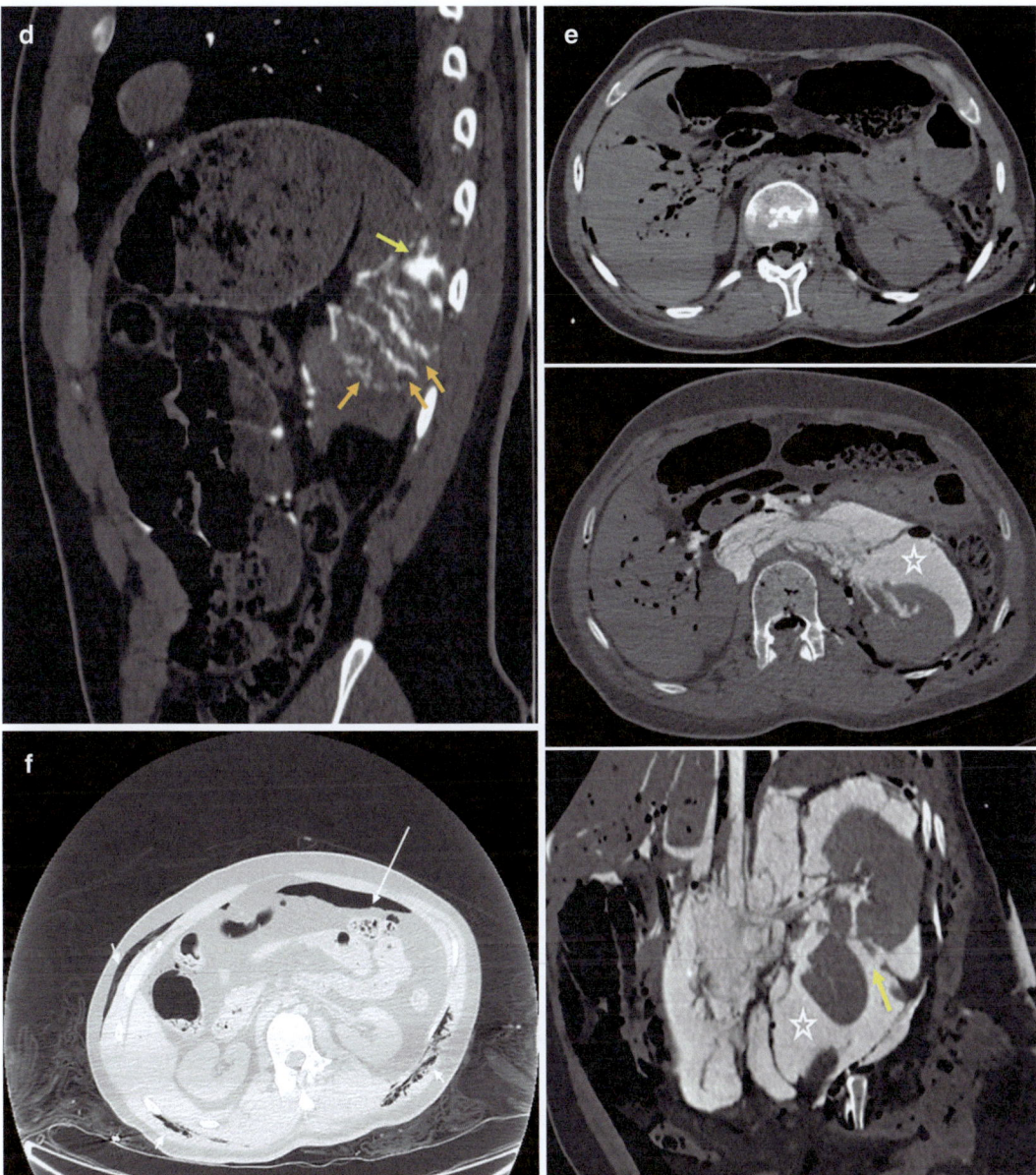

Fig. 3.16 (continued)

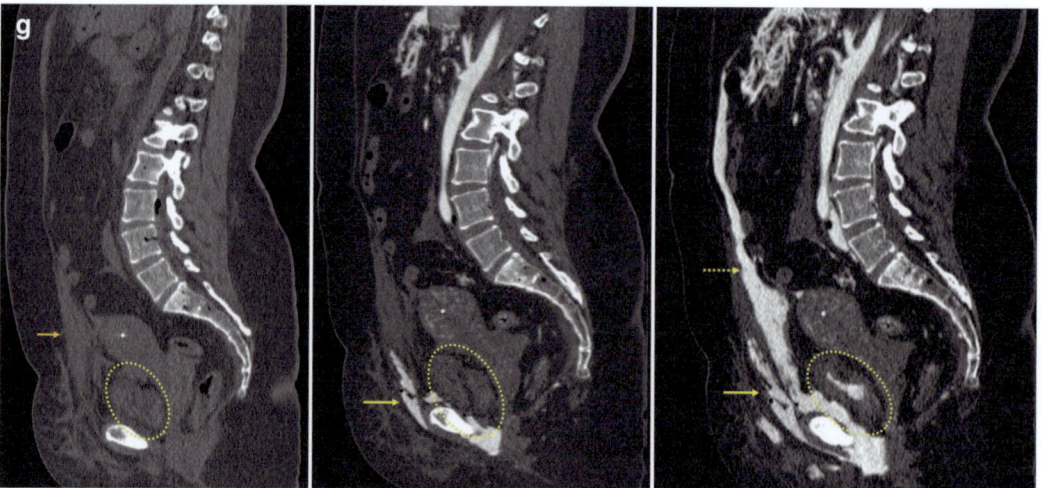

Fig. 3.16 (continued)

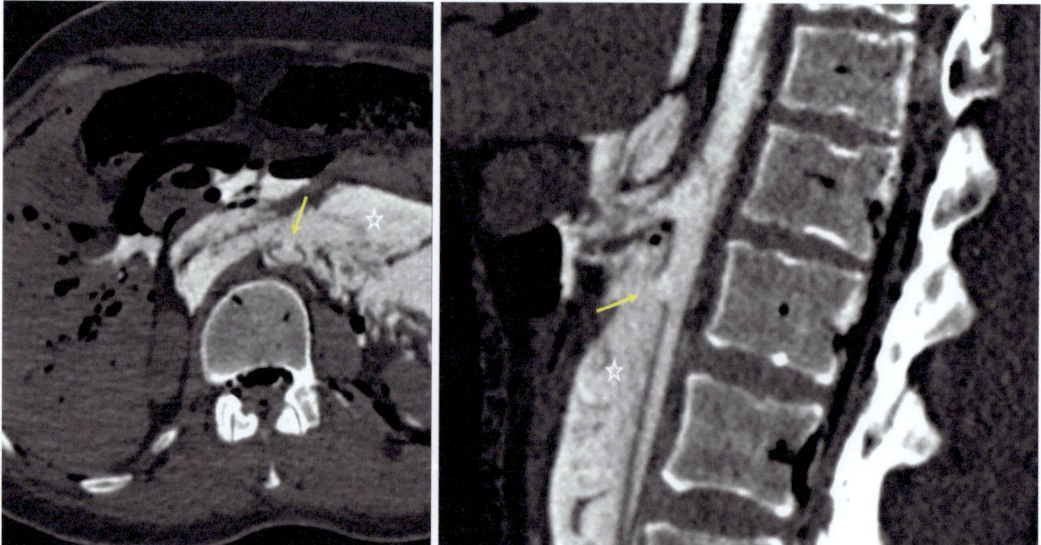

Fig. 3.17 MPMCTA of the abdomen, dynamic phase, soft tissue filter. Context of a fall from great height. Superior mesenteric artery rupture (yellow arrows), asso- ciated with retroperitoneal contrast agent extravasation (white stars); left image, axial view; right image, coronal view)

Defence wounds can be sustained from attacks by fists, feet, blunt or sharp instruments. The classic position for them is on the forearms and hands, which are instinctively raised to protect the eyes, face and head. Under superficial lesions as abrasions and bruises, some bone fractures of the carpal bones, metacarpals and digits may occur. Other defence injuries may be inflicted on the thighs, when attempts are made to shield the genitals [4].

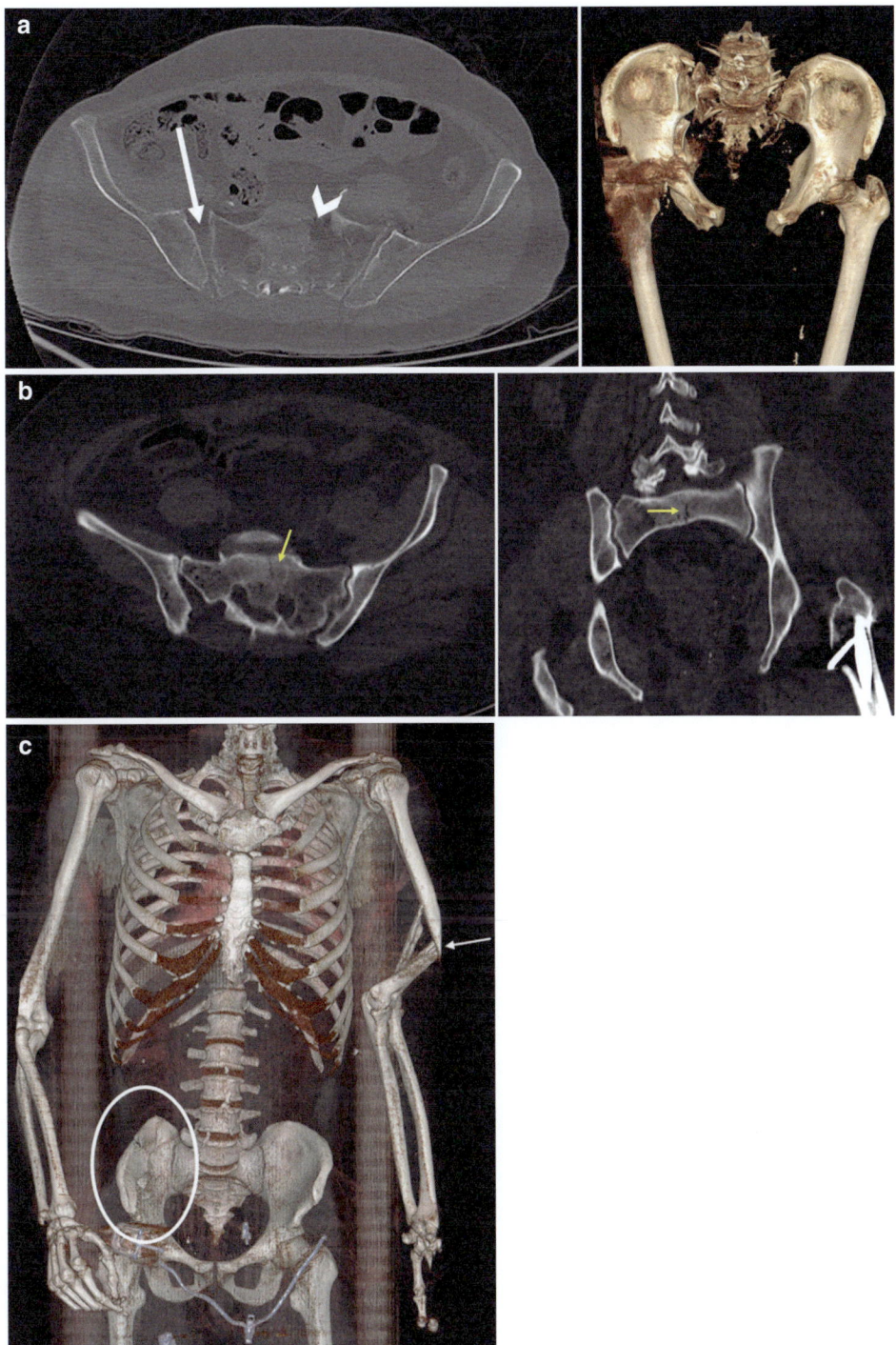

Fig. 3.18 (**a**) PMCT of a cyclist hit by a car. Left image: axial view of the pelvis, bone filter. Disjunction of the right sacroiliac joint (arrow) and fracture of the left ala of the sacrum (arrowhead); right image: 3D VRT reconstruction of the pelvis, anterior view. Major disjunction of the pubic symphysis. (**b**) PMCT of the pelvis, bone filter. Context of a fall from great height. S1 vertical fracture (yellow arrows). Left image, axial view of the pelvis; right image, coronal view of the pelvis. (**c**) PMCT 3D VRT reconstructions of the body, anterior view. Context of a hang-gliding fall. Fracture of the right ilium of the innominate bone (circle). Left displaced humeral fracture (arrow)

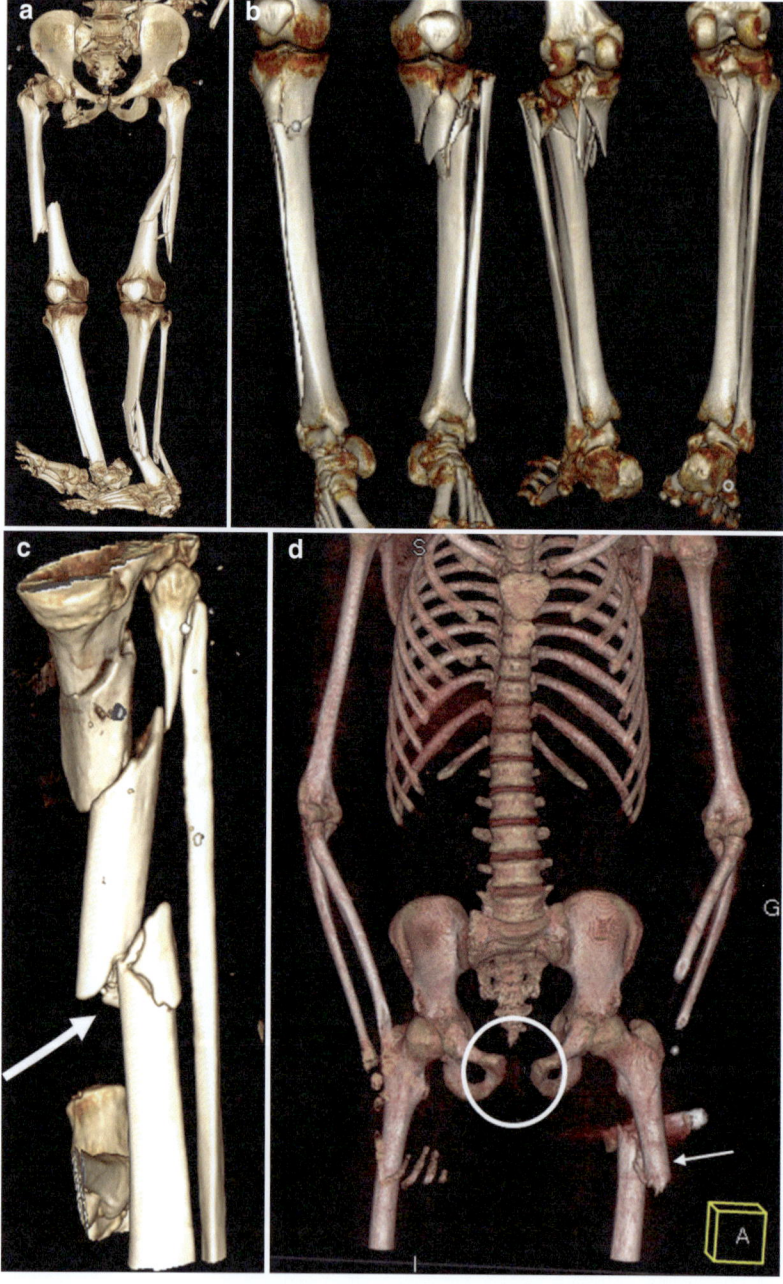

Fig. 3.19 (**a**) PMCT, 3D VRT reconstruction of the lower limbs, anterior view. Context of a crash of a private aircraft. Bilateral multiple fractures of long bones of the lower limbs. (**b**) PMCT, 3D VRT reconstructions of the lower limbs, anterior (left image) and posterior (right image) views. Context of a fall from great height. Important lower limbs displaced fractures, concerning the proximal extremity. (**c**) PMCT, 3D VRT reconstruction of the left lower limb, posterior view. Context of a pedestrian hit by a car on a highway. Tibial wedge-shaped fracture with biconcave side edges (called "Messerer fracture"), with the apex pointing in the direction opposite to the travel direction of the car. (**d**) PMCT, 3D VRT reconstruction of the lower limbs, anterior view. Context of a fall from great height. Major disjunction of the pubic symphysis (circle) and fracture of the upper third part of the left femur (arrow). (**e**) PMCT, context of a plain level fall. Pelvic exploration, coronal MPR reconstruction: fracture of the left femoral neck

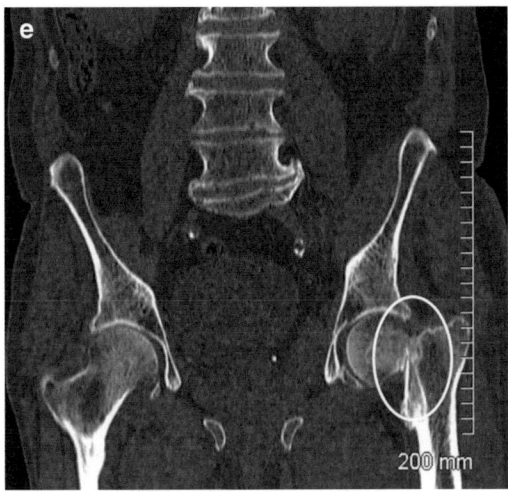

Fig. 3.19 (continued)

3.3.6 Injuries to the Spine

Forces acting on the vertebral column are rotational (accounting for flexion, extension, lateral flexion and torsion) and linear (compression, distraction and translation of various parts of the vertebral column) [18, 24]. These forces, acting in isolation or, more commonly, together, are either physiological or, when they exceed the physical limits imposed by various anatomical structures, pathological. Exposure of the spinal column to pathological forces leads to tearing of perivertebral soft tissues, vertebral subluxation, vertebral fractures and spinal cord injury (Fig. 3.20a–h). Vertebral fractures are frequently associated with injuries to the cranium and brain.

Fig. 3.20 (**a**) PMCT, cervical exploration, bone filter. Context of a fall in a nearly empty swimming pool. Left image, sagittal MPR reconstruction: fracture of the body of the sixth cervical vertebra; right image, axial cervical slice, bilateral fracture of the laminae of the sixth cervical vertebra (arrows). (**b**) PMCT, cervical exploration, bone filter. Context of a fall from great height. Left image, coronal MPR reconstruction: fracture of the body of the fifth cervical vertebra (short arrow); right image, sagittal MPR reconstruction, fracture of the body of the fifth cervical vertebra (short arrow) and fracture of the spine processes of the sixth and seventh cervical vertebrae (arrows). (**c**) PMCT, sagittal MPR reconstruction of the head and the neck, brain filter. Context of a traffic accident. Occipito-cervical dissociation associated with subdural haematoma with severe injuries of the brainstem and the cervical spine. (**d**) PMCT, 3D reconstruction, cervical spine. Context of a facial impact and a fall to the ground. Left image, left lateral view: subluxation of the articular facets between the first (C1) and the second (C2) cervical vertebra (star). Right image, inferior view: rotatory subluxation between C1 and C2, with an abnormal angle between the sagittal orientation of C1 (dotted arrow) and C2 (arrow). (**e**) PMCT, sagittal MPR reconstruction of the chest, bone filter. Context of a traffic accident. Major trauma of the chest with complete dislocation of the upper part of the thoracic spine and fracture of the sternum. (**f**) PMCT, sagittal MPR reconstruction, bone filter. Context of a fall beneath a train. Spinal disjunction between the ninth and tenth thoracic vertebra, with a medullar section. (**g**) PMCT, axial slice of the lumbar spine, bone filter. Context of a fight with punching and kicking. Fracture of the right lateral process of the second lumbar vertebra (arrow). Presence of gas due to alteration of the body. (**h**) MPMCTA of the chest, axial view, soft tissue filter. Context of a fall from great height. T7 burst vertebral fracture (light orange arrows and yellow-dotted circles), with several bone fragments (dark orange arrows), responsible of perivertebral contrast agent extravasation (yellow arrow), which leads further to haemothorax and pleural contrast agent extravasation (white stars). Superior left image: PMCT; superior middle image, MPMCTA, arterial phase; superior right image, MPMCTA, venous phase; inferior left image, MPMCTA, venous phase, sagittal reconstruction; inferior right image, PMCT, 3D VRT reconstruction

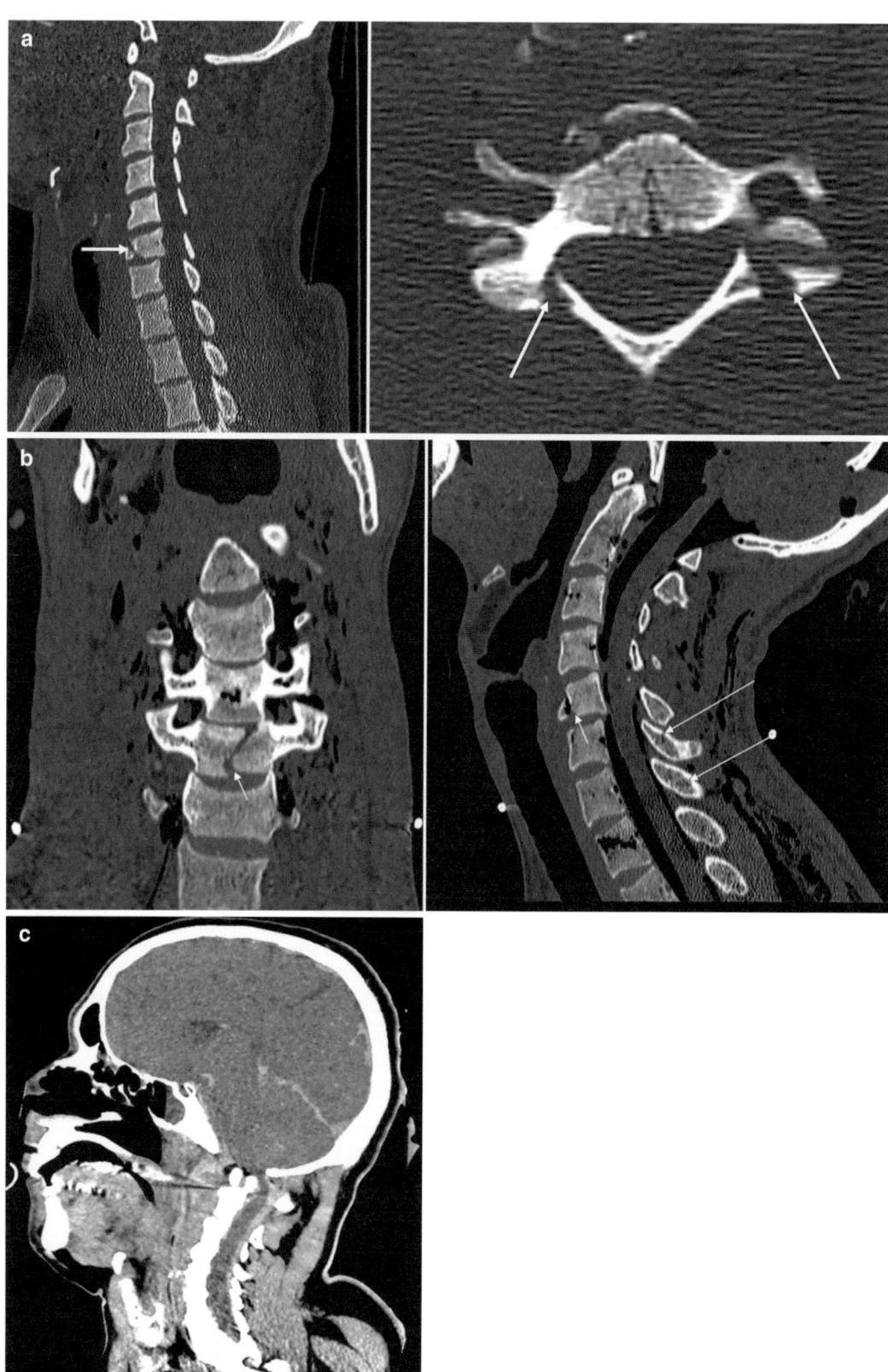

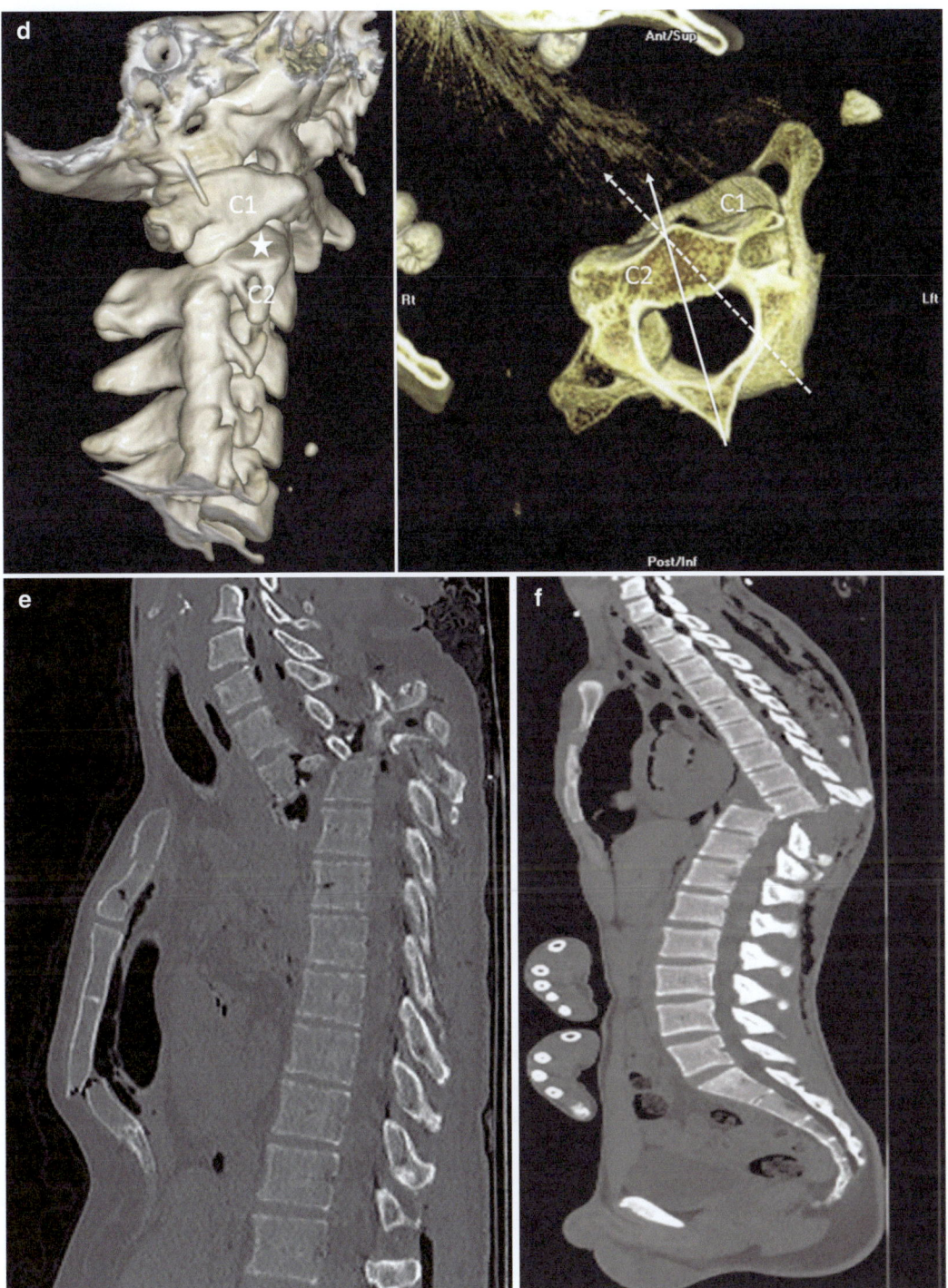

Fig. 3.20 (continued)

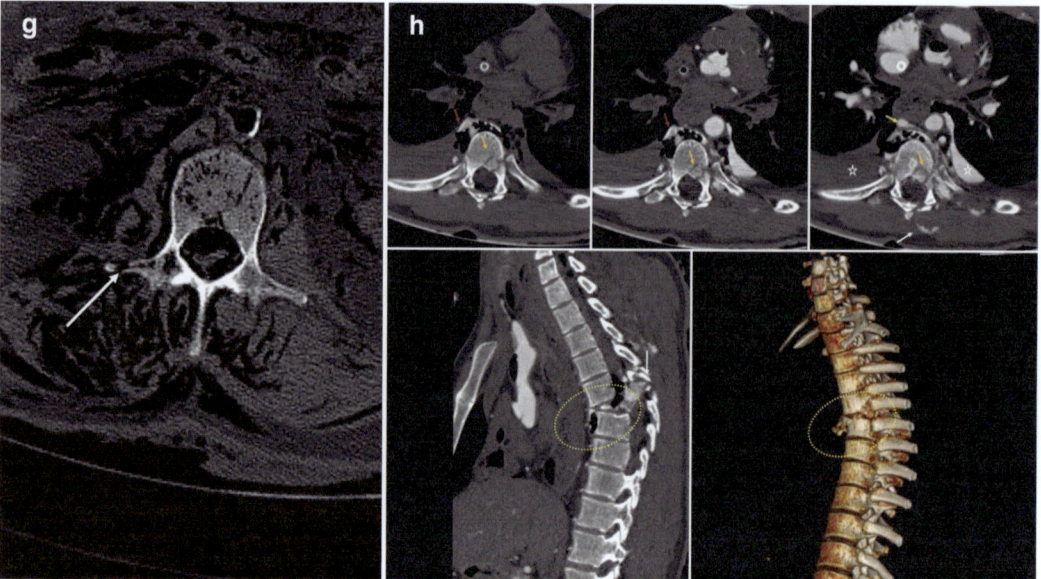

Fig. 3.20 (continued)

In general, vertebral and spinal injuries are more common in the cervical and lumbar regions than in the thoracic area because of the additional support provided to this area by the ribcage.

There are numerous classification schemes for vertebral fractures. Here is a summary of important elements dealing with vertebral and spinal trauma, even if, in practice, the different pattern may be mixed [18, 24]:

- Pure flexion injuries may cause:
  - Compression of the ventral components of the vertebral column (compression fracture)
  - And distraction of the dorsal elements (leading to tearing of the interspinous ligaments and posterior longitudinal ligament and facet dislocation or fracture)
- Extension injuries may cause:
  - Tearing of the anterior longitudinal ligament
  - Avulsion of the intervertebral disk
  - Tearing of the posterior longitudinal ligament
  - Fracture or dislocation of the articular facets
  - And fracture of the pedicle, leading to a fracture dislocation (Fig. 3.20a)

- Compression injuries through axial loading of the vertebral column may cause:
  - A compressive fracture of the vertebral body
  - A comminution fracture of the vertebral body
  - And fractures of the pedicles (burst fractures) (Fig. 3.20b)

Some specificities concerning post-mortem imaging and cervical spine trauma have been recently published:

- Kudo et al. performed a study in order to evaluate retrospectively the correlation between the PMC findings and autopsy results of cervical intervertebral separation [59]. Approximately 70% of the cases with cervical intervertebral separations had various abnormal findings on CT imaging. The most common finding in cases of cervical intervertebral separation in this study was intervertebral gas, with a low sensitivity (33.9%) and a high specificity (99.7%). Other findings were forward intervertebral widening, backward intervertebral widening, anteroposterior misalignment, spur fracture and haematoma in front of a vertebral body.

– Kawasumi et al. performed also a study to evaluate the post-mortem computed tomography (PMCT) findings of intervertebral separation, focused also mainly on cervical spine trauma [60]. Useful radiological criteria retained by the authors for intervertebral separations were vertebral misalignment, intervertebral widening, intra-disc gas and haemorrhage.

3.4 Some Forensic Particularities Important to Know for the Correct Radiological Interpretation of Falls from Height

Situations frequently encountered are jumpers, workplace accidents and other accidental falls [6, 18, 24]. All manners of death are possible.

Many factors will influence the extent and distribution of lesions, which are classically defined as:

– The height of the fall
– The force/area ratio, which is high in feet-first impact, but usually associated with less injuries, contrary to head-first impact, which are most likely fatal
– Falling on a deformable surface
– The age of the victim (generally children tolerate falls better than adults)

Injuries from falls arise from vertical deceleration forces during direct impact, secondary impacts from objects intervening during the descent or after initial impact and energy transfer to sites remote from the impact site [6, 24, 61–63]. Vertical deceleration causes severe chest (aortic rupture, cardiac rupture) and abdomen visceral trauma. Bouncing on impact occurs from falls from great heights. Direct impacts occur on the head, buttocks, lateral body and lower extremities, but the determination of the primary impact is not always obvious. One study of suicides showed that feet-first impacts are common in jumps from lower floors (up to the 12th floor), side-first up to the 13th floor and head-first in free falls from greater heights [24, 64].

Regarding the literature data [3, 5–8, 24, 61]:

– **Concerning the head level** (Figs. 3.2, 3.3 and 3.7):
  • Fatal head injuries dominate, regardless of heights.
  • Dominated below 7–10 m and above 25–30 m [65, 66].
– **Concerning the buttocks** (Fig. 3.18) [6, 24, 61, 63]:
  • Pelvic and thoracolumbar fractures and retroperitoneal bleeding are common.
  • Vertebral fractures by compression and ring fracture of the occipital bone are possible.
– **Concerning the chest** (Fig. 3.11) [6, 24, 61, 63]:
  • Rib fractures can directly tear viscera.
  • The number of rib fractures increases with the height of the fall and above 40 m fractures are the rule [67].
– **At the lower extremities**, when feet touch the floor first (Fig. 3.19) [3, 5–8, 24]:
  • Fractures of the feet, ankles and tibias are frequent.
  • Force is transmitted to the femur, thoracolumbar spine and the base of the skull.

Generally, injuries are seen on the impacted side [5, 24].

Upper-extremity fractures are possible if the victim is struck by objects while falling or attempts to brace the fall when landing.

Hyoid and laryngeal fractures are also possible [24].

3.5 Some Forensic Particularities Important to Know for the Correct Radiological Interpretation of Falls from Plain Level or from Standing Height

Low-energy falls (LEF) occur in one-third of adults over the age of 65 each year, and are a leading cause of death in developed nations [68]. Low-energy falls are associated with significant morbidity and mortality, which appear to increase with age [69]. Low-energy falls are defined as a fall from standing height or less and include falls while transferring, sitting or from the bed [69]. Lee et al. showed that severe injuries from low-height falls in the elderly population occurred in about 7% of the total injuries [70]. In the United States of America, 20–30% of older people who have fallen suffer moderate to severe injuries, such as bruises, hip fractures or head trauma (Figs. 3.8c and 3.19e) [68]. Generally low-energy falls are the predominant trauma mechanism of older individuals leading to injury severities similar to high-energy mechanisms in younger patients [68].

3.5.1 Head Trauma

Lampart et al. studied the prevalence and severity of traumatic intracranial haemorrhage in a large cohort of older adults presenting with low-energy falls and the association with anticoagulation or antiplatelet medication (Figs. 3.10a and 3.21a) [71]. In this study, medication with anticoagulants or antiplatelet agents was not associated with higher prevalence and severity of traumatic intracranial haemorrhage in older patients with low-energy falls undergoing CT examination. In addition to CT-detected skull fractures, visible injuries above the clavicles were the strongest clinical predictors for traumatic intracranial haemorrhage [71].

3.5.2 Other Anatomical Sites of Trauma

Haemorrhage at fracture sites may also lead to death. Some cases have been described concerning pelvic fractures and also the extremities [72]. Rau et al. reported that the most common injury regions caused by falls were the extremities at all adult ages, including the hip and pelvis, regardless of the height of the fall [73]. In this study, the most common injury regions were the head and neck followed by the hip and thigh in the elderly population.

The presence of a pelvic ring fracture is an independent risk factor for mortality in the blunt trauma population [72]. Broek et al. identified 22 cases of massive haemorrhage secondary to pubic rami fractures [74]. Of the 14 elderly patients, 12 of these pubic rami fractures occurred from a fall from standing. Patients with minimally displaced pubic rami fractures could however have laceration of the obturator artery or the inferior epigastric artery which may anastomose with branches from the obturator artery, and a huge vascular injury and blood loss after an apparently minor pelvic trauma [72].

3.5.3 Vascular Trauma

Although the incidence of vascular injuries is rare in the context of low-energy falls and upper-extremity fractures or dislocation, they may be deadly. For example, an axillary artery injury accompanying anterior shoulder dislocation is a rare but serious condition which may result in limb loss or death [75]. Most of these injuries occur in advanced age due to the decreased elasticity of an atherosclerotic artery, and 90% of the cases are above the age of 50 years.

3.5.4 The Potential Influence of Drugs

Some authors study a possible link between some drugs and the severity of the injuries after a simple fall. Alcohol-related falls are more often associated with severe craniofacial injuries [76]. Falls with alcohol consumption were associated with more severe maxillofacial fractures and more mandibular fractures than falls without alcohol consumption [77]. The severity of both, limb and head injuries, is greater and correlates directly with blood alcohol concentration [76]. In alcohol-related falls, the greater incidence of craniofacial injuries and the greater severity of the injuries were explained by the inhibition of protective reflexes and the inability to put the outstretched hand to break the fall [76].

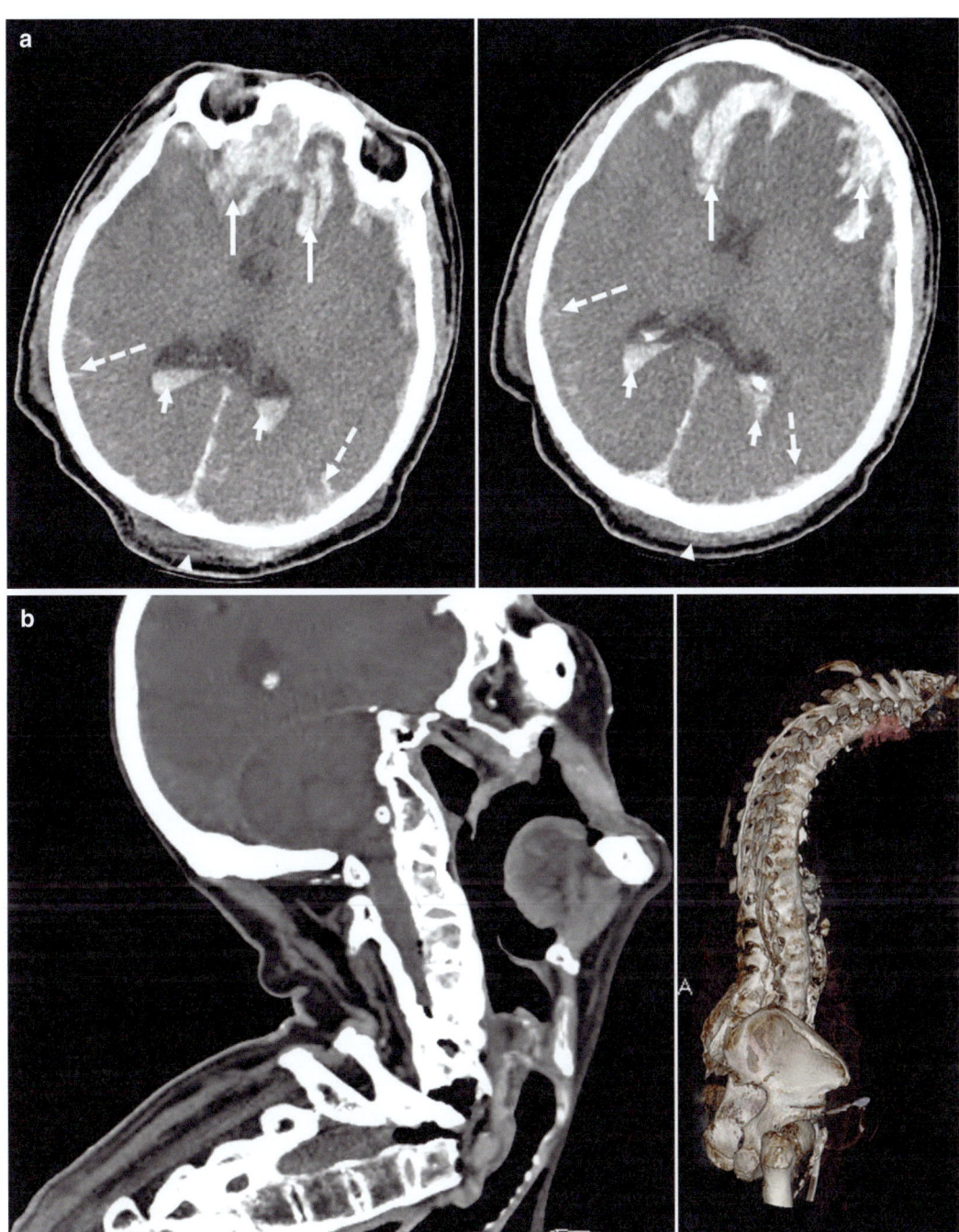

Fig. 3.21 (a) Clinical head CT, axial view of the brain, soft tissue filter. Context of fall from standing height. Clinical subcutaneous occipital haematoma. Intraparenchymal bifrontal haematomas (contrecoup) (arrows), subarachnoid haemorrhage (dotted arrows), intraventricular haemorrhage (short arrows), subcutaneous occipital haematoma (arrowhead). (b) PMCT, context of a plain level fall. Post-mortem diagnosis of ankylosis spondylitis. Left image, sagittal MPR reconstruction: disjunction between the sixth and the seventh cervical verte-bra; right image, 3D VRT reconstruction, right view, ossification of the anterior longitudinal ligament through-out the entire spine and osseous bridging with characteristic bamboo spine configuration. (c) PMCT, context of a plain level fall. Post-mortem diagnosis of ankylosis spondylitis. Left image, 3D VRT reconstruction, fracture of the superior endplate of the eighth thoracic vertebra and a discontinuity of the disk between the seventh and the eighth thoracic vertebra; right image, coronal MPR reconstruction, osseous fusion of both sacroiliac joints

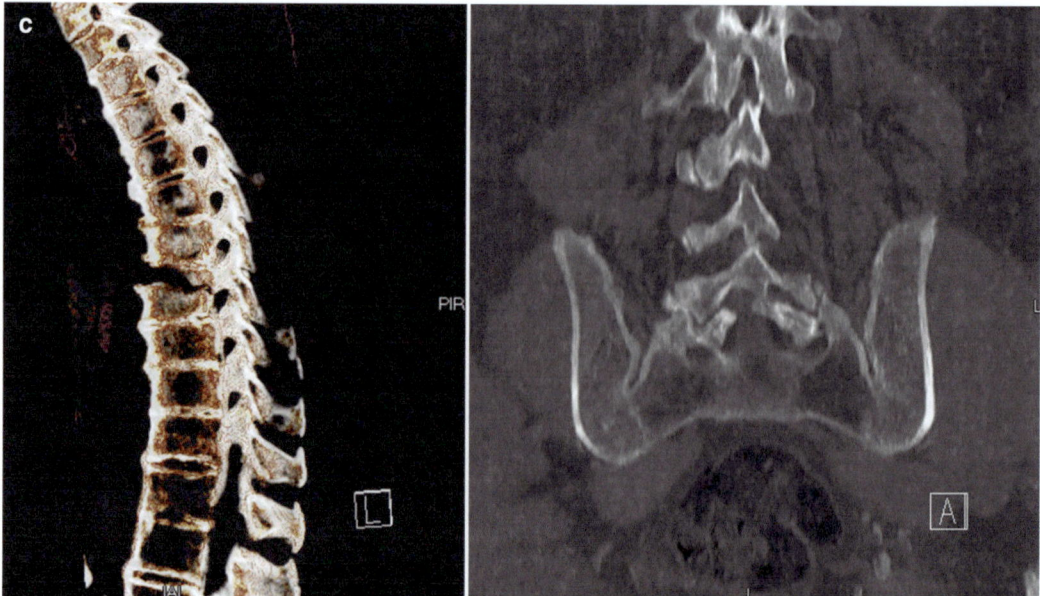

Fig. 3.21 (continued)

3.5.5 Examples of Important Potential Pre-existing Diseases

In cases of serious mismanagement such as delayed diagnosis of entire injury patterns, life-threatening haemorrhage from missed low-energy fractures of the pelvic ring or predisposition to highly unstable spine injuries due to pre-existing pathologies may lead to death [69].

Chronic rheumatic diseases like **ankylosing spondylitis** and **DISH** (diffuse idiopathic skeletal hyperostosis) with a fatal outcome of spinal injuries after a low-energy fall [78, 79]:

- **Ankylosing spondylitis** is a chronic systemic inflammatory disease with a variable course, which causes spinal rigidity with an increased risk of spinal fractures (Fig. 3.21b, c). The disease is characterised by ossification of the spinal joints and ligaments which may lead to progressive rigidity of the spine. The increased risk of injury in the ankylosed spine is well

known. Because of the spinal ankylosis, the fractures are often unstable and might cause spinal cord lesions.
- **Diffuse idiopathic skeletal hyperostosis [DISH]** may lead to spinal injuries equivalent with high-energy trauma, like a traumatic occipito-cervical dissociation, which is an uncommon and fatal injury [80]. DISH makes the spine more prone to fracture after trivial trauma as it causes ankylosis of the spinal column.

In those cases, PMCT is crucial, because it permits to diagnose unknown pre-existing skeletal diseases. For low-energy fall cases, it may explain why a spine injury occur after a "benign" low-energy trauma, which is otherwise from a forensic point of view unusual and could be suspicious [79].

Some **rare cranial conditions** may also lead to major traumatic injuries after a low-energy fall. Mann described a fatal case of trauma in an elderly man that resulted from a backward fall from a standing height and led to severe craniocerebral injuries [81]. At autopsy he found a single blunt-force injury to the right parietal bone that induced a fragmentation of the crania with concentric and radiating fractures which extended across the left parietal bone with an oval-shaped central resorptive depression (biparietal thinning). The biparietal thinning, with a decrease in bone thickness in the parietal bones, would likely reduce their ability to adequately absorb and transmit daily stresses and tolerate acute local trauma, thereby increasing their susceptibility to fracture.

3.6 Examples of Forensic Particularities Important to Know for the Correct Radiological Interpretation of Combined Trauma: Blunt-Sharp Trauma

Cases of combined blunt and sharp force trauma to the head caused by one striking tool are rare [82]:

– **Chop wounds** are represented by sharp force combined with blunt force. Instruments causing such injuries are numerous: hatchets, swords (small), axes, claws of crowbars, machetes, meat cleavers, etc. [4].
– Chop wounds are often severe and can include extensive soft tissue and bone damage.
– They represent a combination of sharp and blunt-force trauma; the sharpness of the cutting edge influences how clean the wound edges are.
– Chop wounds are due to accident or homicide. Suicide by chop wounds is rather the exception.
– The skin injury is a long laceration with quite regular edges. On bones the diagnosis is often typical: one edge is regular; the opposite edge

is often irregular and the bone lesion is an open "V" [83] (Fig. 3.22).

The forensic pathologist may be requested to clarify [19, 20, 84]:

– The type and the identification of the weapon used
– The number of blows
– The directions and angles of the impact(s)
– The mechanism of infliction (accidental or non-accidental)
– The presence and absence of life-threatening injuries are further typical questions raised by the investigating authorities

By applying classical forensic traumatology to surviving victims, 3D CT reconstructions in clinical cases of severe head trauma have several advantages, especially for the forensic pathologist in evaluating those cases because:

– There is an "autopsy-like" appearance of fracture patterns
– It is possible to make length measurements
– It is sometimes possible to assume a reconstruction of the sequence of events
– It may be possible to match the inflicting instruments, particularly with 3D-surface scanner explorations [9, 10]

A common limitation of a clinical CT examination used for forensic purposes is the slice thickness, overlap and field of view used in the scan [84]. Clinical CT scans are tailored to apply low radiation dosages while still enabling the diagnosis of clinical disease entities. Therefore, in many cases clinical CT scans can be insufficient for the best possible forensic 3D reconstruction. However, even imperfect data, for example, with thick slices, can give a chance to answer some judiciary authorities' questions.

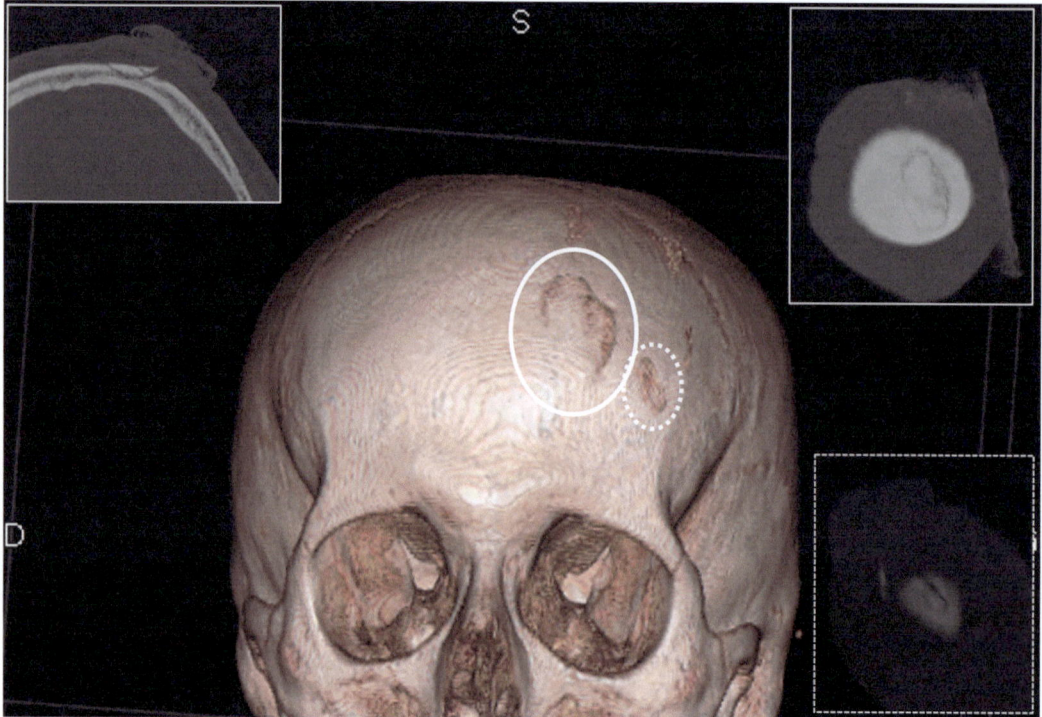

Fig. 3.22 Clinical head CT: context of cranial trauma with a sabre. 3D VRT reconstruction, anterior view: two bone fractures at the frontal bone, one superior and medial (circle), one inferior and lateral (dotted circle). Left upper inlay: 2D axial view of the medial lesion, superficial fracture at the external table and the diploe. Right upper inlay: 3D MIP reconstruction of the medial lesion, oval-shaped bone fragment, more detached at its left and upper side. Right inferior inlay: 3D MIP reconstruction of the lateral lesion, irregular oval-shaped bone fragment, more detached at its left and upper side. It can allow the determination of the lesion trajectory, from the left to the right, from up to down

3.7 Conclusion

Forensic autopsy, even if still considered as the forensic gold standard, must include radiological data to correctly reconstruct the medico-legal cases.

The forensic report is consequently a synthesis of autoptical, biochemical, genetical, toxicological, anthropological and radiological data illustrating the interdisciplinary collaboration which contributes to the progress of forensic pathology.

As illustrated in this chapter, clinical and post-mortem forensic radiology has a major role for assessment of blunt-force trauma. Blunt trauma injuries are sometimes complex forensic events, and imaging may help to better understand the nature and the consequences of the trauma.

Even "minor" traumas, such as falls from standing height, can be documented, revealing unsuspected lesions even after a meticulous external examination. Of course, high kinetic traumas, such as falls from a great height with potentially fatal circumstances, give major added value to imaging.

Post-mortem radiology contributes to:

- The correct diagnostic of blunt-force trauma
- Differentiation between normal and pathological aspects
- Diagnosis of lethal injuries

– Diagnosis of some vital signs (like gas embolism, bloody pulmonary inhalation)
– Highlight some pre-existing medical diseases, which must be included in the forensic way of thinking to understand the severity of lesions, although a minor trauma occurred
– Understanding of how the trauma potentially occurred
– Checking of the specificity and compatibility of the radiological lesions diagnosed with the death context

Some lesions may be diagnosed with imaging and autopsy; some others might exclusively diagnose with imaging, like gas effusions.

All radiological modalities are not equivalent!

PMCT is essentially indicated for detection and diagnosis of gas bubbles and effusions, fluid effusions and bone trauma in general. The possibility to measure objectively Hounsfield units of the effusion is useful to differentiate aqueous and bloody effusions.

MPMCTA and PMCTA will allow the detection of the site of vascular injuries or parenchymal injuries. This can be useful for superficial and profound wounds (subcutaneous, muscular or organ injuries).

PMMR allows the detection of parenchymal injuries. It has a high interest for cardiac and neuro-radiological injuries (particularly for the brain, and spine).

3D-surface scanning permits documentation of skin lesions, and also dry bones.

Furthermore, the possibilities of image fusion (between different tools like the PMCT and 3D-surface scanner data) can also be of major interest for the understanding of the mechanism of the trauma.

Post-mortem radiology permits imaging of many "classical" forensic autoptical aspects and concepts from the most common to the rarest. Reinterpretation of clinical radiological exploration has also a major interest for the forensic pathologist who examines victims of violence and may be sometimes the single element of objective documentation. Post-mortem and clinical forensic radiology improves the completeness and quality of the post-mortem and clinical data.

Besides the huge interest of forensic radiology for the forensic speciality and experts' reports, forensic radiology can easily be visualised or demonstrated or explained in court, facilitating the understanding of medical laypeople. This may increase its impact and highlight the fact that, today, forensic radiology is now an indispensable complementary tool for the evaluation of patients in clinical forensic medicine and cadavers in forensic pathology.

References

1. Beauthier JP. Traité de médecine légale. Bruxelles: De Boeck; 2008, 837 p.
2. Catanese CA. Color atlas of forensic medicine and pathology. Boca Raton: CRC Press; 2009, 424 p.
3. Dolinak D, Matshes EW, Lew EO. Forensic pathology: principles and practice. London, Amsterdam: Elsevier, Academic Press; 2005, xxii, 690 p.
4. Knight B, Knight BFP, Saukko PJ. Knight's forensic pathology. 3rd ed. London: Arnold; 2004, ix, 662 p.
5. Spitz WU. In: Spitz WU, editor. Medicolegal investigation of death. 3rd ed. Springfield: Charles C Thomas; 1993.
6. Dedouit F, Mokrane FZ, Savall F, Faruch M, Grimm J, Grabherr S, et al. Blunt trauma. In: Grabherr S, Grimm J, Heinemann A, editors. Atlas of postmortem angiography. Springer; 2016. p. 107 26.
7. Pollak S, Saukko PJ. Blunt injury. In: Siegel J, Saukko P, Knupfer G, editors. Encyclopedia of forensic sciences. Academic Press; 2000. p. 316–25.
8. Di Maio DJ, Di Maio VJM. Forensic pathology. 2nd ed. Boca Raton: CRC Press; 2001.
9. Fahrni S, Campana L, Dominguez A, Uldin T, Dedouit F, Delemont O, et al. CT-scan vs 3D surface scanning of a skull: first considerations regarding reproducibility issues. Forensic Sci Res. 2017;2(2):93–9.
10. Fahrni S, Delemont O, Campana L, Grabherr S. An exploratory study toward the contribution of 3D surface scanning for association of an injury with its causing instrument. Int J Legal Med. 2019;133(4):1167–76.
11. Ross S, Ebner L, Flach P, Brodhage R, Bolliger SA, Christe A, et al. Postmortem whole-body MRI in traumatic causes of death. AJR Am J Roentgenol. 2012;199(6):1186–92.
12. Grabherr S, Grimm J, Dominguez A, Vanhaebost J, Mangin P. Advances in post-mortem CT-angiography. Br J Radiol. 2014;87(1036):20130488.
13. Chevallier C, Doenz F, Vaucher P, Palmiere C, Dominguez A, Binaghi S, et al. Erratum to: postmor-

tem computed tomography angiography vs. conventional autopsy: advantages and inconveniences of each method. Int J Legal Med. 2013;128:577.

14. Grabherr S, Egger C, Vilarino R, Campana L, Jotterand M, Dedouit F. Modern post-mortem imaging: an update on recent developments. Forensic Sci Res. 2017;2(2):52–64.

15. Schnider J, Thali MJ, Ross S, Oesterhelweg L, Spendlove D, Bolliger SA. Injuries due to sharp trauma detected by post-mortem multislice computed tomography (MSCT): a feasibility study. Legal Med (Tokyo). 2009;11(1):4–9.

16. Dedouit F, Otal P, Costagliola R, Loubes Lacroix F, Telmon N, Rouge D, et al. [Role of modern cross-sectional imaging in thanatology: a pictorial essay]. J Radiol. 2006;87(6 Pt 1):619–38.

17. Jonsson H Jr, Bring G, Rauschning W, Sahlstedt B. Hidden cervical spine injuries in traffic accident victims with skull fractures. J Spinal Disord. 1991;4(3):251–63.

18. Shkrum MJ, Ramsay DA. In: Shkrum MJ, Ramsay DA, editors. Forensic pathology of trauma: common problems for the pathologist. Totowa: Humana Press; 2007.

19. Wittschieber D, Beck L, Vieth V, Hahnemann ML. The role of 3DCT for the evaluation of chop injuries in clinical forensic medicine. Forensic Sci Int. 2016;266:e59–63.

20. Grassberger M, Gehl A, Puschel K, Turk EE. 3D reconstruction of emergency cranial computed tomography scans as a tool in clinical forensic radiology after survived blunt head trauma-report of two cases. Forensic Sci Int. 2011;207(1–3):E19–23.

21. Grabherr S, Grimm J, Heinemann A. Atlas of post-mortem angiography. Springer; 2016.

22. Montoriol R, Guilbeau-Frugier C, Chantalat E, Roumiguie M, Delisle MB, Payre B, et al. Detection of glass particles on bone lesions using SEM-EDS. Int J Legal Med. 2017;131(5):1347–54.

23. Metzdorff MT, Miller SH, Smiley P, Klabacha ME. Blunt traumatic rupture of the abdominal wall musculature. Ann Plast Surg. 1984;13(1):63–6.

24. Shkrum MJ, Ramsay DA. Forensic pathology of trauma—commons problems for the pathologist. Humana Press; 2007.

25. Guyomarc'h P, Campagna-Vaillancourt M, Kremer C, Sauvageau A. Discrimination of falls and blows in blunt head trauma: a multi-criteria approach. J Forensic Sci. 2010;55(2):423–7.

26. Kremer C, Racette S, Dionne CA, Sauvageau A. Discrimination of falls and blows in blunt head trauma: systematic study of the hat brim line rule in relation to skull fractures. J Forensic Sci. 2008;53(3):716–9.

27. Kremer C, Sauvageau A. Discrimination of falls and blows in blunt head trauma: assessment of predictability through combined criteria. J Forensic Sci. 2009;54(4):923–6.

28. Lefevre T, Alvarez JC, Lorin de la Grandmaison G. Discriminating factors in fatal blunt trauma from low level falls and homicide. Forensic Sci Med Pathol. 2015;11(2):152–61.

29. Viel G, Gehl A, Sperhake JP. Intersecting fractures of the skull and gunshot wounds. Case report and literature review. Forensic Sci Med Pathol. 2009;5(1):22–7.

30. Gomez Rosello E, Quiles Granado AM, Artajona Garcia M, Juanpere Marti S, Laguillo Sala G, Beltran Marmol B, et al. Facial fractures: classification and highlights for a useful report. Insights Imaging. 2020;11(1):49.

31. Rhea JT, Novelline RA. How to simplify the CT diagnosis of Le fort fractures. AJR Am J Roentgenol. 2005;184(5):1700–5.

32. Yen K, Lovblad KO, Scheurer E, Ozdoba C, Thali MJ, Aghayev E, et al. Post-mortem forensic neuroimaging: correlation of MSCT and MRI findings with autopsy results. Forensic Sci Int. 2007;173(1):21–35.

33. Bintz M, Gall WE, Harbin D. Blunt myocardial disruption: report of an unusual case and literature review. J Trauma. 1992;33(6):933–4.

34. Wanek S, Mayberry JC. Blunt thoracic trauma: flail chest, pulmonary contusion, and blast injury. Crit Care Clin. 2004;20(1):71–81.

35. Kessel B, Alfici R, Ashkenazi I, Risin E, Moisseev E, Soimu U, et al. Massive hemothorax caused by intercostal artery bleeding: selective embolization may be an alternative to thoracotomy in selected patients. Thorac Cardiovasc Surg. 2004;52(4):234–6.

36. Irgau I, Fulda GJ, Hailstone D, Tinkoff GH. Internal mammary artery injury, anterior mediastinal hematoma, and cardiac compromise after blunt chest trauma. J Trauma. 1995;39(5):1018–21.

37. Madoff DC, Brathwaite CE, Manzione JV, Bilaniuk JW, Giron F, Char D, et al. Coexistent rupture of the proximal right subclavian and internal mammary arteries after blunt chest trauma. J Trauma. 2000;48(3):521–4.

38. Relihan M, Litwin MS. Morbidity and mortality associated with flail chest injury: a review of 85 cases. J Trauma. 1973;13(8):663–71.

39. Mordehai J, Kurzbart E, Kapuller V, Mares AJ. Tracheal rupture after blunt chest trauma in a child. J Pediatr Surg. 1997;32(1):104–5.

40. Tomlanovich MC. Pulmonary parenchymal injuries. Emerg Med Clin North Am. 1983;1(2):379–92.

41. Salehian O, Teoh K, Mulji A. Blunt and penetrating cardiac trauma: a review. Can J Cardiol. 2003;19(9):1054–9.

42. Dueholm S, Fabrin J. Isolated coronary artery rupture following blunt chest trauma. A case report. Scand J Thorac Cardiovasc Surg. 1986;20(2):183–4.

43. Clark DE, Wiles CS 3rd, Lim MK, Dunham CM, Rodriguez A. Traumatic rupture of the pericardium. Surgery. 1983;93(4):495–503.

44. Levine AJ, Collins FJ. Blunt traumatic pericardial rupture. J Accid Emerg Med. 1995;12(1):55–6.

45. Burkhart HM, Gomez GA, Jacobson LE, Pless JE, Broadie TA. Fatal blunt aortic injuries: a review of 242 autopsy cases. J Trauma. 2001;50(1):113–5.

46. Shkrum MJ, McClafferty KJ, Green RN, Nowak ES, Young JG. Mechanisms of aortic injury in fatalities occurring in motor vehicle collisions. J Forensic Sci. 1999;44(1):44–56.

47. Yoak MB, Beaver BL, Denning DA. Blunt traumatic subclavian artery injury. W V Med J. 2000;96(2):403–4.

48. Le Guyader A, Bertin F, Laskar M, Cornu E. Blunt chest trauma: a right pulmonary vein rupture. Eur J Cardiothorac Surg. 2001;20(5):1054–6.

49. van de Wal HJ, Draaisma JM, Vincent JG, Goris RJ. Rupture of the supradiaphragmatic inferior vena cava by blunt decelerating trauma: case report. J Trauma. 1990;30(1):111–3.

50. Shkrum MJ, Green RN, Shum DT. Azygos vein laceration due to blunt trauma. J Forensic Sci. 1991;36(2):410–21.

51. Sofocleous CT, Hinrichs CR, Hubbi B, Doddakashi S, Bahramipour P, Schubert J. Embolization of isolated lumbar artery injuries in trauma patients. Cardiovasc Intervent Radiol. 2005;28(6):730–5.

52. Rubikas R. Diaphragmatic injuries. Eur J Cardiothorac Surg. 2001;20(1):53–7.

53. Evers K, DeGaeta LR. Abdominal trauma. Emerg Med Clin North Am. 1985;3(3):525–39.

54. Krause KR, Howells GA, Bair HA, Glover JL, Madrazo BL, Wasvary HJ, et al. Nonoperative management of blunt splenic injury in adults 55 years and older: a twenty-year experience. Am Surg. 2000;66(7):636–40.

55. Baylis SM, Lansing EH, Glas WW. Traumatic retroperitoneal hematoma. Am J Surg. 1962;103:477–80.

56. Tejerina Alvarez EE, Holanda MS, Lopez-Espadas F, Dominguez MJ, Ots E, Diaz-Reganon J. Gastric rupture from blunt abdominal trauma. Injury. 2004;35(3):228–31.

57. Roth SM, Wheeler JR, Gregory RT, Gayle RG, Parent FN 3rd, Demasi R, et al. Blunt injury of the abdominal aorta: a review. J Trauma. 1997;42(4):748–55.

58. Chattopadhyay S, Sukul B. Pattern of defence injuries among homicidal victims. Egypt J Forensic Sci. 2013;3:81–4.

59. Kudo S, Kawasumi Y, Usui A, Arakawa M, Yamagishi N, Igari Y, et al. Post-mortem computed tomography of cervical intervertebral separation: retrospective review and comparison of the autopsy results of 57 separations. J Forensic Radiol Imaging. 2018;12:57–63.

60. Kawasumi Y, Usui A, Yoshiyuki Y, Sato M, Hayashizaki Y, Saito H, et al. PMCT findings of intervertebral separation. J Forensic Radiol Imaging. 2014;2:182–7.

61. Goonetilleke UK. Injuries caused by falls from heights. Med Sci Law. 1980;20(4):262–75.

62. Lowenstein SR, Yaron M, Carrero R, Devereux D, Jacobs LM. Vertical trauma: injuries to patients who fall and land on their feet. Ann Emerg Med. 1989;18(2):161–5.

63. Warner KG, Demling RH. The pathophysiology of free-fall injury. Ann Emerg Med. 1986;15(9):1088–93.

64. Isbister ES, Roberts JA. Autokabalesis: a study of intentional vertical deceleration injuries. Injury. 1992;23(2):119–22.

65. Atanasijevic TC, Savic SN, Nikolic SD, Djoki VM. Frequency and severity of injuries in correlation with the height of fall. J Forensic Sci. 2005;50(3):608–12.

66. Turk EE, Tsokos M. Pathologic features of fatal falls from height. Am J Forensic Med Pathol. 2004;25(3):194–9.

67. Atanasijevic TC, Popovic VM, Nikolic SD. Characteristics of chest injury in falls from heights. Legal Med (Tokyo). 2009;11(Suppl 1):S315–7.

68. Lampart A, Arnold I, Mader N, Niedermeier S, Escher A, Stahl R, et al. Prevalence of fractures and diagnostic accuracy of emergency X-ray in older adults sustaining a low-energy fall: a retrospective study. J Clin Med. 2019;9(1):97.

69. Pedersen V, Lampart A, Bingisser R, Nickel CH. Accuracy of plain radiography in detecting fractures in older individuals after low-energy falls: current evidence. Trauma Surg Acute Care Open. 2020;5(1):e000560.

70. Lee H, Kim SH, Lee SC, Kim S, Cho GC, Kim MJ, et al. Severe injuries from low-height falls in the elderly population. J Korean Med Sci. 2018;33(36):e221.

71. Lampart A, Kuster T, Nickel CH, Bingisser R, Pedersen V. Prevalence and severity of traumatic intracranial hemorrhage in older adults with low-energy falls. J Am Geriatr Soc. 2020;68(5):977–82.

72. Rich C, Raynor J, Raukar N. Nondisplaced pubic ramus fracture associated with exsanguination and death. Am J Emerg Med. 2018;36(2):342.e1–2.

73. Rau CS, Lin TS, Wu SC, Yang JC, Hsu SY, Cho TY, et al. Geriatric hospitalizations in fall-related injuries. Scand J Trauma Resusc Emerg Med. 2014;22:63.

74. Ten Broek RP, Bezemer J, Timmer FA, Mollen RM, Boekhoudt FD. Massive haemorrhage following minimally displaced pubic ramus fractures. Eur J Trauma Emerg Surg. 2014;40(3):323–30.

75. Eyler Y, Yilmaz Kilic T, Turgut A, Hakoglu O, Idil H. Axillary artery laceration after anterior shoulder dislocation reduction. Turk J Emerg Med. 2019;19(2):87–9.

76. Johnston JJ, McGovern SJ. Alcohol related falls: an interesting pattern of injuries. Emerg Med J. 2004;21(2):185–8.

77. Hino S, Yamada M, Iijima Y, Araki R, Kaneko T, Horie N. Effects of alcohol consumption on maxillofacial fractures in simple falls. Clin Exp Dent Res. 2020;6(5):544–9.

78. Thomsen AH, Jurik AG, Uhrenholt L, Vesterby A. Traumatic death in ankylosing spondylitis. J Forensic Sci. 2010;55(4):1126–9.

79. Savall F, Mokrane FZ, Dedouit F, Capuani C, Guilbeau-Frugier C, Rouge D, et al. Spine injury following a low-energy trauma in ankylosing spondylitis: a study of two cases. Forensic Sci Int. 2014;241:123–6.

80. Alahmadi BH, Alalawi HH, Alahmadi AH, Alshammari AN. Atypical occipitocervical dissociation associated with ossification of the posterior longitudinal ligament and diffuse idiopathic skeletal hyperostosis in low-energy trauma. J Orthop Case Rep. 2020;10(8):11–4.

81. Mann RW, Kobayashi M, Schiller AL. Biparietal thinning: accidental death by a fall from standing height. J Forensic Sci. 2017;62(5):1406–9.

82. Kunz SN, Gorges N, Fischer F, Adamec J. Beer stein blast to the head a rare case of combined blunt and sharp force trauma. Int J Legal Med. 2020;134(5):1791–6.

83. Quatrehomme G, Alunni V. The link between traumatic injury in soft and hard tissue. Forensic Sci Int. 2019;301:118–28.

84. Wozniak K, Rzepecka-Wozniak E, Moskala A, Pohl J, Latacz K, Dybala B. Weapon identification using antemortem computed tomography with virtual 3D and rapid prototype modeling—a report in a case of blunt force head injury. Forensic Sci Int. 2012;222(1–3):e29–32.

Sharp Trauma

4

Coraline Egger and Pia Genet

4.1 Introduction

Examining cases of sharp force injury is an important part of the routine work of the forensic pathologist, whether the victim deceased or survived. During his work, he can be asked to examine victims of sharp force injury or perpetrators presenting lesions provoked during the manipulation of a sharp weapon. In forensic medicine, different lesion types can be described. Depending on the weapon used, the wounds can present the characteristics of lesions induced by a cutting or a stabbing object or a combination of both of them, e.g., knives, scissors, cutters, arrows, spears, and daggers. There exist objects which can have the characteristic of a sharp as well as the characteristic of a blunt weapon, e.g., axe, broken glass, ice picks, and screwdrivers.

In general, lesions provoked by a cutting object are more superficial as lesions provoked by a stabbing object; they are producing an injury that is longer than deep [1–4]. The wound edges are generally straight depending of the weapon and the anatomical location of the lesion. However, a special type of incised wound is the throat cut, where deeper structures can be involved (e.g., vessels, laryngeal structures, and trachea). On the opposite, per definition, a stabbing wound is deeper than its length on the skin. It may reach all the different tissues and organs of the body. In case of death, the most common cause is an internal or external hemorrhage, and in rare cases it can result from cardiac tamponade, gas embolism, asphyxia, central paralysis, or infection [1–4].

Concerning the interpretation of the injury, it is important to determine the wound track and to describe its direction and its depth. In general, it is possible for stabbing wounds; however, for incised wounds this may be more difficult or impossible, as they are usually superficial or tangential. Moreover, the forensic pathologist may be able to differentiate offensive from defensive lesions, as well as accidental and self-inflicted lesions [5]. It is important to lay out that defensive lesions are often more superficial than offensive lesions, and frequently situated on the forearms and/or hands [1–3]. In case of death, it is important to determine if the deceased person was alive during the assault, and therefor to search for vitality signs (gas embolism, blood volume depletion, and large hemorrhagic infiltration of the surrounding tissues).

As radiological methods, especially multidetector computed tomography (MDCT) and

C. Egger (✉)
Unit of Forensic Imaging and Anthropology, University Center of Legal Medicine Lausanne-Geneva, University and University Hospital of Geneva, Geneva, Switzerland
e-mail: coraline.egger@hcuge.ch;

P. Genet
Unit of Forensic Imaging and Anthropology, University Center of Legal Medicine Lausanne-Geneva, Lausanne, Switzerland
e-mail: pia.genet@chuv.ch;
piapatricica.baumann@hcuge.ch

MDCT-angiography, are gaining in importance in forensic medicine, these methods are getting more and more involved in the process of managing cases correlated to sharp trauma [6–11]. Combined with a conventional forensic autopsy or a forensic clinical examination, those methods permit to explore a forensic case related to sharp trauma in detail by analyzing the wound track and the damaged surrounding tissues and organs. As these radiological methods are performed before the autopsy, they have the advantage to be able to "guide" the physician during his examination [12]. This permits the forensic pathologist to be attentive to certain damages and correlations which otherwise could have been missed. Additionally, radiological methods allow to illustrate forensic findings by the mean of imaging catalogs for the mandatory authorities.

In this chapter, we discuss the advantages of using radiological methods in cases of sharp trauma especially MDCT and MDCT-angiography for postmortem cases and clinical forensic cases. Moreover, we will highlight their benefit and their additional value to a conventional forensic autopsy and the evaluation of a clinical forensic case.

In this chapter, we will explain several findings, which can be found in MDCT and MDCT-angiography in the different kinds of sharp trauma, as incised and stab wounds.

4.2   Incised Wounds

Incised wounds are usually superficial lesions and often only involve the skin and the subcutaneous tissues [1–3]. Therefore, they may be difficult to visualize by radiological methods.

The most suitable radiological methods for analyzing this kind of lesions are MDCT and MDCT-angiography [7]. Conventional X-ray and MRI can have an additional value, but they are not the modality of choice. Indeed conventional X-ray has a low resolution for soft tissues and is concerned by the problematic of superposition in two dimensions of all the structures present in the field of view. MRI is an expensive, time-consuming, and not overall available technique. Moreover, as

in clinics, incised wounds can be visualized by MDCT, which is faster, less expensive, and easily accessible in comparison with MRI.

Incised wounds can be visualized by MDCT through a cutaneous and/or a subcutaneous poss. Muscular defect, which can be associated with an infiltration or with the presence of gas (emphysema) in the soft tissues (Figs. 4.1 and 4.2) [13]. Furthermore, MDCT-angiography permits to visualize a leakage of contrast medium nearby the lesion (Fig. 4.3) [14]. In cases of throat cut, MDCT enables to visualize an eventual damage of the laryngeal structures and of the trachea. On the other hand, MDCT-angiography allows in these cases to analyze the vascular structures in details and to find also small lesions of the vessels as lesions of very small vessel that can be difficult to detect during conventional autopsy.

As incised wounds are most often superficial and/or tangential, the wound track is unfortunately mostly not reconstructable, and no trajectory can be established.

One of the advantages of MDCT is the possibility to perform a three-dimensional reconstruction of the surface of the skin (Fig. 4.4) [15]. This can

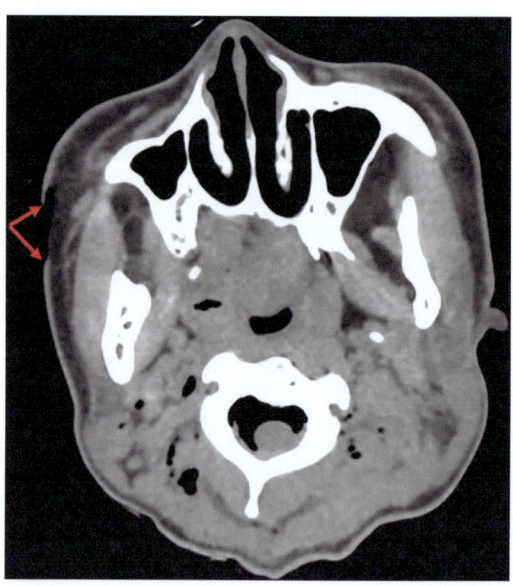

Fig. 4.1 Axial view of a MDCT of the head in soft tissue window showing a superficial cutting wound of the right cheek (red arrows) without subcutaneous infiltration and/or emphysema

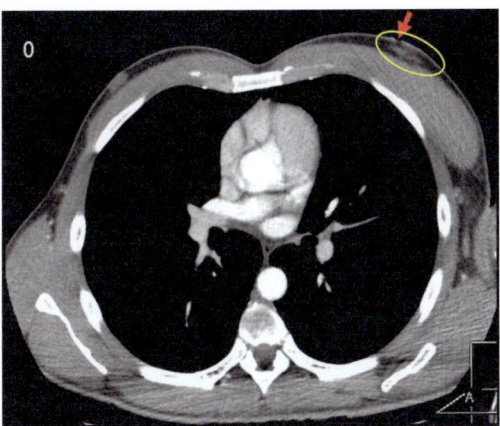

Fig. 4.2 Axial view of a MDCT of the thorax in soft tissue window showing a superficial cutting wound of the left pectoral region (red arrow) associated with a subcutaneous infiltration (yellow circle)

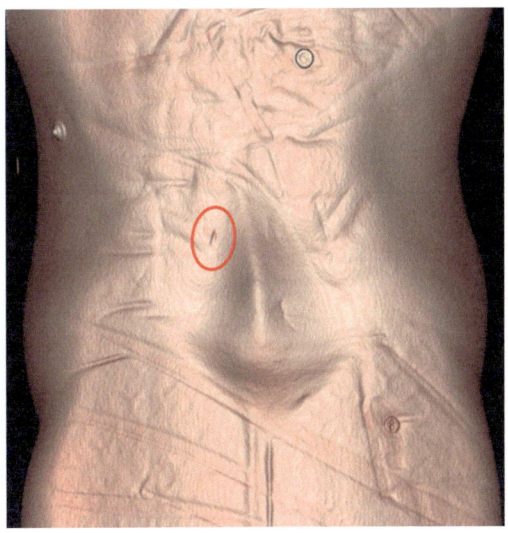

Fig. 4.4 3D reconstruction of a MDCT of the surface of the skin of the back showing a superficial cutting wound of the right lumbar region (red circle)

characteristics of the lesion in detail. However, it has to be stated that image resolution of MDCT is probably not sufficient to document in details the lesions on the surface of the skin. Photography, photogrammetry, and 3D-surface scanner are much more appropriated for this purpose.

4.3 Stab Wounds

In contrast to incised wounds, stab wounds are, per definition, deeper than they are long. They can involve inner tissues and organs, and affect not only the surface of the body [1–3]. Therefore, imaging techniques are suited for the complete evaluation of the injury extent.

MDCT is useful for the assessment of the different layers along the wound track (skin, subcutaneous tissues, muscles, bones, and organs) [16–19]. The wound can be represented by a skin defect, and an infiltration and/or emphysema of the subcutaneous and muscular tissues can show their damage (Fig. 4.5a, b). Without injection of contrast medium, lesions of the organs or big vessels can only be suspected, respectively, by infiltrations and/or emphysema, and effusions surrounding the injured structure. Damages of the skeleton may be visible by straight cuts

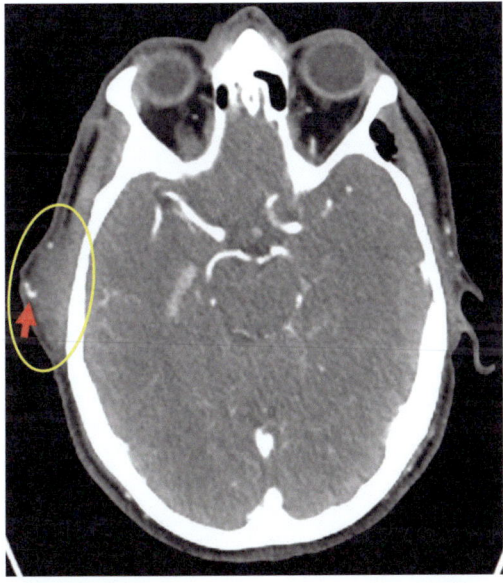

Fig. 4.3 Axial view of a MDCT-angiography of the head in soft tissue window showing a superficial cutting wound of the right temporal region (yellow circle) associated with a leakage of contrast medium (red arrow)

be very helpful in clinical forensic cases where the lesions have been already sutured or where the edges of the wound have already been excised during surgical/medical care. The morphology of the wound and of its edges is of primordial importance for the forensic interpretation, and with the help of MDCT, it is therefore possible to evaluate the

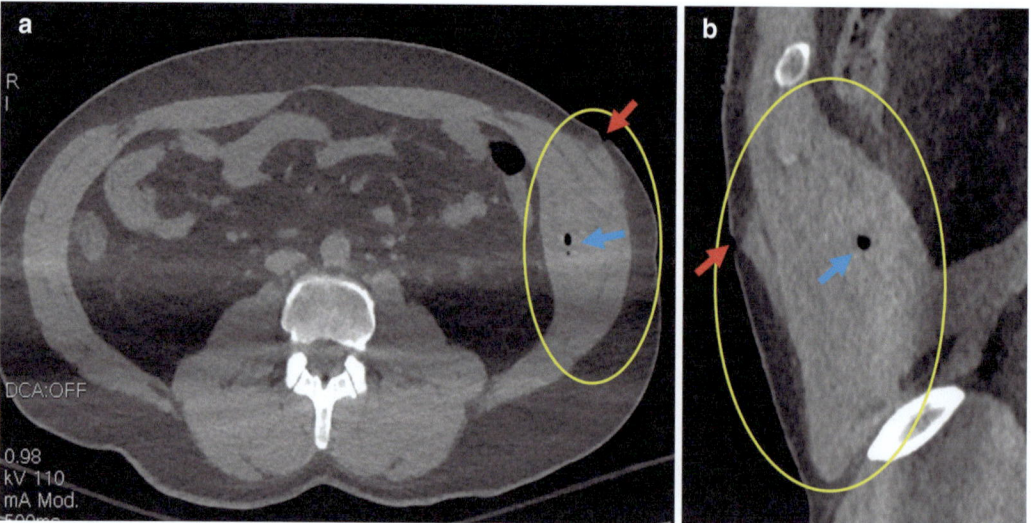

Fig. 4.5 (**a**) Axial view of a MDCT of the abdomen in soft tissue window showing a sharp wound on the skin of the left low abdominal region (red arrow) associated with a subcutaneous infiltration, a muscular hematoma (yellow circle), and an emphysema (blue arrow). (**b**) Sagittal view of a MDCT of the abdomen in soft tissue window showing a sharp wound on the skin of the left low abdominal region (red arrow) associated with a subcutaneous infiltration, a muscular hematoma (yellow circle), and an emphysema (blue arrow)

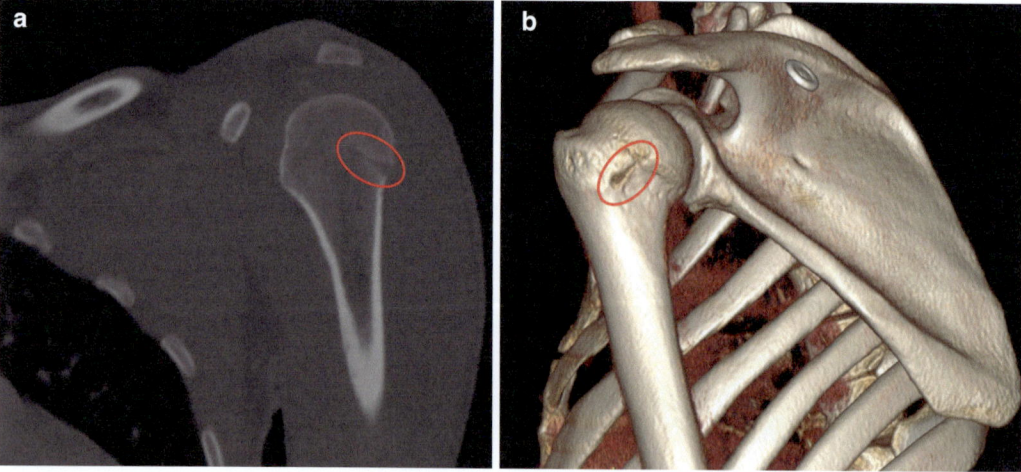

Fig. 4.6 (**a**) Oblique coronal view of a MDCT of the right shoulder in bone window showing a straight cut through the humerus (red circle). (**b**) Latero-posterior view of a 3D VRT (volume rendering technique) recon-struction of a MDCT of the skeleton of the right shoulder in bone window showing a straight cut through the humerus (red circle)

through the bones or fractures with straight edges (Fig. 4.6a, b). A pneumothorax and pneumoperitoneum can indirectly indicate a lesion of the thoracic or abdominal cavity without observing a direct damage of the pleura or abdominal wall (Fig. 4.7).

MDCT-angiography is the method of choice for analyzing stab wounds [7, 20, 21]. It permits a good contrast of the different organs and inner structures of the body, in particular the vessels, veins, and arteries, depending on the opacification of the venous or the arterial system. By the

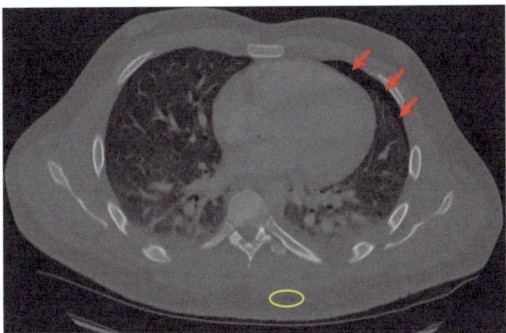

Fig. 4.7 Axial view of a MDCT of the thorax in bone window showing a dorsal subcutaneous emphysema (yellow circle) indirectly indicating a stabbing wound and a left pneumothorax (red arrows) without any visible lesion of the lung and of the parietal pleura. The lesion of the skin is not visible on this radiological image

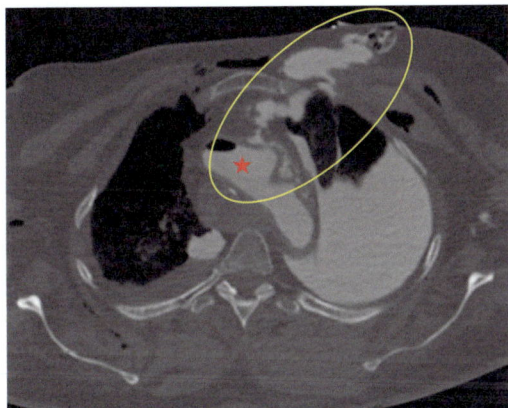

Fig. 4.8 Oblique axial view of the arterial phase of a MDCT-angiography showing a lesion of the thoracic aorta (red star) by a leakage of contrast medium highlighting the wound track (yellow circle)

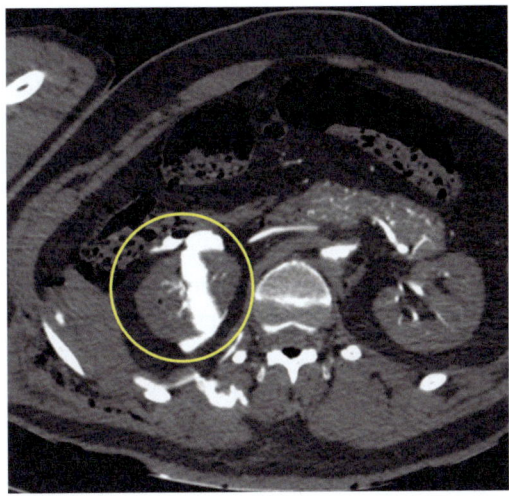

Fig. 4.9 Axial view of the arterial phase of a MDCT-angiography showing a lesion of the right kidney with a leakage of contrast medium through the organ (yellow circle)

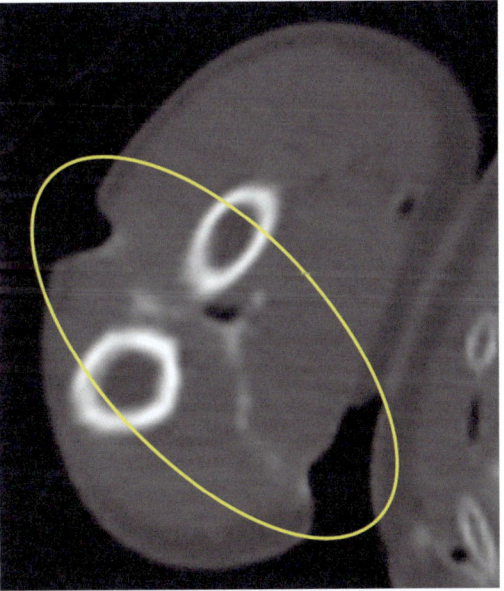

Fig. 4.10 Oblique axial view of the dynamic phase of a MDCT-angiography showing a leakage of contrast medium between two skin and subcutaneous tissue defects highlighting their connection (yellow circle)

mean of the leakage of contrast medium, a lesion of a vessel can be easily identified, as well as damages of soft tissues and parenchyma of solid organs (Figs. 4.8 and 4.9) [22]. Besides, lesions of the solid organs can be better visualized with an opacification of the venous system. Thanks to small vascular lesions all along the trajectory, the whole trajectory is getting enhanced by the contrast agent and can therefore be visualized by MDCT-angiography. The leakage can also, for example, define whether two lesions communicate with each other or not, especially at upper and lower extremities (Fig. 4.10).

As previously mentioned, MDCT enables to perform three-dimensional reconstructions of the surface of the skin, which can be also useful for stab wounds [15]. Moreover, it permits 3D reconstruction of the vessels and therefore to show the leakage of the contrast medium in a tridimensional way. For the forensic pathologist, it is important to be able to determine the direction and the angle of the trajectory and its depth [22, 23]. A three-dimensional reconstruction of MDCT-angiography images permits to reconstruct the direction and the angle of the trajectory of most of the cases (Fig. 4.11). Furthermore, it allows the measurement of the minimum and/or maximum depth of the wound track depending on the case (Fig. 4.12). Ideally, the measurement should be carried out in two of the three dimensions (axial, coronal, and sagittal) in order to avoid a bias of measurement and to assure the correct measurement of the wound track. The measurements are easy to perform in the case of a lesion of a fix structure (organ or bone) (Fig. 4.13a, b), but can be trickier to conduct if only the soft tissues are damaged. In these cases, only diffused infiltration and emphysema may be visible, and at best only a minimum depth can be given. In case of pneumothorax and pneumoperitoneum without a visible damage of internal organs, the measurement of the depth of the path has to be done between the skin surface and the internal thoracic or abdominal wall.

It is also to highlight that during the reconstruction of the wound path, it has to be considered that in postmortem in particular, but also in the living, the position of the organs can change due to hemorrhages, pneumothorax, and collapse of the lungs. Moreover, the absence of respiratory movements and heartbeats can influence the position of the organs compared to the moment when the person was alive and suffered the trauma (Figs. 4.14 and 4.15) [24, 25]. Additionally, the movement and position of the protagonists during the assault have to be considered. An important emphysema related to the sharp trauma has also to be considered when measuring the wound track, as it can falsify the measurement of the depth, making it seem longer than it really is (Fig. 4.16). It has to be kept in mind that the length of the measured trajectory doesn't correspond to the length of the weapon used. The elasticity and the compression of the tissue during the stabbing can influence the wound channel. Furthermore, the blade of the knife is not always thrusted until the handle of the knife.

It may happen that a sharp object breaks during the hit of hard structures (e.g., bones) and that fragments remain inside the body [26–28]. They

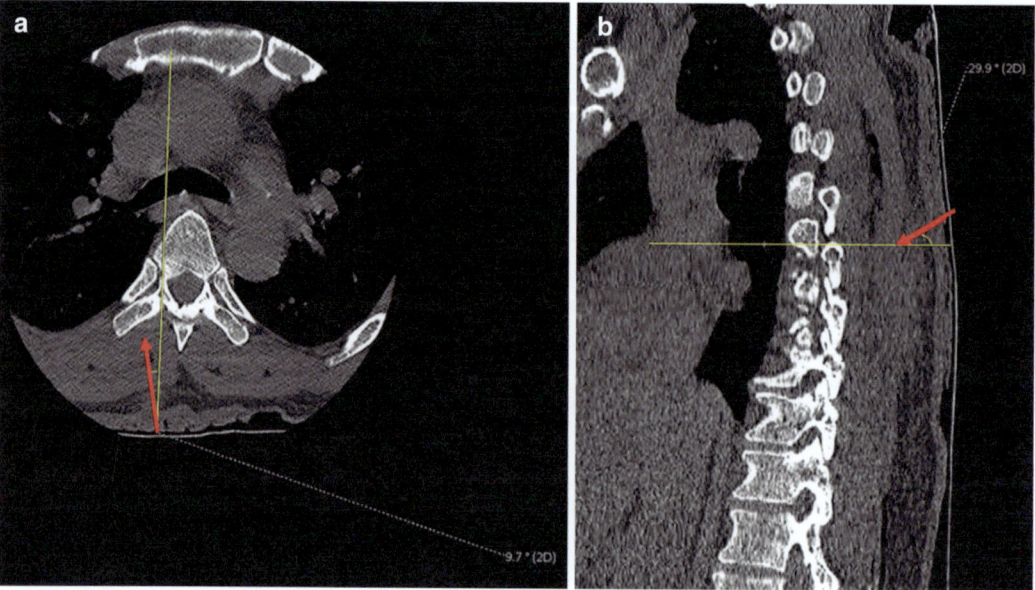

Fig. 4.11 Axial (**a**) and sagittal (**b**) view of a MDCT of the thorax showing the angles (red arrows) of the respective wound track

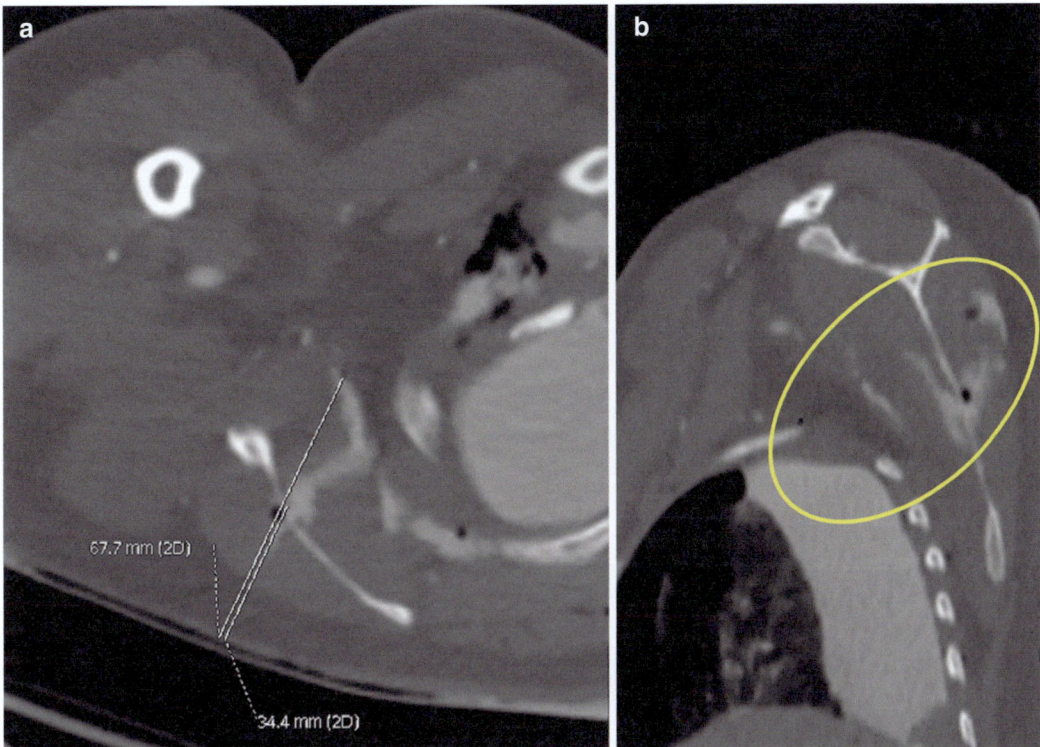

Fig. 4.12 Oblique axial (**a**) and oblique sagittal (**b**) view of the venous phase of a MDCT-angiography showing a leakage of contrast medium in the muscle tissues of the right shoulder going through the right scapula (yellow circle). (**a**) Measurement of the minimum (until the fracture of the scapula) and maximum (until the deepest penetration of the contrast medium) depth of the wound track

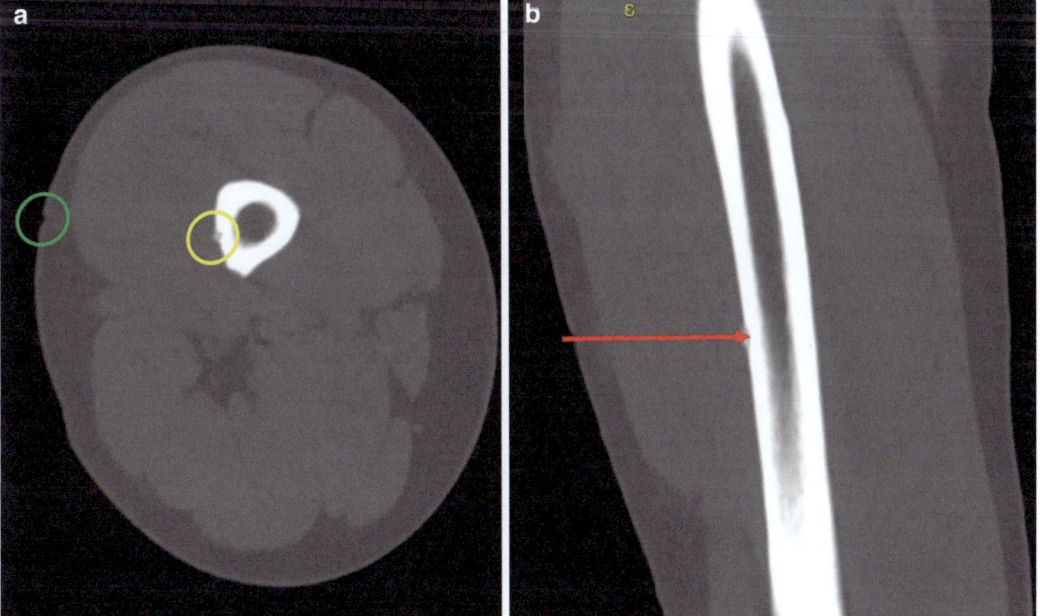

Fig. 4.13 Axial (**a**) and coronal (**b**) view of a MDCT showing a skin defect on the lateral side of the proximal right thigh (green circle) and bone defect on the proximal femur (yellow circle) allowing to define a trajectory and its maximal depth (red arrow)

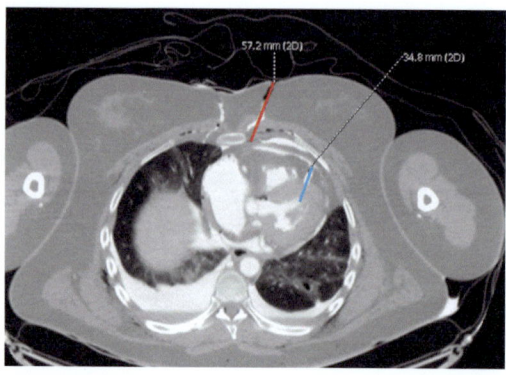

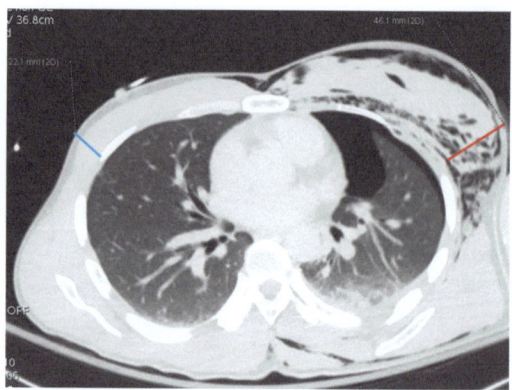

Fig. 4.14 Axial view of the dynamic phase of a MDCT-angiography showing a sharp trauma wound track from the left pectoral region to the left chamber of the heart, with visualization of a misalignment between the superficial (red line) and deep (blue line) part of the wound track due to multifactorial reasons (e.g., respiratory movements and heartbeats during lifetime and a postmortem shift of organs)

Fig. 4.16 Axial view of a MDCT of the thorax showing a sharp trauma wound at the left pectoral region associated with an important subcutaneous emphysema leading to an enlargement of the subcutaneous tissues (red line versus blue line) and falsifying the depth of the wound track

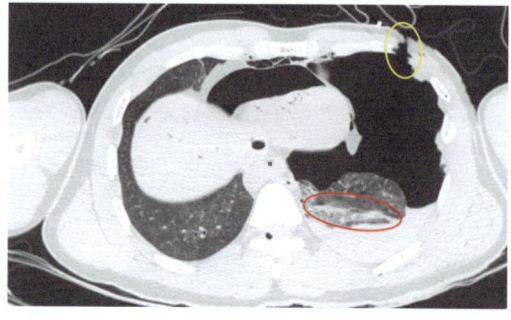

Fig. 4.15 Axial view of a MDCT showing a sharp trauma wound track from the left anterior thoracic wall (yellow circle), penetrating the left pleural cavity with lesion of the left lung (red circle). The left lung is collapsed and the trajectory is not aligned

By the use of 3D reconstructions, it is possible to determine whether the wound track passes next to vital structures or not, and to measure the distance between the wound path and the structure of interest (Fig. 4.19) [15]. This can be of major importance for classifying the dangerousness of the lesion.

MRI is not the modality of choice, but it can be valuable in case of cerebral or spinal cord injury (Fig. 4.20) [29].

The use of conventional X-ray is limited but can make bone fractures visible (Fig. 4.21). It is not suited for 3D analysis.

can be visible on the X-rays and on the MDCT. Depending on their size, they can be hard to find during the autopsy (Fig. 4.17a–c).

Sometimes corpses are admitted to forensic institutes with the sharp object still in the body, allowing a full forensic imaging with the detailed visualization of the whole trajectory based on the foreign object (Fig. 4.18a, b) [23].

Due to the complexity of the radiological assessment of stab wounds, it is recommended that the interpretation of those images should be performed by a radiologist with experience in that field in collaboration with a forensic pathologist. The results of the conventional autopsy and/or of the clinical examination should always be considered for the interpretation of the images.

Regarding three-dimensional reconstruction, 3D-surface scanner can be interesting in case of stab trauma. If the wound is associated with a

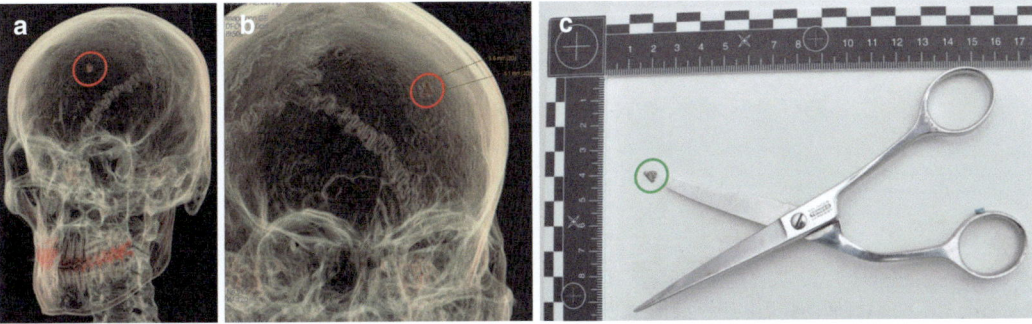

Fig. 4.17 3D reconstructions of a MDCT of the skull (**a**, **b**) with visualization of a triangular foreign body of metallic density at the frontal left region (red circles). (**c**) Photograph of a broken pair of scissors (suspected weapon), with a triangle fragment missing (green circle) at one of its extremity

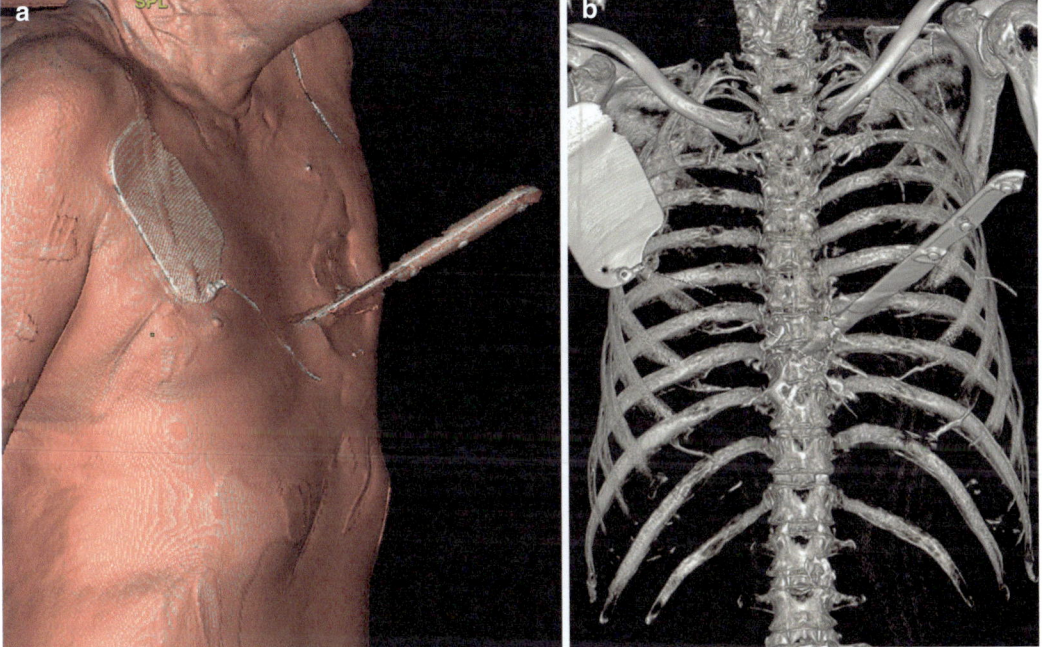

Fig. 4.18 (**a**) 3D reconstruction of a MDCT of the surface of the body showing the presence of a knife penetrating the thoracic cavity on the left side. (**b**) 3D reconstruction of the thoracic skeleton with visualization of the penetration of the knife between the ribs

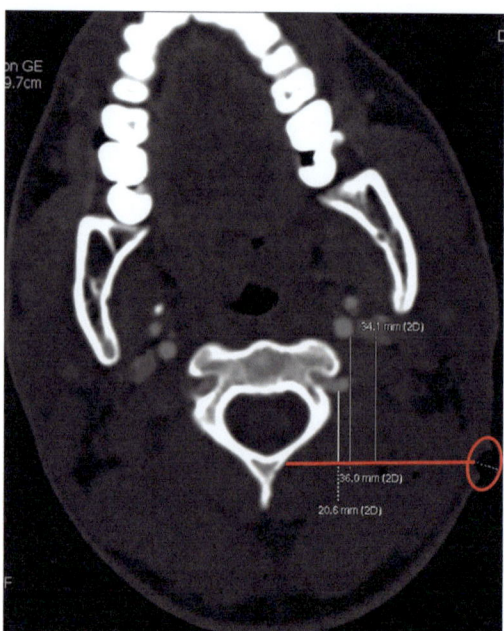

Fig. 4.19 Axial view of a MDCT of the neck showing the distance (white lines) between the wound track (red line) on the left side of the neck and the major vessels (vertebral and carotid arteries, jugular vein). The red circle shows the skin defect

bruise or abrasion representing the handle of the knife, the 3D-surface scanner can give additional information about the weapon, by comparing the shape of the surrounding lesion (bruises, abrasion) and the shape of the handle of the weapon. Moreover, it can be useful to perform a 3D-surface scanner of the victim, in order to reconstruct the position of the victim and of the perpetrator during the assault.

Literature reports also the usefulness of micro-CT for analyzing the morphological characteristics of the cut marks induced by knife blades on the bones, in order to be able to link a suspected weapon to the induced lesion on a bone [30–33].

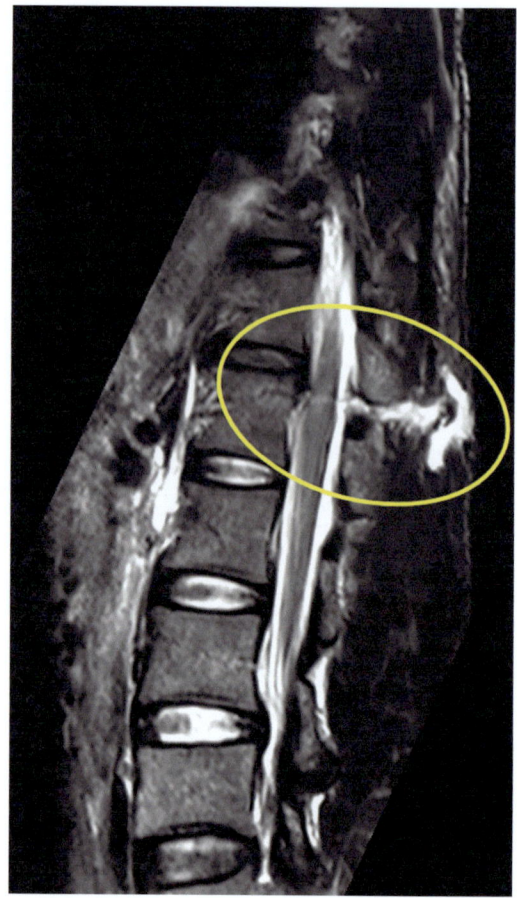

Fig. 4.20 Sagittal view of an injected MRI showing a wound track with a lesion of the spinal cord and of a vertebral corps (yellow circle)

All the previously mentioned radiological methods can be used together or independently to illustrate the lesions and the trajectory for the juridical authorities. In postmortem, the best way to show the trajectories is to perform a MDCT-angiography. Depending on the structures, which are affected, images that illustrate the venous system, the arterial system, or both vascular systems have to be used.

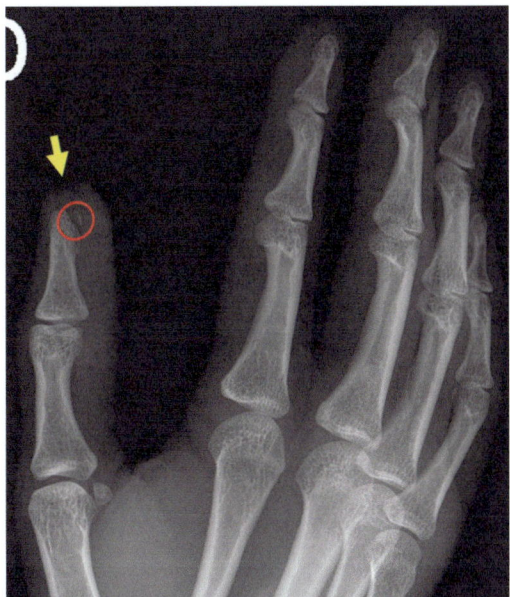

Fig. 4.21 Conventional X-ray of the right hand with visualization of a sharp trauma wound of the thumb, with a skin defect (yellow arrow) and a fracture of the distal phalange (red circle)

4.4   Conclusion

In summary, the following recommendations can be made for forensic practice:

1. The most suitable imaging modality for sharp trauma is MDCT-angiography.
2. 3D VRT (volume rendering technique) reconstructions permit a detailed analysis and illustration of the injury extent and of the trajectory (direction, angle, depth, etc.).
3. Stab wounds are radiologically more easily assessable than incised wounds.
4. Priority should be given to interdisciplinary work between radiologist and forensic pathologist because of the complexity of the subject.

References

1. Spitz WU. Sharp force injury. In: Spitz WU, Spitz DJ, editors. Spitz and Fisher's medicolegal investigation of death: guidelines for the application of pathology to crime investigation. 4th ed. Springfield, IL: Charles CT; 2006. p. 532–606.
2. Brinkmann B. Spitze, scharfe und halbscharfe Gewalt. In: Brinkmann B, Madea B, editors. Handbuch gerichtliche Medizin. Springer; 2004. p. 571–91.
3. Madea B. Mechanical trauma and classification of wounds. In: Handbook of forensic medicine. Wiley Blackwell; 2014. p. 313–23.
4. Saukko P, Knight B. The pathology of wounds: incised wounds. In: Ueberberg A, editor. Knight's forensic pathology. 3rd ed. London: Arnold Publishers; 2004. p. 153–66.
5. Schmidt U. Sharp force injuries in "clinical" forensic medicine. Forensic Sci Int. 2010;195(1–3):1–5.
6. Grabherr S, Egger C, Vilarino R, Campana L, Jotterand M, Dedouit F. Modern post-mortem imaging: an update on recent developments. Forensic Sci Res. 2017;2(2):52–64.
7. Chevallier C, Doenz F, Vaucher P, Palmiere C, Dominguez A, Binaghi S, Mangin P, Grabherr S. Postmortem computed tomography angiography vs. conventional autopsy: advantages and inconveniences of each method. Int J Legal Med. 2013;127(5):981–9.
8. Schnider J, Thali MJ, Ross S, Oesterhelweg L, Spendlove D, Bolliger SA. Injuries due to sharp trauma detected by post-mortem multislice computed tomography (MSCT): a feasibility study. Legal Med (Tokyo). 2009;11(1):4–9.
9. Dirnhofer R, Thali M, Vock P. The virtopsy approach: 3D optical and radiological scanning and reconstruction in forensic medicine. London NW: CRC Press; 2009.
10. Thali MJ, Viner MD, Brogdon BG. Brogdon's forensic radiology. 2nd ed. London NW: CRC Press; 2010.
11. Jeffery AJ. The role of computed tomography in adult post-mortem examinations: an overview. Diagn Histopathol. 2010;16:546–51.
12. Poulsen K, Simonsen J. Computed tomography as routine in connection with medico-legal autopsies. Forensic Sci Int. 2007;171(2–3):190–7.
13. Garetier M, Deloire L, Dédouit F, Dumousset E, Saccardy C, Ben SD. Postmortem computed tomography findings in suicide victims. Diagn Interv Imaging. 2017;98(2):101–12.
14. Moskała A, Woźniak K, Kluza P, Bolechała F, Rzepecka-Woźniak E, Kołodziej J, Latacz K. [Validity of post-mortem computed tomography angiography (PMCTA) in medico-legal diagnostic management of stab and incised wounds]. Arch Med Sadowej Kryminol. 2012;62(4):315–26.
15. Takahashi Y, Sano R, Hayakawa A, Fukuda H, Kubo R, Okawa T, Tokue H, Takei H, Kominato Y. Superimposed CT imaging using fusion function to visualize the relationship between the knife and the wound path in a stabbing victim. J Forensic Sci. 2021;66(3):1148–53.
16. Reginelli A, Pinto A, Russo A, Fontanella G, Rossi C, Del Prete A, Zappia M, D'Andrea A, Guglielmi G, Brunese L. Sharp penetrating wounds: spectrum of

imaging findings and legal aspects in the emergency setting. Radiol Med. 2015;120(9):856–65.

17. Peschel O, Szeimies U, Vollmar C, Kirchhoff S. Postmortem 3-D reconstruction of skull gunshot injuries. Forensic Sci Int. 2013;233(1–3):45–50.

18. Jalalzadeh H, Giannakopoulos GF, Berger FH, Fronczek J, van de Goot FRW, Reijnders UJ, Zuidema WP. Post-mortem imaging compared with autopsy in trauma victims—a systematic review. Forensic Sci Int. 2015;257:29–48.

19. Schmitt-Sody M, Kurz S, Reiser M, Kanz KG, Kirchhoff C, Peschel O, Kirchhoff S. Analysis of death in major trauma: value of prompt post mortem computed tomography (pmCT) in comparison to office hour autopsy. Scand J Trauma Resusc Emerg Med. 2016;29(24):38.

20. Minoiu AC, Genet P, Mirea I, Covaliu B, Minoiu E, Popa BV, Grabherr S. Augmenting autopsy through MPMCTA in cases involving stabbing wounds. Romanian J Legal Med. 2019;27:22–7.

21. Grabherr S, Grimm J, Heinemann A. Sharp trauma. In: Atlas of post-mortem angiography. Springer; 2016. p. 411–51.

22. Woźniak K, Moskała A, Rzepecka-Woźniak E. Imaging for homicide investigations. Radiol Med. 2015;120(9):846–55.

23. Winskog C. Precise wound track measurement requires CAT scan with object in situ: how accurate is post-mortem dissection and evaluation? Forensic Sci Med Pathol. 2012;8(1):76–7.

24. Hainsworth SV, Delaney RJ, Rutty GN. How sharp is sharp? Towards quantification of the sharpness and penetration ability of kitchen knives used in stabbings. Int J Legal Med. 2008;122(4):281–91.

25. Ruder TD, Ketterer T, Preiss U, Bolliger M, Ross S, Gotsmy WF, Ampanozi G, Germerott T, Thali MJ, Hatch GM. Suicidal knife wound to the heart: challenges in reconstructing wound channels with post mortem CT and CT-angiography. Legal Med (Tokyo). 2011;13(2):91–4.

26. Ebner L, Flach MP, Schumann K, Gascho D, Ruder T, Christe A, Thali M, Ampanozi G. The tip of the tip of the knife: stab sequence reconstruction using postmortem CT in a homicide case. J Forensic Radiol Imaging. 2014;2(4):205–9.

27. Kawasumi Y, Hosokai Y, Usui A, Saito H, Ishibashi T, Funayama M. Postmortem computed tomography images of a broken piece of a weapon in the skull. Jpn J Radiol. 2012;30(2):167–70.

28. Sano R, Takahashi Y, Hayakawa A, Murayama M, Kubo R, Hirasawa S, Tokue H, Shimada T, Awata S, Takei H, Yuasa M, Uetake S, Akuzawa H, Kominato Y. Use of postmortem computed tomography to retrieve small metal fragments derived from a weapon in the bodies of victims in two homicide cases. Legal Med (Tokyo). 2018;32:87–9.

29. Ruder TD, Thali MJ, Hatch GM. Essentials of forensic post-mortem MR imaging in adults. Br J Radiol. 2014;87(1036):20130567.

30. Pounder DJ, Sim LJ. Virtual casting of stab wounds in cartilage using micro-computed tomography. Am J Forensic Med Pathol. 2011;32(2):97–9.

31. Thali MJ, Taubenreuther U, Karolczak M, Braun M, Brueschweiler W, Kalender WA, Dirnhofer R. Forensic microradiology: micro-computed tomography (micro-CT) and analysis of patterned injuries inside of bone. J Forensic Sci. 2003;48(6):1336–42.

32. Norman DG, Watson DG, Burnett B, Fenne PM, Williams MA. The cutting edge—micro-CT for quantitative toolmark analysis of sharp force trauma to bone. Forensic Sci Int. 2018;283:156–72. https://doi.org/10.1016/j.forsciint.2017.12.039. Epub 2017 Dec 30.

33. Komo L, Grassberger M. Experimental sharp force injuries to ribs: multimodal morphological and geometric morphometric analyses using micro-CT, macro photography and SEM. Forensic Sci Int. 2018;288:189–200. https://doi.org/10.1016/j.forsciint.2018.04.048. Epub 2018 May 1.

Gunshot Trauma

5

Jean-Loup Gassend, Fabiano Riva,
and Virginie Magnin

5.1 Introduction

The characteristics of gunshot wounds are intimately linked to the type of ammunition and weapon used. Rifled weapons, in which the projectile spins on its long axis in order to remain stable, can be broadly divided into handheld (pistol, submachine gun) and shoulder weapons (rifles, machine guns, assault rifles). Generally, shoulder weapons fire projectiles at a higher speed, imparting a greater amount of energy—and thus a greater wounding potential—to them. Another type of weapon that is often encountered is the smooth bore gun, in which the bullet is not stabilized by spinning.

Ammunition can also be broadly categorized into types that are fitted with bullets that are jacketed and not meant to deform (e.g., full metal jacket, FMJ), and types that are designed to deform upon hitting their target (e.g., jacketed

J.-L. Gassend (✉)
Unit of Forensic Medicine, University Center of Legal Medicine Lausanne-Geneva, University of Lausanne, University Hospital of Vaud, Lausanne, Switzerland
e-mail: Jean-Loup.Gassend@chuv.ch

F. Riva · V. Magnin
Unit of Forensic Imaging and Anthropology, University Center of Legal Medicine Lausanne-Geneva, University of Lausanne, University Hospital of Vaud, Lausanne, Switzerland
e-mail: Fabiano.Riva@chuv.ch;
Virginie.Magnin@chuv.ch

soft point (JSP) or jacketed hollow point (JHP)), modifying the manner in which they transmit their energy to the target. A large variety of bullet types are also designed to be used in smoothbore weapons, for example, multiple projectiles (e.g., birdshot and buckshot), monobloc projectiles (e.g., slug), or projectiles designed for less-lethal use (e.g., beanbag).

5.2 General Characteristics and Morphology of Gunshot Lesions

5.2.1 Entry Wounds

Bullet entry wounds have several characteristic that the forensic pathologist will try to identify in order to differentiate them from exit wounds. Bullets tend to produce an actual skin defect as the entry site, which is round or oval. This defect is surrounded by an abrasion ring and may also be surrounded by a contusion ring. If the bullet did not travel through any intermediate targets such as clothes, the margins of the entry defect may be soiled by bullet wipe [1]. If the shot was fired from short range, powder tattooing and burns may be visible on the skin around the entry. When a shot is fired in contact with the skin, gases from the muzzle can penetrate the wound, inflating it, typically resulting in localized tissue destruction accompanied by stellate skin lesions. When a rifle

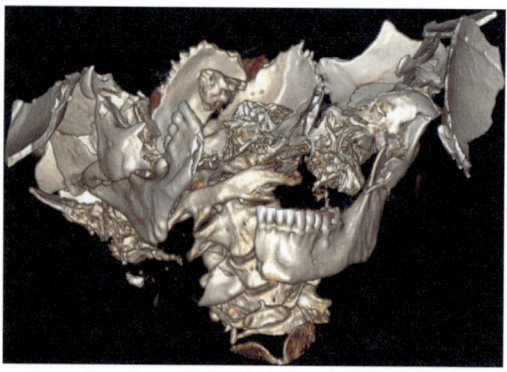

Fig. 5.1 Mandibular fractures and complete disruption of the cranium in consequence of a contact rifle gunshot to the area under the chin, illustrating the explosive-like effect that high-powered bullets can have

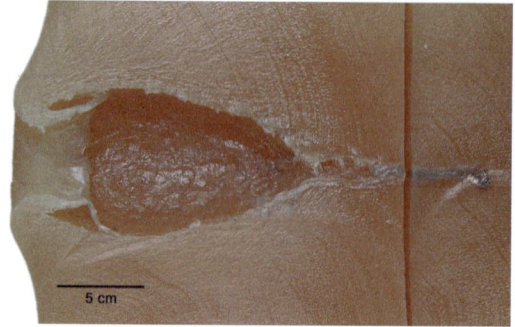

Fig. 5.2 Damage caused to ballistic soap by a .223 Remington JSP projectile. The damage visible in the ballistic soap corresponds to the temporary cavity, illustrating how disproportionately large it can be. In a human body, the temporary cavity collapses after a few milliseconds, leaving only the permanent cavity to be seen by the forensic radiologist and pathologist. The temporary cavity however can leave visible sequelae, such as lacerations radiating from the permanent cavity, or even the complete disruption of an organ

is fired in contact with the head, the gases in combination with the direct effects of the bullet (see next paragraph) can result in the destruction of the cranial vault accompanied by the evisceration of all or part of the brain (Fig. 5.1).

5.2.2 Wounding Process and Projectile Dynamics

Within the body, a bullet causes wounds mainly through two mechanisms: (a) by crushing and shredding tissue on the projectile's path and (b) by creating a temporary cavity (Fig. 5.2). The temporary cavity is created by the projection of tissues away from their contact surface with the projectile. The tissues are accelerated radially away from the wound channel and undergo deformation (elastic, plastic, or both, depending on the organ) [1, 2]. The temporary cavity collapses after reaching its maximum size, the whole process only lasting in the order of a millisecond. For high-velocity bullets, the temporary cavity can be highly destructive, particularly on tissues with little elasticity such as the liver and brain. The maximum size of the temporary cavity depends on the drag opposed to the projectile's movement and therefore on its velocity and its contact surface with respect to the direction of travel [2, 3]. The emplacement in the wound track where the maximal temporary cav-

ity takes place will depend on the type and the speed of the projectiles. Any increase of a bullet's forward-facing surface results in a greater loss of kinetic energy and therefore in a greater energy transfer and thus in a more severe wound. Such an increase in surface can be caused by loss of stability (a bullet traveling sideways presents a greater surface) or by the projectile's deformation. Hunting projectiles (like JSP and JHP), for example, are normally designed to deform and mushroom as soon as they penetrate (Fig. 5.3). As can be seen on the intact specimen, the soft lead core of the bullet is exposed at its tip, causing the bullet to deform and mushroom rapidly when it reaches its target. The deformed projectile presents a larger surface than the intact bullet, causing more energy release and therefore a greater temporary cavity and wounding potential, in order to maximize their wounding potential [1].

If a bullet strikes a bone with sufficient speed, it will perforate the bone, and even cause a comminuted fracture if traveling at high velocity. The bullet may also be deformed, destabilized, and fragmented by such an encounter. The location where the bone was perforated will classically display a beveled appearance, with the hole being

1 cm

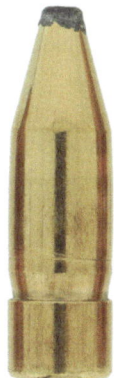
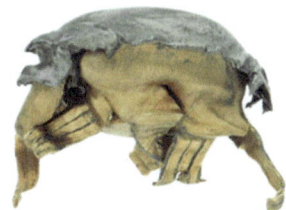
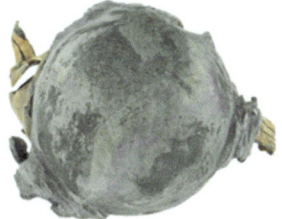

Fig. 5.3 Comparison of an unfired (at left) caliber .308 Winchester JSP projectile with a specimen fired into a soft tissue simulant (lateral view at center and superior view at right)

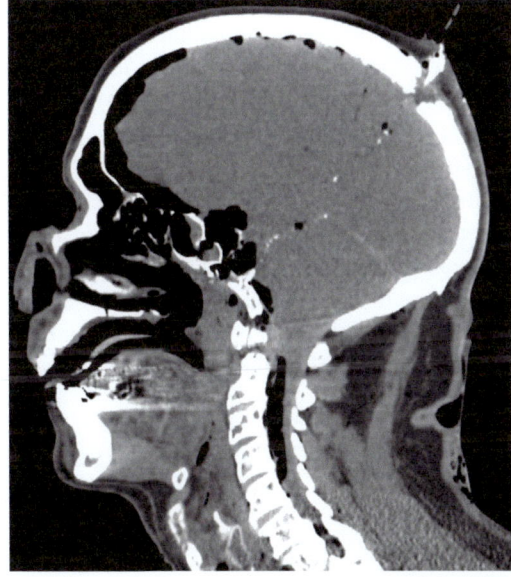

Fig. 5.4 Classical beveled appearance of an exit hole in the posterior parietal bone, the bullet having been fired in the mouth. The bony defect is smaller where the bullet penetrated the bone and larger where it exited, indicating the direction of travel

smaller at the site of penetration and becoming larger following the bullet's path (some notable exceptions to this rule have been described). Such a beveled appearance is best visualized on the flat bones of the skull (Fig. 5.4). If a bullet has

fragmented, fragments can be found along the wound path, and some large fragments may remain within the body despite the presence of an exit hole [1].

Some of the most resistant elements a bullet comes across when hitting a human are the skin, bones, and heavy clothing. If the bullet lacks sufficient energy to exit the body, it will therefore often be found lodged in areas of higher resistance, in other words against a bone, or in the subcutaneous tissue opposite the site of entry (Fig. 5.5). Similarly, it is not uncommon for a bullet or bullet fragments to remain lodged in a person's clothing.

5.2.3 Exit Wounds

The exit wound differs from the entrance wound, mainly because it is created by a bullet that has lost some of its energy and is often deformed and destabilized, and because the exit wound is not exposed to the powder or gases coming from the muzzle. The exit wound usually takes the form of an irregular skin laceration. As there is normally no actual skin defect, the margins of the wound can be approximated. There is no powder tattooing and no burns. There is no "classical" abrasion ring around the exit; however, if the skin was supported at the time the bullet exited, for example, by a belt or chair, an abrasion may be present around the exit wound.

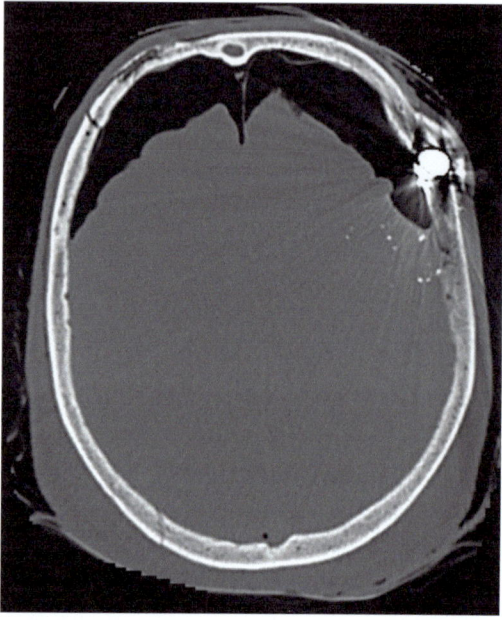

Fig. 5.5 This bullet entered the skull, traveled through the brain, fractured the skull a second time, but did not possess sufficient kinetic energy to pierce through the skin and exit the victim's head, therefore remaining lodged under the skin and bone fragments. The bone and skin are among the most resistant tissues a bullet encounters when traveling through the body

5.2.4 Difficulties and Pitfalls

Performing an autopsy of a gunshot wound victim without the assistance of radiology can be tricky. Even basic information, such as knowing how many gunshot wounds are present, may be difficult to determine before the body is actually opened. Superficial lesions, caused, for example, by fragments of bullets or intermediary targets (such as glass or the body of a car), may appear to be entrance or exit wounds to both laymen and medical personnel (Fig. 5.6a, b). Skin lacerations caused by compound fractures can also be mistaken for bullet wounds. On the other hand, small-caliber bullet wounds, or wounds in areas that are difficult to observe (e.g., inside the mouth or under thick hair), may be overlooked or passed off as minor injuries. Similarly, in cases where a body is mangled, burned, or badly decomposed, it may be completely impossible to suspect the presence of a bullet based only on the external appearance of the corpse. Radiological examination is therefore strongly recommended in all such cases.

Intracorporeal trajectories can be very difficult to predict, as people are rarely in "anatomical position" at the time they are shot. Linear trajectories in a hunched over person will become curved once the body is lying flat on an autopsy table. Furthermore, bullet trajectories are not

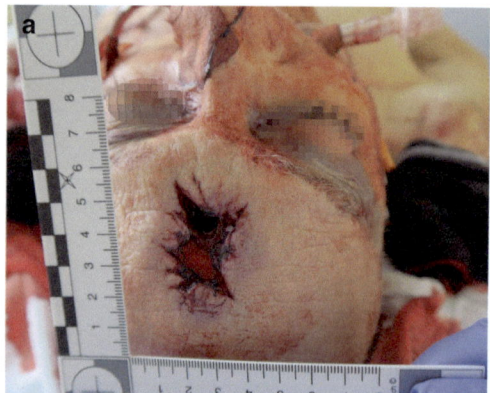
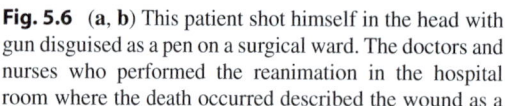
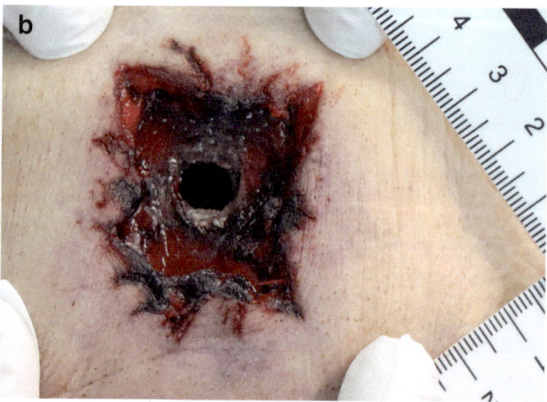

Fig. 5.6 (**a**, **b**) This patient shot himself in the head with gun disguised as a pen on a surgical ward. The doctors and nurses who performed the reanimation in the hospital room where the death occurred described the wound as a simple "laceration" and removed the pengun from the scene without recognizing its true nature. There was no suspicion that a firearm was involved until a forensic pathologist was fortuitously called to the scene

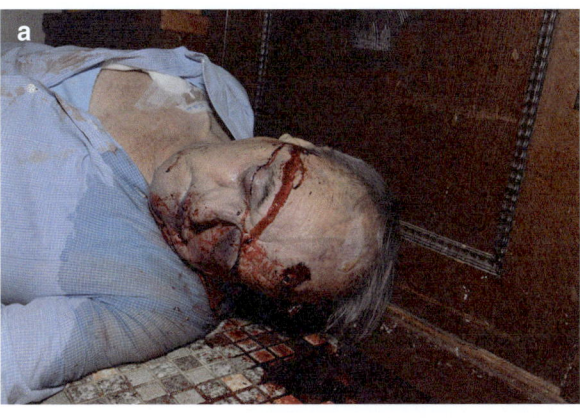
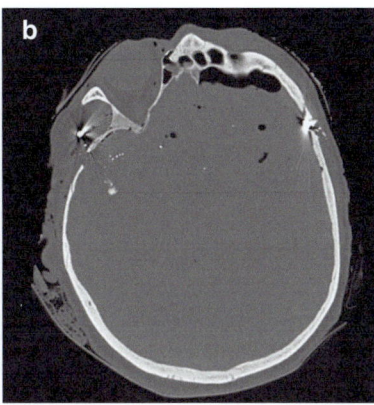

Fig. 5.7 (**a**, **b**) Man discovered at home with a pistol shot in the area of the right temple. The police called to the scene assumed that lesion visible in the left frontal area was an exit hole and were puzzled not be find the spent bullet at the scene despite a spirited search. Once the body was scanned, it was quickly revealed that the fragmented bullet was in fact still present within the skull and that the frontal wound was a superficial lesion presumably caused by the victim falling to the ground after shooting himself

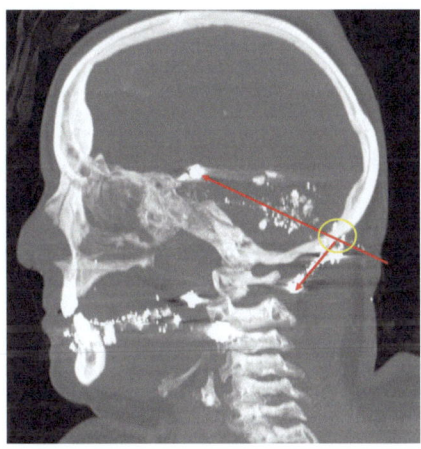

Fig. 5.8 This person was shot with a pistol in the occipital area. The bullet fragmented, one large fragment entering the skull, while another traveled downward toward the cervical vertebra. A second bullet was fired into the mouth. Imaging greatly assisted in understanding the trajectories followed by the various fragments so that they could be retrieved

necessarily linear, and bullets can ricochet on, or follow the surfaces of bones. Occasionally, what were thought to be an entrance and exit hole may turn out being two entrance holes, or what looked like a bullet wound will turn out being a superficial wound (Fig. 5.7a, b).

During the autopsy, the abovementioned problems can be clarified, though in a much more painstaking manner than if a radiological examination has already been performed. Locating bullets or bullet fragments can however be notoriously difficult at autopsy, not only in the body itself but also in the clothing worn by the victim. In the case of fragmented bullets, it is to be expected that certain large fragments will be missed if the autopsy is performed without the aid of a radiological examination (Fig. 5.8).

5.3 Imaging of Ballistic Trauma

A CT scan enables a quick and efficient overview of the body, differentiating superficial wounds from actual bullet tracks, and enabling the precise location of bullets or radiolucent projectile components [4]. Special filters can reduce metal artifact around the bullet, enabling an approximation of its shape and size to be made and revealing construction characteristics [5]. This may rapidly reveal information that is vital to the police investigation, such as the use of more than one type of projectile. It must be noted however that only a gross differentiation of bullet classes can be achieved radiologically and not an exact caliber/type identification [6].

The body should be scanned fully dressed, in order to document bullets or fragments that have remained caught in clothing, where they may occasionally end up in the lining of a jacket or similar tricky locations.

The characteristics of the entrance and exist holes that are so precious to the forensic pathologist, such as the abrasion ring or powder tattooing, are not visible radiologically. In fact, the entrance and exit wounds themselves may not even be visible radiologically. Other signs however, such as beveling of the bone and the location of small bone and bullet fragments, are good indicators of the direction of travel of the projectile within the body. Bone fragments are often extruded as subcutaneous bone chips near the exit wound. While these can unintentionally be dislodged at autopsy, they are easily documented with CT imaging [6] (Fig. 5.9). For gunshots fired at very close range, gunshot residue may be identifiable radiologically around the entrance wound [7] (Fig. 5.10a, b).

The direction, shape, and extent of single wound tracks is usually fairly obvious radiologically, particularly if bone or bullet fragments are present (Fig. 5.11). Interpretation can become much more complicated if several wound tracks are present. High-velocity or unjacketed/partially jacketed bullets may leave a trail behind them in the form of a "lead snowstorm." Bone fragments or air within a wound track are also readily visible radiologically [6]. The radiologist should brief the forensic pathologist on the number and orientation of wound tracks that are visible, and on the location of all bullets or major fragments. This will enable the pathologist to have a clear picture in his mind during the autopsy, and not to overlook any important frag-

ments (Figs. 5.12 and 5.13a, b). Postmortem angiography can identify small vascular lesions that are difficult to identify at autopsy, as well as highlight wound tracks.

Puppe's rule states that a new fracture line will stop when it reaches a pre-existing fracture line. In forensic medicine this rule can be used to determine the order in which gunshot or other injuries were inflicted, particularly to the head [2]. Such fractures are much more readily visible on CT scan images than on the actual skull during autopsy.

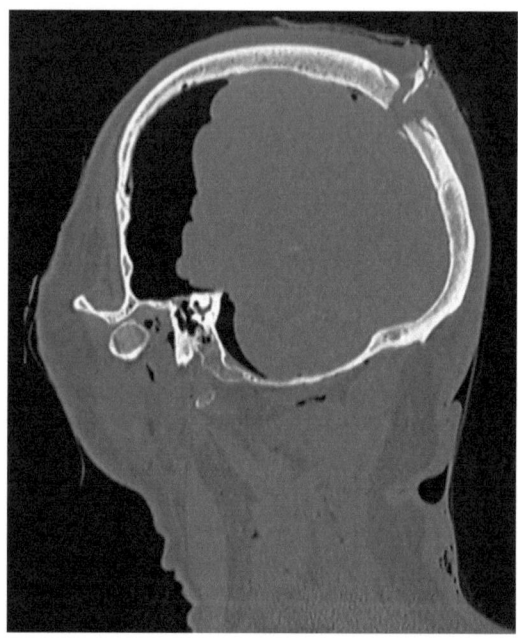

Fig. 5.9 Small bone fragments in the subcutaneous tissue that (along with the beveled appearance of the bony defect) are clear evidence of an exit wound

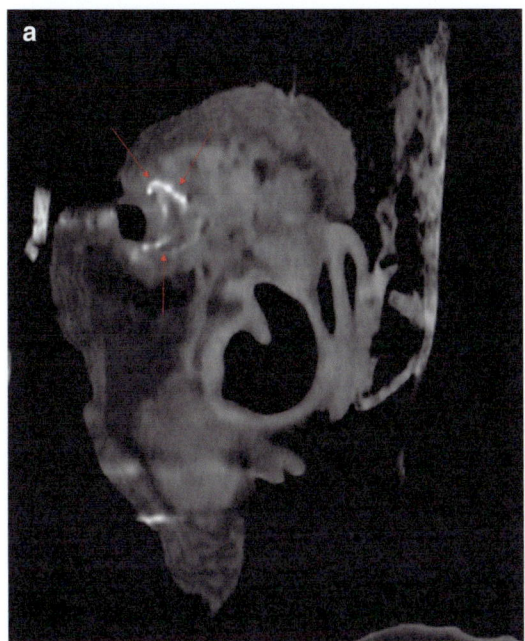
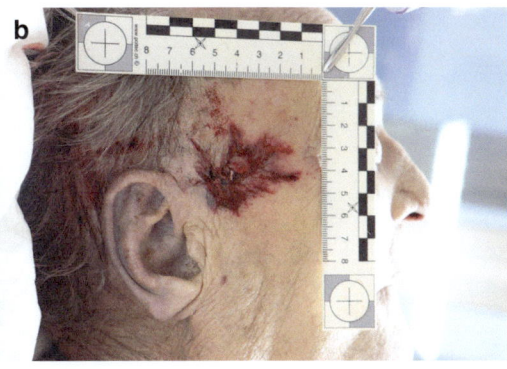

Fig. 5.10 (**a**, **b**) Gunshot residue visible radiologically around an entrance wound (red arrows)

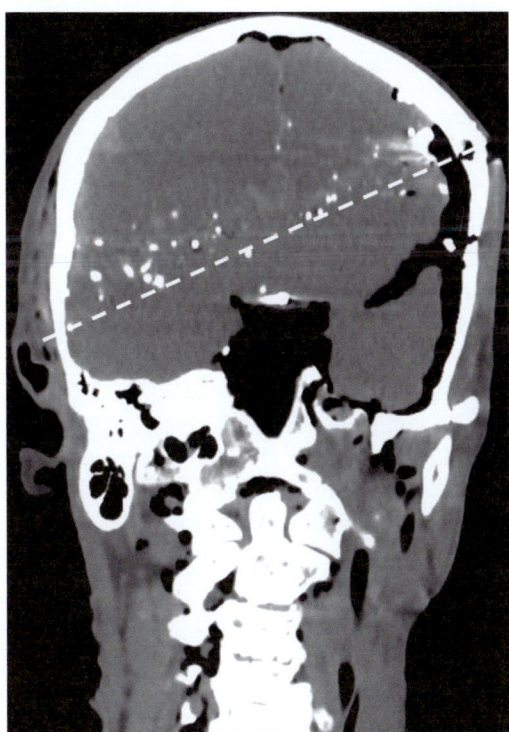

Fig. 5.11 Intracranial trajectory of a bullet, marked as clearly by numerous bone and lead fragments ("lead snowstorm") as was Hansel and Gretel's trail with bread crumbs

5.3.1 Limitations

In countries where there is widespread gun violence, it is not uncommon for a patient presenting with a fresh gunshot wound to also have old bullets related to previous episodes of violence still embedded in his body (Fig. 5.14). Such cases demand a certain level of suspicion on the part of the radiologist.

Bullet trajectories are not necessarily linear when fired into test materials. Moreover, within the human body, a wound track can be influenced by ricochets on bones, by body movements, or by movements of various organs with respect to each other. The radiologist should therefore not be surprised by wound tracks that may be very far from linear, and should try to understand the reason for this based on the possible influencing factors mentioned above (Figs. 5.15, 5.16, and 5.17). If required, ballistics tests can be performed in order to correctly interpret the radiological and autopsy findings [8].

Because numerous types of bullets share very similar sizes and characteristics, because bullets are often deformed after penetrating their target, and because of imaging resolution limitations, no

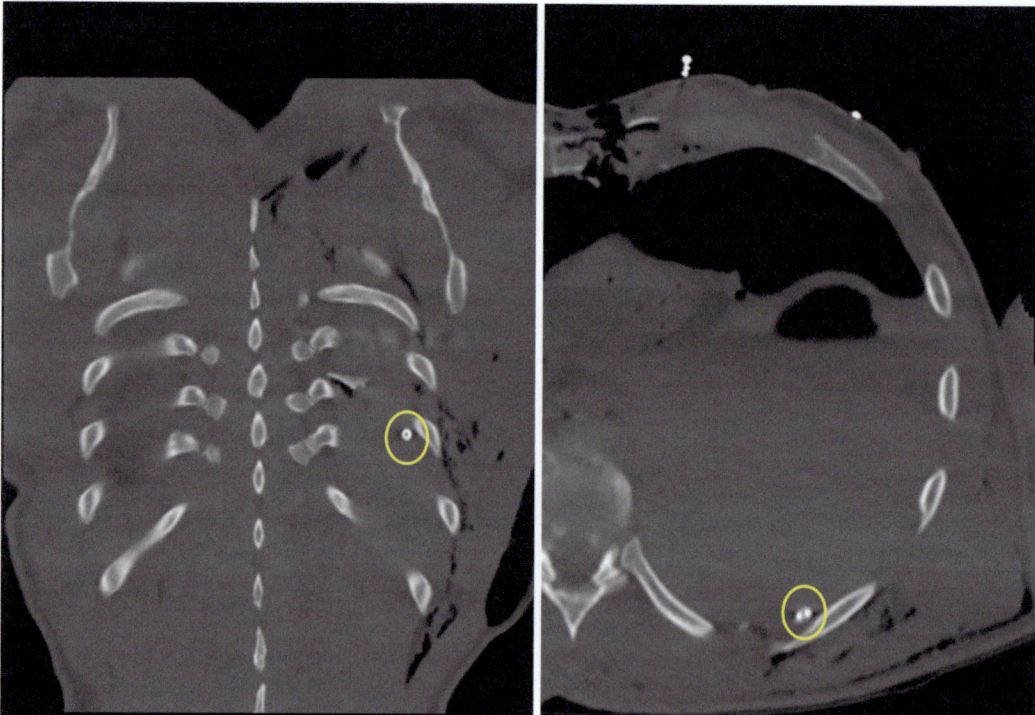

Fig. 5.12 CT scan of a person shot with a 9 mm Luger RUAG Action 4 expanding bullet used by the Swiss police. The small plastic cap from the front of the bullet is seen here within a collection of blood in the thoracic cav- ity. The radiologist forgot to inform the forensic patholo- gists of this fact, and the plastic cap was subsequently disposed of down the drain with the hemothorax blood and lost

attempts should be made to determine the exact type and caliber of a bullet based on imaging only [5, 6, 9]. Such attempts have been fraught with error. Similarly, the interpretation of wound tracks should be performed with care if there are multiple bullet wounds in close proximity to each other.

No estimation of distance of shot in cases of shotgun pellets should be performed radiologi- cally, as the rate of spread of pellets in the body is greater than in the air (the so-called billiard ball effect) [6].

Projectiles containing steel can be displaced by MRI [10]. If MRI is available, it must there- fore first be excluded that the bullet contains any steel components before the decision to perform an MRI is taken. Dual-energy CT may help dis- tinguish between various materials a bullet is made of. Elements with a considerable difference in their atomic number can be characterized with the dual-energy index [11]. Information on bullet composition represents additional information that can be used for ammunition identification purposes.

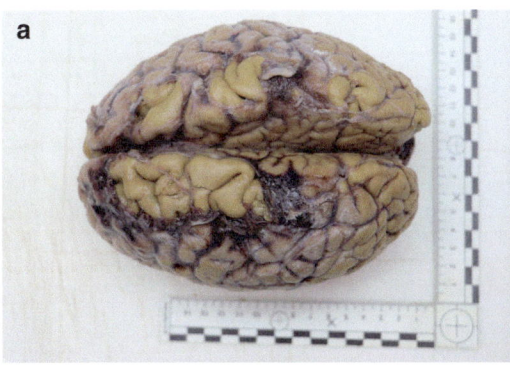

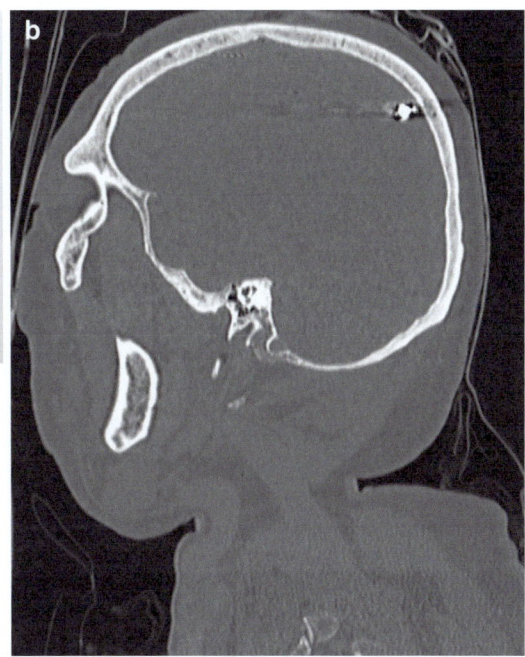

Fig. 5.13 (**a**, **b**) Brain fixed in formalin of a victim who shot himself in the mouth with a small-caliber pistol. Although the location of the bullet looks very obvious on the CT, it took several minutes of exploring before the forensic pathologist finally managed to locate it within a small hematoma under the arachnoid. Without the imaging, locating the bullet would have been even more difficult, and one might even had assumed the bullet had somehow gotten lost during the autopsy or fixation process

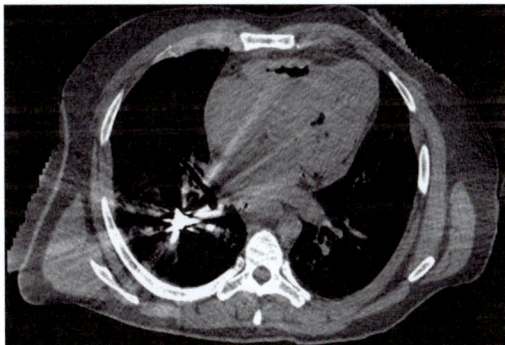

Fig. 5.14 An "old" bullet discovered in the right lung of a patient having died of unrelated causes

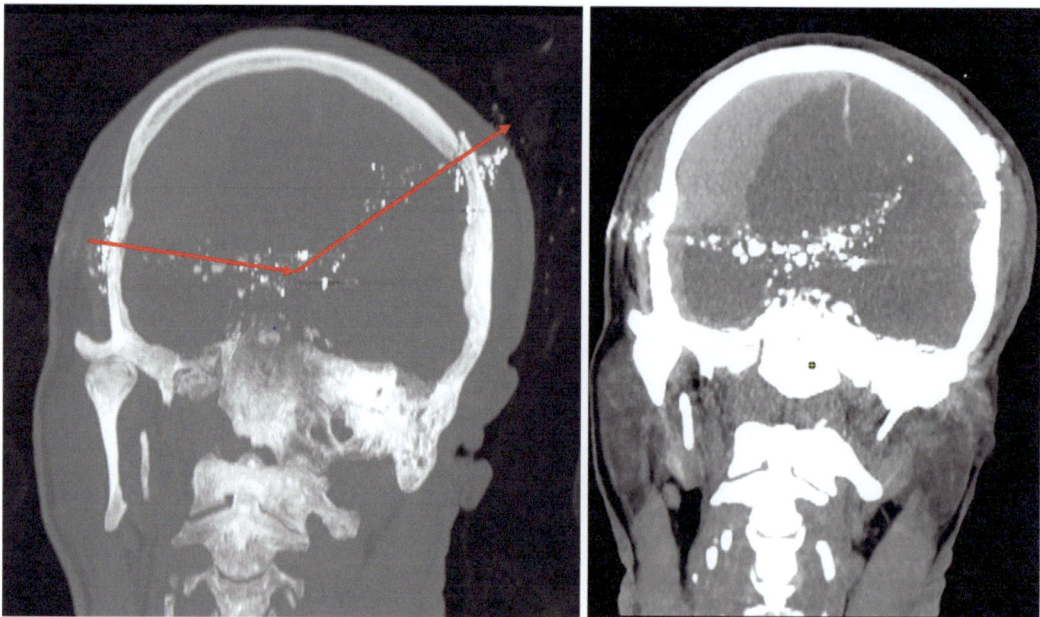

Fig. 5.15 Lead fragments from a transcranial gunshot, revealing what appears, in bone window, to be a rather puzzling, curved trajectory (red arrows). Images from the cerebral window reveal that the brain is severely deformed by a subdural hemorrhage that formed after the passage of the bullet, explaining the curved appearance of the trajectory

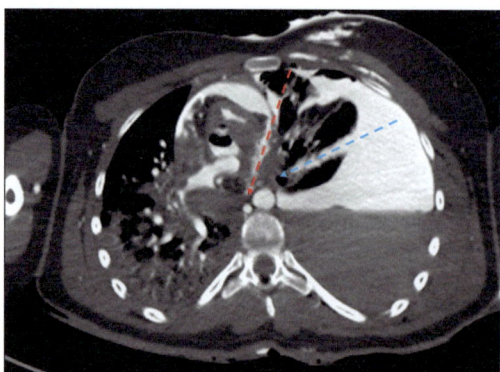

Fig. 5.16 Postmortem angiography images of a patient who shot herself in the left breast with a pistol, the bullet exiting under the left scapula. Contrast medium clearly highlights bullet tracks in the heart (red arrow) and left lung (blue arrow), as well as a massive hemothorax. Both bullet tracks do not line up with each other at all, and seem to indicate the bullet was traveling backward and to the right. These apparent discrepancies are explained by the facts that the collapse of the left lung and the formation of the hemothorax caused both the lung and heart to considerably change position and orientation after the passage of the bullet

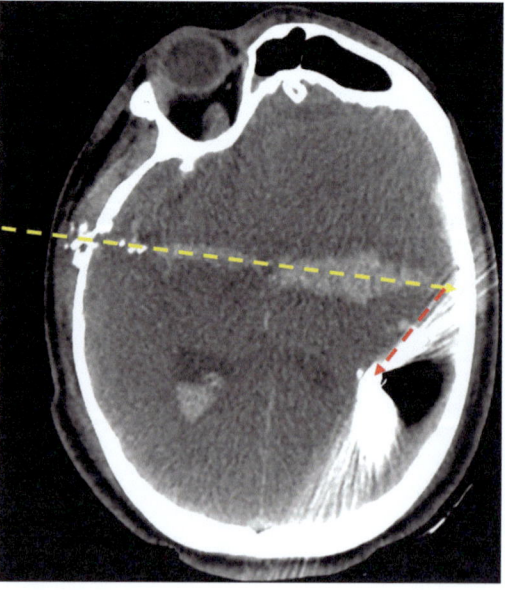

Fig. 5.17 A classical trajectory for a ricochet bullet caliber 6.35 mm Browning that first traveled through the brain (yellow arrow) and then bounced off the inside of the skull, causing it to travel back into the brain in a different direction (red arrow)

References

1. DiMaio VJM. Gunshot wounds—practical aspects of firearms, ballistics, and forensic techniques. 2nd ed. Boca Raton: CRC Press; 1999.
2. Kneubuehl BP, Coupland RM, Rotschild MA, Thali MJ. Wound ballistics—basics and applications. Berlin: Springer; 2011.
3. MacPherson D. Bullet penetration: modeling the dynamics and the incapacitation resulting from wound trauma. 2nd ed. Ballistic Publications; 2005.
4. Miller CR, Haag M, Gerrard C, Hatch GM, Elifritz J, Simmons MC, Lathrop S, Nolte KB. Comparative evaluation of potentially radiolucent projectile components by radiographs and computed tomography. J Forensic Sci. 2016;61(6):1563–70.
5. Marais AAS, Dicks HJ. Utilization of X-ray computed tomography for the exclusion of a specific caliber and bullet type in a living shooting victim. J Forensic Sci. 2019;64(1):264–9.
6. Giorgetti A, Giraudo C, Viero A, Bisceglia M, Lupi A, Fais P, Quaia E, Montisci M, Cecchetto G, Viel G. Radiological investigation of gunshot wounds: a systematic review of published evidence. Int J Legal Med. 2019;133(4):1149–58.
7. Schweitzer W, Verster J, Aldomar E, Ebert L, Bolliger SA, Thali MJ, Ampanozi G. Forensic volumetric visualization of gunshot residue in its anatomic context in forensic post mortem computed tomography: development of transfer function preset. Forensic Imaging. 2021;25:200451. https://doi.org/10.1016/j.fri.2021.200451.
8. Colard T, Delannoy Y, Bresson F, Marechal C, Raul JS, Hedouin V. 3D-MSCT imaging of bullet trajectory in 3D crime scene reconstruction: two case reports. Legal Med (Tokyo). 2013;15(6):318–22.
9. Bixler RP, Ahrens CR, Rossi RP, Thickman D. Bullet identification with radiography. Radiology. 1991;178(2):563–7.
10. Dedini RD, Karacozoff AM, Shellock FG, Xu D, McClellan RT, Pekmezci M. MRI issues for ballistic objects: information obtained at 1.5-, 3- and 7-tesla. Spine J. 2013;13(7):815–22.
11. Winklhofer S, Stolzmann P, Meier A, Schweitzer W, Morsbach F, Flach P, Kneubuehl BP, Alkadhi H, Thali MJ, Ruder T. Added value of dual-energy computed tomography versus single-energy computed tomography in assessing ferromagnetic properties of ballistic projectiles: implications for magnetic resonance imaging of gunshot victims. Investig Radiol. 2014;49(6):431–7.

Traffic Accidents

6

Pia Genet, Lorenzo Campana, and Coraline Egger

6.1 Introduction

Traffic accidents happen daily and are often lethal in particular if they happen at high velocity or if pedestrians are included. As such deceases are consisting in a violent cause of death, they are a fix part of the medicolegal routine. They often arise a lot of questions, from a penal and civil law as an insurance point of view. In order to answer those questions, a reconstruction of the accident is frequently necessary. For the reconstruction of a traffic accident, the pattern of injury and the dynamic of the accident are crucial. The latter are influenced by the type of accident, the type of vehicle and/or person involved, the speed of the accident, and the behavior of the protagonists. An important question that has often to be answered is whether the accident was preventable or not. To elucidate those questions, an autopsy of the corpse or a clinical examination of the survived person is essential, as the pattern of injury is often related to a certain mechanism or dynamic of accident. The traffic accidents can be divided into three main categories: two-wheel accidents (bicycle, motor-

cycle, etc.), four-wheel accidents (car, bus, truck, etc.), and pedestrian accidents [1–6].

As radiological methods are gaining importance in forensics, they should have a fix part in solving traffic accident cases. Indeed, the gold standard in those cases is the use of the multidetector computed tomography (MDCT), as it permits an overview of the major pattern of lesions [7–10]. In case of traffic accidents, bones fractures in different anatomical regions are often observed, and there exist typical types and localizations of fractures. Indeed, MDCT is the method of choice to visualize the skeleton and consequently fractures in general. Most of the lesions are caused by a blunt trauma; however, lesions due to a combined trauma (blunt-sharp) may be found, especially in cases where sharp objects are involved, e.g., glass fragments of the windshield and windows or metal fragments of vehicles. MDCT enables also to highlight those foreign objects.

Although magnetic resonance imaging (MRI) is not the modality of choice for examining traffic accidents, it can be useful, especially in cases of trauma of the brain and the spine [11]. Conventional X-ray can be useful in the evaluation of fractures, but with a lower resolution than MDCT. It should be used when MDCT is not available.

To evaluate the pattern of lesions of inner organs and vessels, a MDCT-angiography can be very helpful [12, 13]; however, the contrast medium used should be taken into account.

P. Genet (✉) · L. Campana · C. Egger
Unit of Forensic Imaging and Anthropology,
University Center of Legal Medicine
Lausanne-Geneva, University of Lausanne, University
Hospital of Vaud, University and University Hospital
of Geneva, Lausanne, Switzerland
e-mail: pia.genet@chuv.ch;
lorenzo.campana@chuv.ch; coraline.egger@hcuge.ch

© The Author(s), under exclusive license to Springer Nature Switzerland AG 2024
S. Grabherr et al. (eds.), *Forensic Imaging of Trauma*, https://doi.org/10.1007/978-3-031-48381-3_6

Indeed, in cases where fat embolism has to be searched as a sign for vitality of the trauma, lipophilic liquids are not recommended. In those cases, the possibility of an MDCT-angiography with hydrosoluble and hygroscopic carrier's substances should be considered [14].

Generally, in cases of trauma, signs of vitality concerning the lesion are searched for to prove that the victim was alive at the time of the trauma [15]. Those signs are different depending of the type of trauma. Forensic pathologists can find, for example, cardiac gas embolism and blood aspiration in cases of trauma (sharp and blunt) toward the head and neck, pulmonary fat embolism in case of blunt trauma, petechiae in case of violence against the neck or thoracic compression, and subendocardial hemorrhagic infiltrations of the left ventricle of the heart in case of trauma (e.g., head trauma and hemorrhage). Gas embolism is the only sign of vitality which can be surely detected by radiological methods, in particular by MDCT [16]. Furthermore, it can be punctured and sampled under MDCT guidance to be further analyzed to ensure the diagnosis of vital gas embolism [17].

The radiological methods have the benefit to be able to "lead" the physician during his examination, as they are performed before the autopsy, and enable the forensic pathologist to find certain lesions, which otherwise he could have missed [9]. Moreover, radiological methods, especially MDCT, allow to illustrate the radiological findings in details by the mean of an imaging catalog. In case of traffic accidents, this can be very useful to show the complete pattern of lesions in a three-dimensional way and to make them comprehensible for nonmedical experts implicated in the investigation (police, prosecutor, lawyer, etc.). Additionally, photogrammetry and the 3D-surface scanner technique can be important tools in solving traffic accident cases. Depending on the country and its standards, the scene of the accident and eventually the involved vehicles are documented by 3D-surface scanners and/or photogrammetry by the police. This permits later on a detailed reconstruction of the accident [18–22].

In this chapter, we will discuss the benefits of the imaging techniques cited above in cases of traffic accidents. Furthermore, we will point out the advantages and the added value of all the different radiological modalities in the investigation of the different types of traffic accidents.

6.2 Two-Wheel Accidents

In general, two-wheel traffic accidents concern collisions between two-wheel vehicles (bicycle, motorcycle, etc.) and four-wheel vehicles (car, bus, truck, etc.). It may also include a collision between two two-wheel vehicles, and an impact between a two-wheel vehicle and a pedestrian. The latter will be discussed in detail in Sect. 6.4 "Pedestrian accidents".

The collisions cited above can be front-end, front to side, side to side, or rear-end. The pattern of lesions depends on the direction of the impact and on the size and the speed of the involved vehicles.

The dynamic of the accident can be divided into three phases: a collision phase (impact between the involved vehicles), a flying phase (projection of the two-wheel rider on, over, or against the four-wheel vehicle), and a sliding phase (projection of the two-wheel rider on the ground). Each phase of impact can provoke typical lesions depending on the direction:

- As a consequence of the collision phase: pelvic and femoral fractures are usually described as well as skull base ring fractures [23, 24], and lower forearm and hand fractures. In case of an impact against the motorcycle handlebars, lesions of the thoracic and abdominal organs can be observed.
- As a consequence of the flying phase: fractures of the lower extremities, of the skull, and of the spine frequently occur [25, 26].
- As a consequence of the sliding phase: cutaneous and soft tissue lesions are predominant.

Besides, the collision and the flying phases can provoke fractures of the scapula, the clavicle, the ribs, and the four extremities, as lesions of inner organs and vessels [2, 3, 5].

All those fractures can be visualized with MDCT (Figs. 6.1, 6.2, 6.3, and 6.4) [7–9]. MDCT

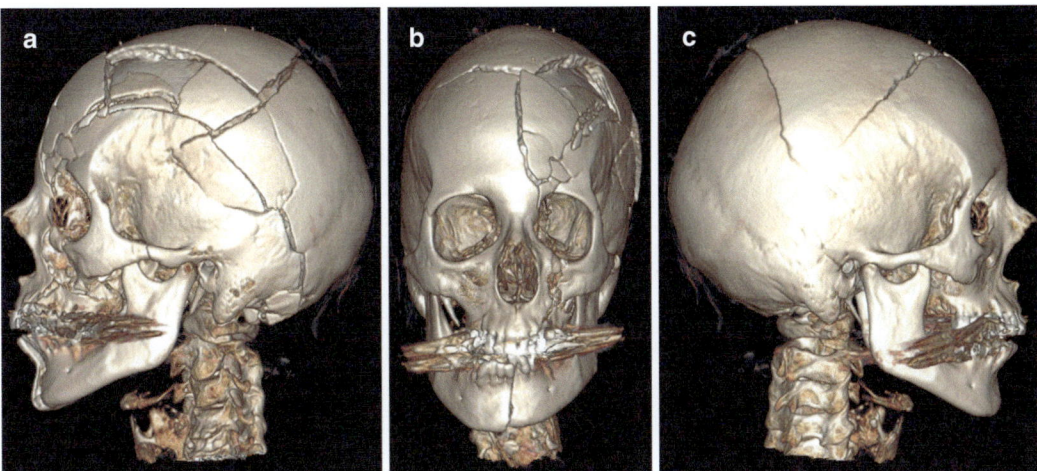

Fig. 6.1 Cyclist without a helmet hit by a car in a front-to-side collision, with impact of the left side of the head on the A pillar of the car. 3D reconstructions of a MDCT of the skull (**a**: left lateral view, **b**: frontal view, and **c**: right lateral view) showing a complex fracture of the cranium and the facial skeleton with an impact zone on the left lateral side

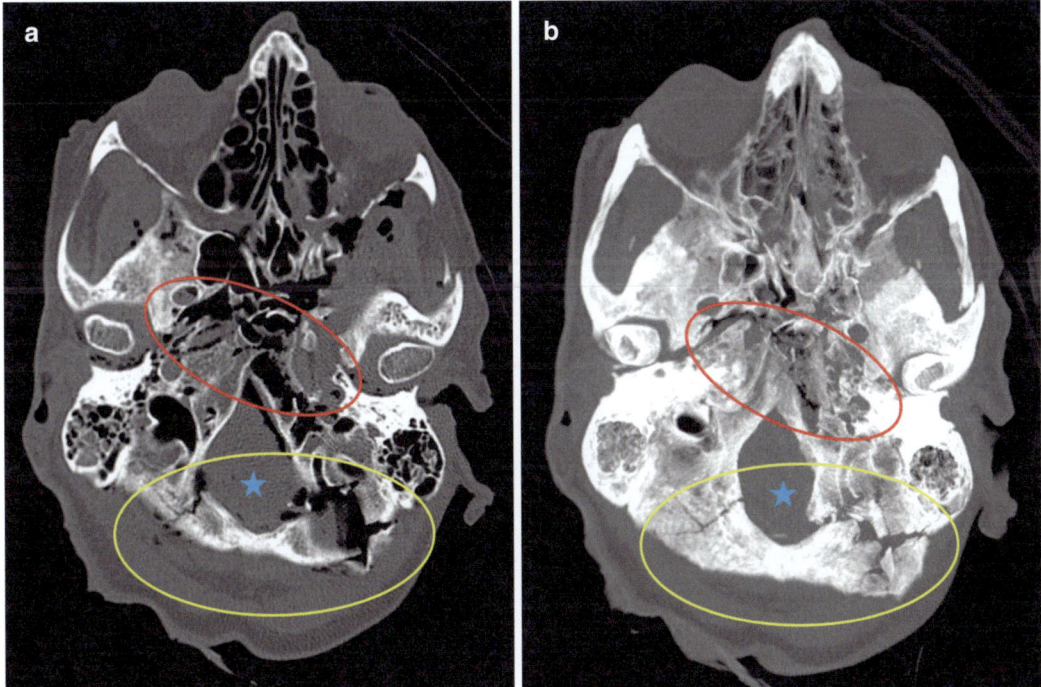

Fig. 6.2 Motorcyclist who lost the control of his vehicle and hit a tree, after being projected from the motorcycle. (**a**) Axial views of a MDCT of the skull in bone window with the visualization of a fracture of the skull base (red circles) and of the occipital bone (yellow circles) passing through the foramen magnum (blue stars). (**b**) Maximum intensity projection (MIP) reconstruction

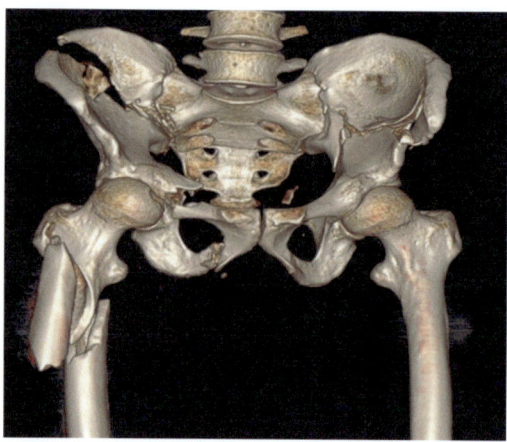

Fig. 6.3 Cyclist hit by a car in a rear-end collision with projection on the ground and impact on the right side of the body. 3D reconstruction of a MDCT of the pelvis in frontal view showing a bilateral complex fracture

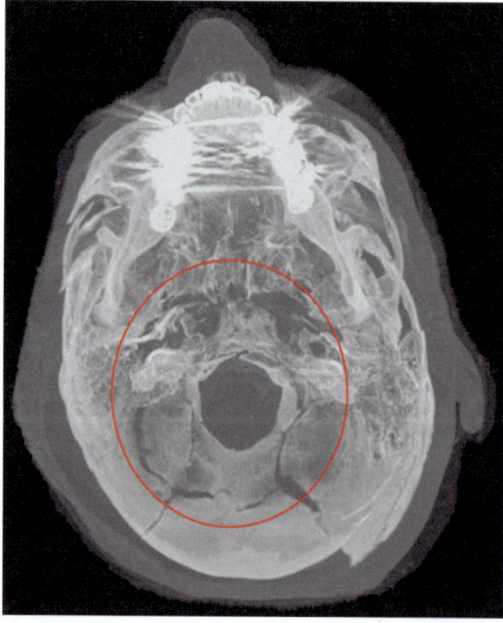

Fig. 6.4 Motorcyclist hit by a bus in a front-to-front collision with impact of the head on the windshield of the bus. 3D MIP (maximum intensity projection) bone reconstruction of a MDCT of the base of the skull in inferior view with the visualization of a skull base ring fracture (red circle)

has the great advantage to be able to localize fractures and anatomical regions which are difficult to access for the forensic pathologist during autopsy (e.g., facial bones, spine, and four extremities). Moreover, it permits to get an overview of all lesions and to represent them in a three-dimensional way, which can be significant for the reconstruction of the accident.

A MDCT-angiography in all those cases allows a visualization of the damages of the inner organs and vessels (Figs. 6.5, 6.6, and 6.7) [12, 13]. MRI can reveal lesions of the spinal cord, which are difficult to impossible to see by MDCT.

However, it has to be noted that cutaneous and soft tissue lesions can be difficult to visualize by MDCT, although lesions of subcutaneous and muscle tissue can be seen through an infiltration of those soft tissues.

Often the direct contact with a certain force, between an object and the skin, leaves an impression of the object structure on the skin. With a detailed surface documentation of the body and the vehicle, morphometric comparisons true to scale between shaped injuries and the structures on the vehicle can be performed, to determine possible contact(s) between the vehicle and the body [20–22]. Even if the lesion doesn't present a specific shape, its localization can be helpful for the reconstruction of the accident. In case of a two-wheel accident, cutaneous lesions which present a specific shape can be found, for example, on the lower part of the body, resulting from an impact with the handlebar structures of the two-wheel in case of a frontal impact (Fig. 6.8). Other typical impressions on the skin can be observed, for example, on the upper part of the body, mainly the head, due to the impact on the other vehicle (Fig. 6.9) [27]. Nevertheless, the skin injuries on the head are limited because two-vehicle driver is usually wearing a helmet.

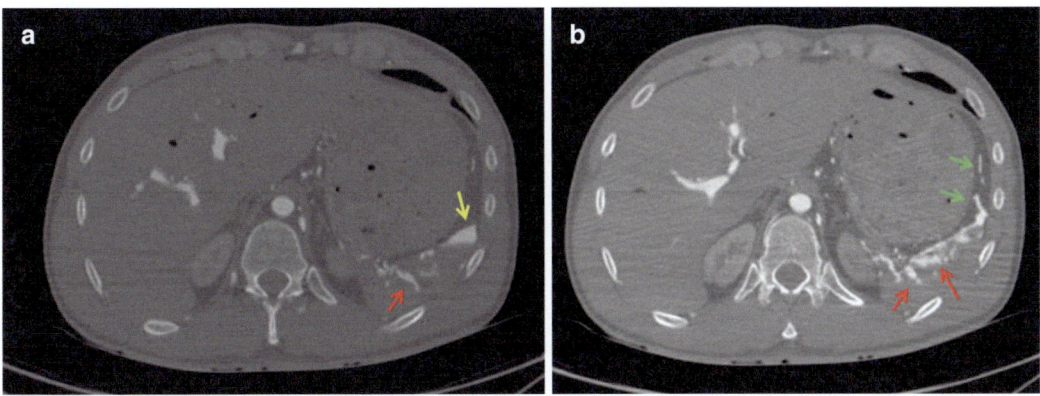

Fig. 6.5 Cyclist hit by a car in a rear-end collision with projection on the ground and impact on the right side of the body. Axial views of a MDCT-angiography of the abdomen in arterial phase showing a damage to the spleen, highlighted by contrast agent leakages: in the parenchyma in (**a, b**) (red arrows), contained in the subcapsular space (yellow arrow) and in the abdominal cavity in (**b**) (green arrows)

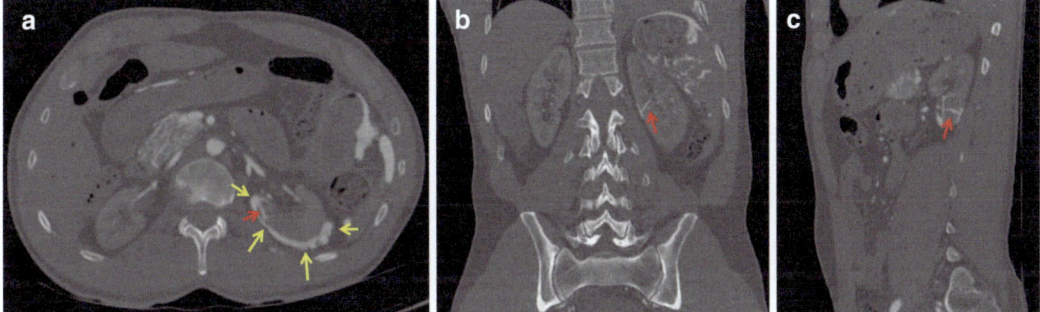

Fig. 6.6 Cyclist hit by a car in a rear-end collision with projection on the ground and impact on the right side of the body. Axial (**a**), coronal (**b**), and sagittal (**c**) views of a MDCT-angiography of the abdomen in arterial phase with visualization of a left kidney damage highlighted by contrast agent leakages: in the parenchyma in (**a–c**) (red arrows) and in the perirenal space (yellow arrows)

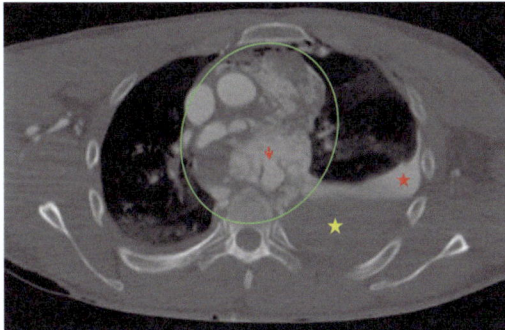

Fig. 6.7 Motorcyclist hit by a car in a rear-end collision. Axial view of a MDCT-angiography of the thorax in dynamic phase showing a transmural rupture of the thoracic aorta (red arrow), with a hemo-mediastinum (green circle) and a left hemothorax (yellow star). This image shows contrast agent leakage in the left pleural cavity (red star), accumulating above the hemothorax (yellow star)

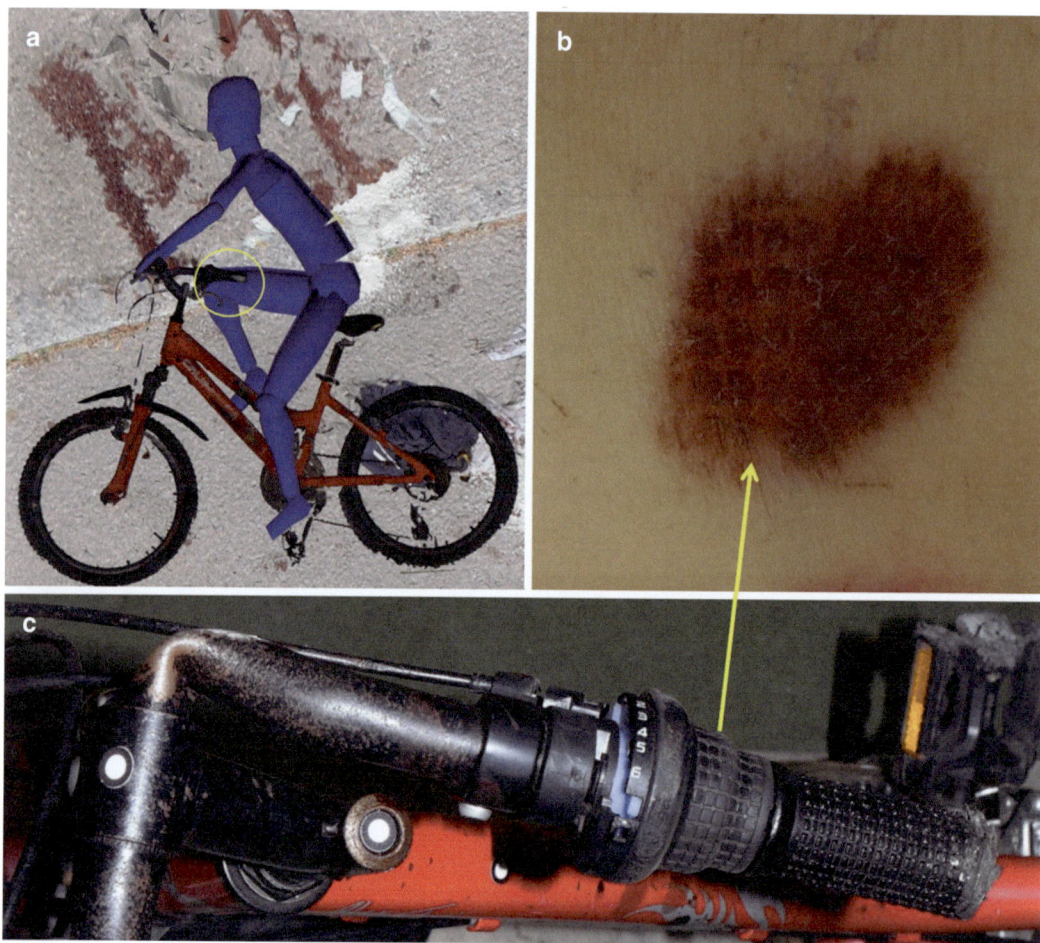

Fig. 6.8 Cyclist hit by a tractor while turning right, with subsequent overrun. Handlebar impression from a bicycle on the right leg of the cyclist. (**a**) Repositioned mannequin representing the victim on the bike with his right leg touching the handlebar (yellow circle). (**b**) Shaped injury on the right leg, close to the knee. (**c**) Handlebar of the bicycle showing the same pattern as the shaped injury found on the skin of the right leg (yellow arrow)

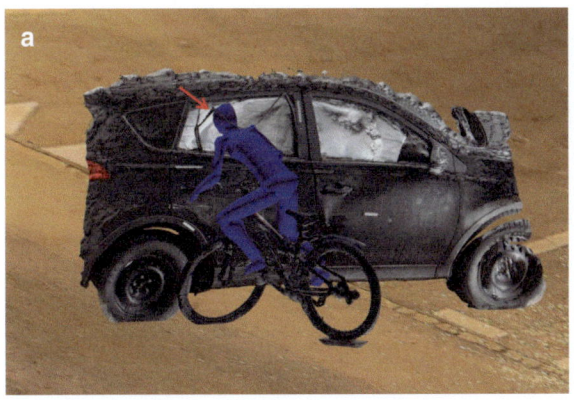 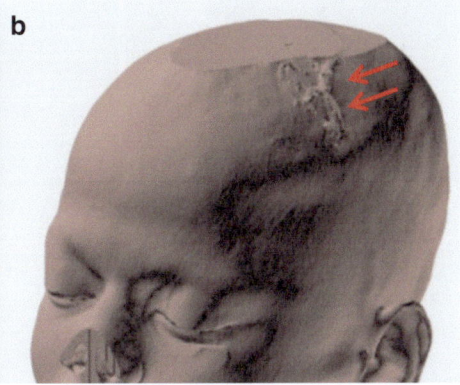

Fig. 6.9 Cyclist who hit a car in a front-to-side collision. Injuries of the upper part of the body due to an impact between the bicycle and the car. (**a**) Impact of the head of the cyclist on a side window/window frame of the car (red arrow). (**b**) 3D model of the head segmented based on CT-scan data showing the corresponding damage to the skin on the left side of the head (red arrows)

6.3 Four-Wheel Accidents

Often, four-wheel traffic accidents concern collisions between four-wheel vehicles (car, bus, truck, etc.) and two-wheel vehicles (bicycle, motorcycle, etc.). It may also include a collision between two four-wheel vehicles, and an impact between a four-wheel vehicle and a pedestrian. The latter will be discussed in detail in Sect. 6.4 "Pedestrian accidents."

However, four-wheel accidents can also involve only one vehicle, for example, if the driver himself is responsible for the accident, under, for example, the effect of alcohol, drugs, or medication or due to a faintness and/or a sudden death.

Those collisions can be front-end, front to side, side to side, or rear-end. They can lead to an overturn or an underrun of the vehicle. The pattern of lesions depends on the direction of the impact and on the size and the speed of the involved vehicles. Moreover, it depends on the structures which are situated in the vehicle (e.g., steering wheel, seat belt, airbag system, pedals, gear stick, etc.) and on the structures which are constitutive of the vehicle (e.g., A, B, C pillars, windshield, windows, dashboard, etc.) [2, 3, 5].

As previously mentioned in "two-wheel accidents," all those fractures can be visualized with MDCT [7–9]. MDCT has the great advantage to be able to localize fractures and anatomical regions which are difficult to access for the forensic pathologist during autopsy (e.g., spine, facial bones, and four extremities) (Figs. 6.10 and 6.11). Moreover, it permits to get an overview of all lesions and to represent them in a three-dimensional way, which can be significant for the reconstruction of the accident (Fig. 6.12).

A MDCT-angiography in all those case allows a visualization of the damages of the inner organs and vessels. MRI can reveal lesions of the spinal cord, which are difficult to impossible to see by MDCT.

6.3.1 Front-End Collision

The lesions depend on the deceleration during the impact and if the driver or the passenger(s) wear a seat belt or not. The more important the deceleration is, the higher the velocity which provokes a force on the person will be and the more important the lesions will be [28, 29]. If the driver or the passenger touches the dashboard, they can

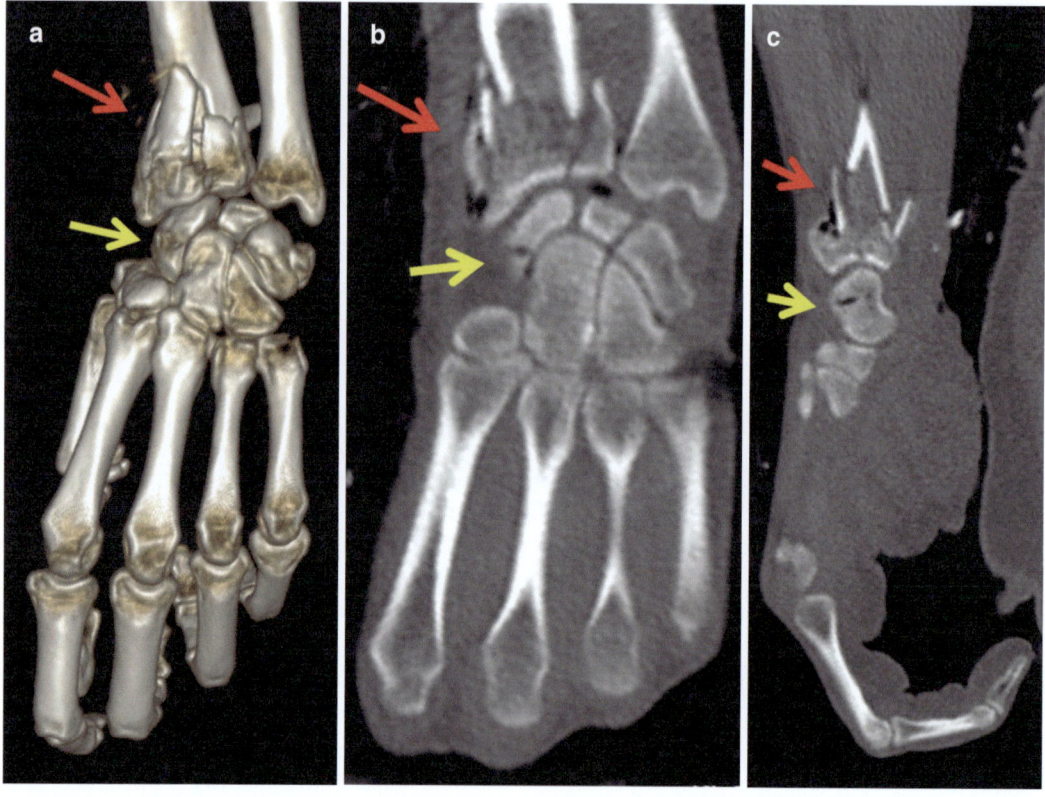

Fig. 6.10 Car driver who hit another car in a rear-end collision. 3D reconstruction (**a**), coronal view in bone window (**b**), and sagittal view in bone window (**c**) of a MDCT of the left hand illustrating a fracture of the distal radius (red arrows) and of the scaphoid bone (yellow arrows)

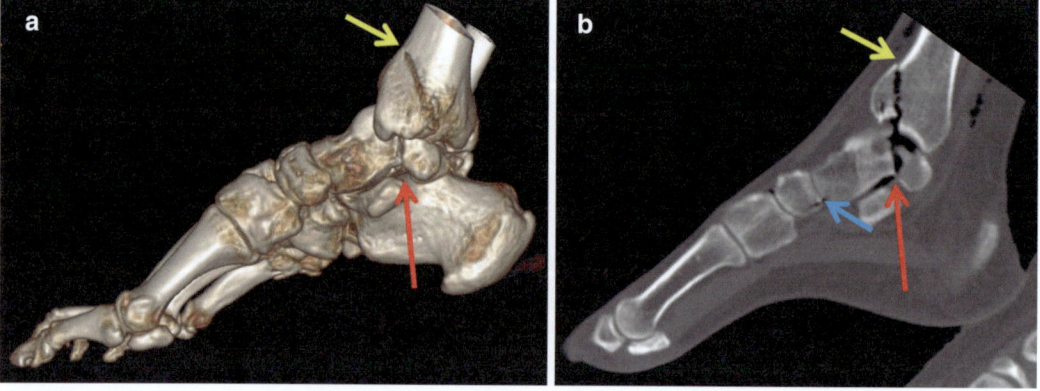

Fig. 6.11 Car driver who was trying to brake as he hit another car in a rear-end collision. 3D reconstruction (**a**) and sagittal view in bone window (**b**) of a MDCT of the right foot showing a fracture of the distal tibia (yellow arrows), a fracture of the talus bone (red arrows), and a fracture of the navicular bone (blue arrow)

present fractures of the knee(s), or the hip joints. If the driver tries to push the footrest or the pedals, fractures of the ankle joints or the feet can appear. In case the driver is holding the wheel or the gear stick, fractures of the hands can be visible. The head of the driver or the passengers can

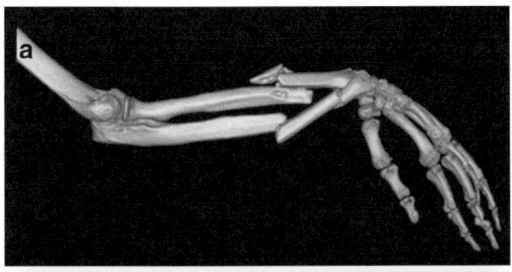

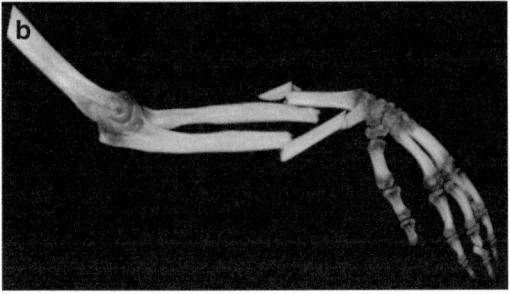

Fig. 6.12 Bus driver who intentionally drove against a wall. 3D reconstruction (**a**) and 3D MIP (maximum intensity projection) (**b**) of a MDCT of the left forearm and hand illustrating a pluri-fragmental fracture of the radius and the ulna

ments can be visible by MDCT on the surface of the body, e.g., the head or in the soft tissues. It has to be mentioned that the ejection of the vehicle during an accident significantly decreases the chance to survive.

6.3.2 Side Collision

In cases of side collisions, the consequence of the impact can be more important as less structures of the vehicle protect the occupants of the vehicle (only side doors and/or windows in the absence of side airbags). Lesions of abdominal organs, such as the liver and spleen, are dominating [2, 3, 5]. Those lesions are ideally visualized by MDCT-angiography. Side collisions may induce contusions of the cervical spine, especially lesions of the ligaments and the spinal cord. The gold standard to highlight such damages is the MRI.

hit the wheel (with possible airbag), the A pillar, the windshield, the dashboard, or the front seats. The different impacts can provoke craniocerebral lesions (cutaneous wounds, fractures, hemorrhage) [2, 3, 5]. Those different lesions are detectable by MDCT.

The seat belts, the airbags, or the wheel can provoke fracture of the ribs as lesions of the thoracic and abdominal organs, which can be suspected by MDCT and confirmed by MDCT-angiography [30, 31]. In addition, ruptures of the vessels, e.g., an aortic rupture, can be found and detected by MDCT-angiography. By MRI it is possible to identify possible myocardial contusions [11]. Moreover the seat belt can induce a typical mark on the skin and the soft tissues of the thorax and abdomen, which can be easily seen during the autopsy, but difficultly by MDCT, although an infiltration of the soft tissues may be visible by MDCT.

If the driver or the passengers don't wear a seat belt, they can be ejected out of the vehicle through the windshield. In this case, glass frag-

6.3.3 Rear-End Collision

In a rear-end collision, the typical observed lesion is the "whiplash" trauma of the cervical spine [2, 3, 5]. Fractures may be observable by MDCT. In case of lesions of the cervical vessels, MDCT-angiography is indicated. If damages of the spinal cord and ligaments are suspected, a MRI should be performed.

6.3.4 Single-Vehicle Accident

Depending on the dynamic and the kinetic of the accident, the panel of lesions can be vast, from minor superficial traumatic lesions (e.g., driver faints or dies suddenly in a parking slot or in general while driving slowly) to important traumatic lesions of the skeleton and the organs like previously mentioned (e.g., driver losing control of the vehicle because of the speed or voluntarily impacting an obstacle in the context of a suicide).

6.3.5 3D Reconstructions of Four-Wheel Accidents

From a medicolegal point of view, 3D documentation of four-wheel occupants can be interesting in cases where it is not clear who drove the vehicle during the accident [32]. Concerning the course of the accident, in case of four-wheel accidents, 3D reconstruction is the responsibility of the police. A lot of structures inside of the vehicle can cause shaped injuries on the skin of the body in cases of impacts between the body and certain structures of the vehicle. In these cases, it is important to document the lesions and the body surface with a 3D scanner, as also the inside of the car for a possible comparison and reconstruction of the accident. Such a reconstruction can permit to find shape lesions which can allow the compatibility of a person as the driver (Figs. 6.13 and 6.14) [32]. The morphometric characteristics of a person can be crucial for such a reconstruction. Indeed, for example, the suspected driver can be sat virtually on the driver seat, to verify if he reaches the pedals and the gear changer with his extremities (cf. Fig. 6.8 in chapter "3D Documentation"). However, those kinds of reconstructions require that during the surface acquisition of the cabin, the seat of the driver is in the same position as during the accident.

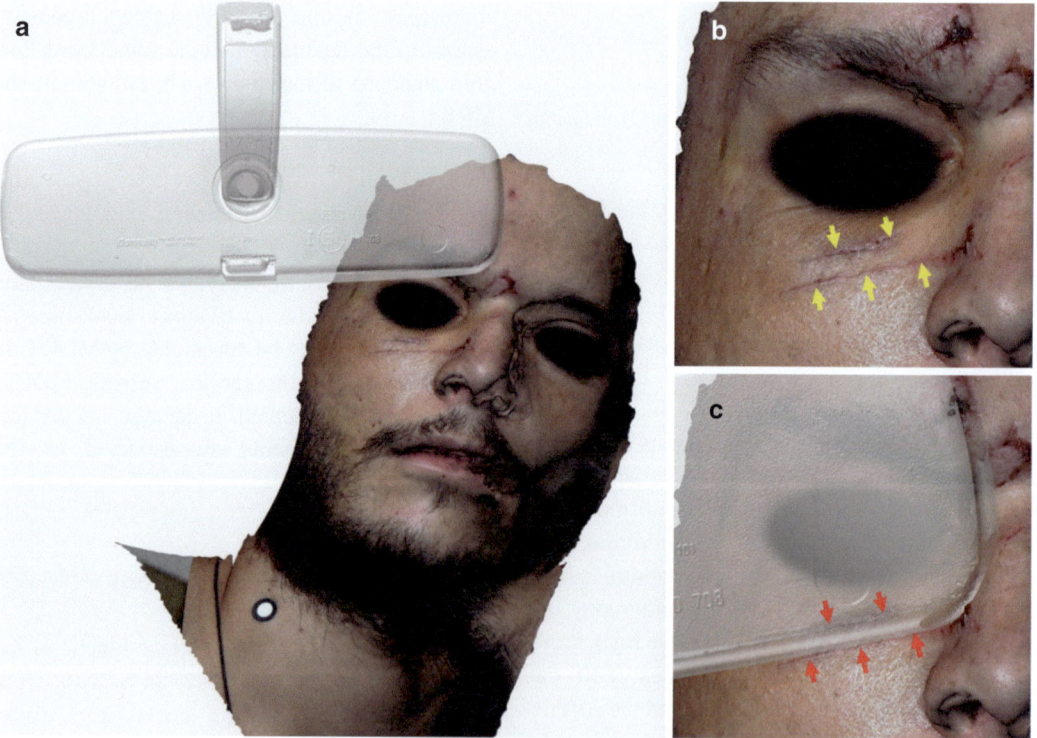

Fig. 6.13 Car accident with several occupants. Reconstruction of the accident with the aim to determine who the driver was. Morphometric comparison of car cabin structures with shaped injuries on the body (**a**). Shaped skin lesions on the face (yellow arrows; **b**) reproducing a part of the car interior rearview mirror edges (red arrows; **c**)

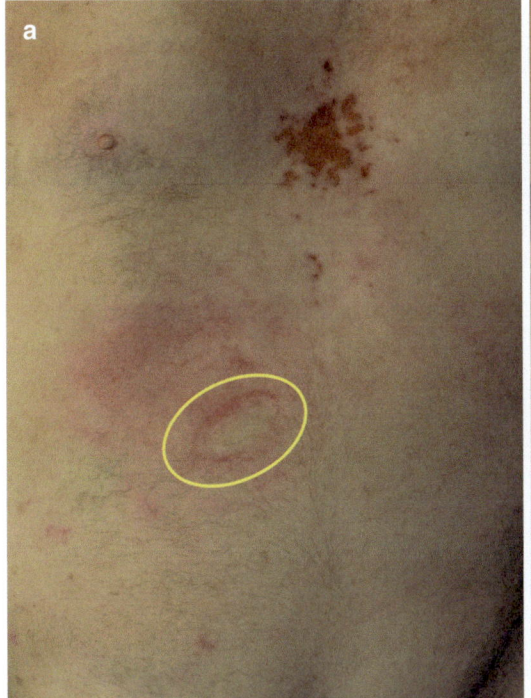 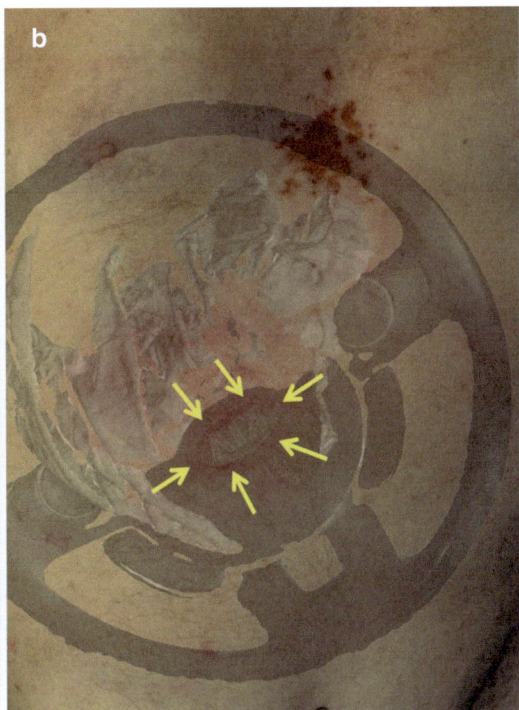

Fig. 6.14 Car accident with two occupants. Reconstruction of the accident with the aim to determine who the driver was. Morphometric comparison of car-cabin structures with shaped injuries on the body. Oval-shaped skin lesion on the anterior part of the abdomen (yellow circle; **a**) corresponding to the car brand logo on the steering wheel (yellow arrows; **b**)

6.4 Pedestrian Accidents

Pedestrians can be involved in collisions with four-wheel vehicles (car, bus, truck, etc.) and two-wheel vehicles (bicycle, motorcycle, etc.).

As in two-wheel accidents, the impact can be frontal, side, or rear-end. In this case, the dynamic of the accident and the pattern of lesions depend on the direction of the impact, the size, and the speed of the involved vehicle, as on the stature of the pedestrian.

In general, the dynamic of the accident can be divided into three major phases: an impact phase (impact between the involved vehicle and the pedestrian), a loading phase (catapulting of the pedestrian on the hood of the car), and a shuffling off phase (projection of the pedestrian on the ground). Depending on the size and the speed of the vehicle, the loading phase may not exist, and the pedestrian is projected directly to the ground [2, 3, 5]. The following lesions can be associated with the different phases:

- As a consequence of the impact phase: the most typical fracture is the so-called Messerer fracture (Fig. 6.15) [33, 34], which can be visible on the lower extremities (femur, tibia, and/or fibula). It consists in a flexion fracture with a triangular bone fragment, which indicates the location and the direction of the impact. However, depending on the size of the vehicle and the pedestrian, fractures of the hip, the vertebral spine, and ribs as lesions of the thoracic and abdominal organs may also result [35–38].

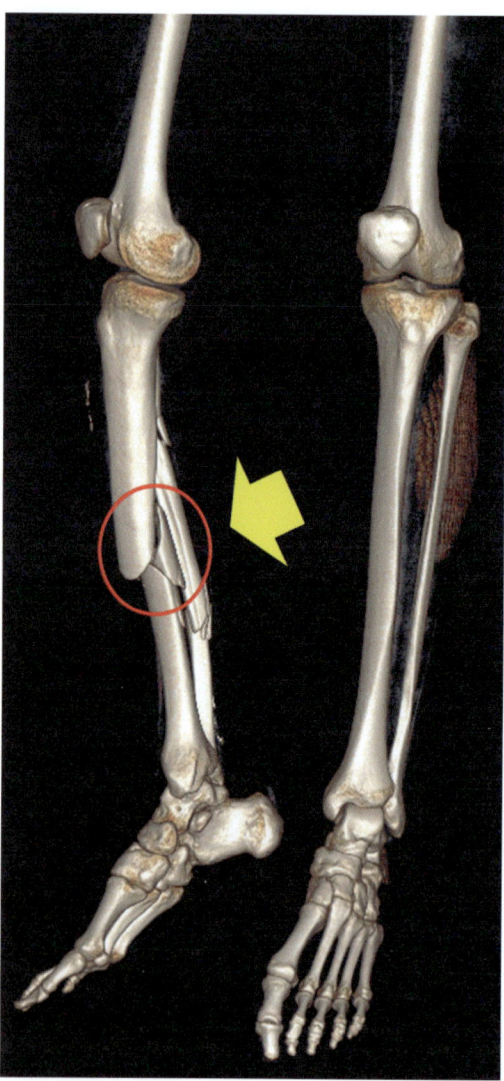

Fig. 6.15 Pedestrian hit by a car while crossing the street, with impact on the posterior side of the right leg. 3D reconstruction of a MDCT of the lower extremities showing complex fractures of the bones of the right leg, with a Messerer fracture of the right tibia (red circle), indicating an impact direction from the back to the front (yellow arrow)

– As a consequence of the loading phase: blunt trauma of the thorax and abdomen is dominating. This phase may result in a craniocerebral trauma (skin, soft tissue, bone, intracranial hemorrhage) (Fig. 6.16), as the head hits the

windshield or the A pillar. Glass fragments can be found on the surface of the skin or in the soft tissues (Fig. 6.17).

– As a consequence of the shuffling off phase: cutaneous and soft tissue lesions are predominant.

Like previously described, the fractures can be visualized with MDCT, including all the advantages of the modality concerning the description of the size and location of the different fracture. Moreover, a MDCT-angiography permits to evaluate the damages of the inner organs and vessels. As mentioned before, MRI can reveal lesions of the spinal cord and the surrounding tissues (Fig. 6.18) [39, 40].

In case of overrun by the vehicle involved in the accident and/or by a vehicle following the involved vehicle, the typical tire tread marks can be seen on the skin, or the clothes, but they are undetectable by all radiological modalities. However, those marks can be associated with widespread avulsions or detachments of the soft tissues, or burst fractures of the skull or fractures of the skeleton [41–43]. MDCT allows the visualization of those damages (Fig. 6.19), though MRI may be able to show the lesions of the soft tissues. After an overrun, the victim can be even dragged by the vehicle on a certain distance and/ or stay stuck under the vehicle. In this case, the victim would mainly present cutaneous and soft tissue lesions.

Typical injuries found on pedestrians, which can be used for a 3D reconstruction, are lesions which can result from an impact between the body and, for example, bumper structures, car headlights, and/or windshield wiper of the vehicle [18, 20–22]. The Messerer fracture can also be very useful for the reconstruction of the respective positions of the pedestrian and the vehicle at the moment of the impact (Fig. 6.20). A powerful element in the case of overrun can be the morphometric comparison between the pattern of the tire and a visible tire tread marks on the skin (Fig. 6.21). This can be of high impor-

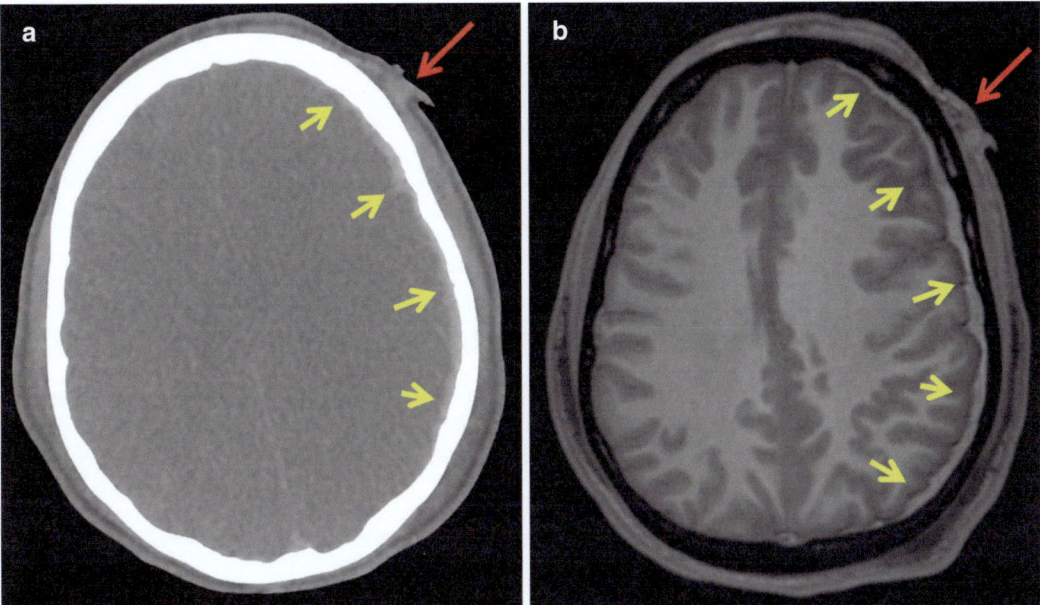

Fig. 6.16 Pedestrian hit by a car with impact on the windshield with the left frontal side of the head. Axial views of a MDCT in soft tissue window (**a**) and of a MRI in T1 TFE MPR (**b**) of the head showing a frontal left skin lesion (red arrows) and a subdural hematoma of the left hemisphere (yellow arrows)

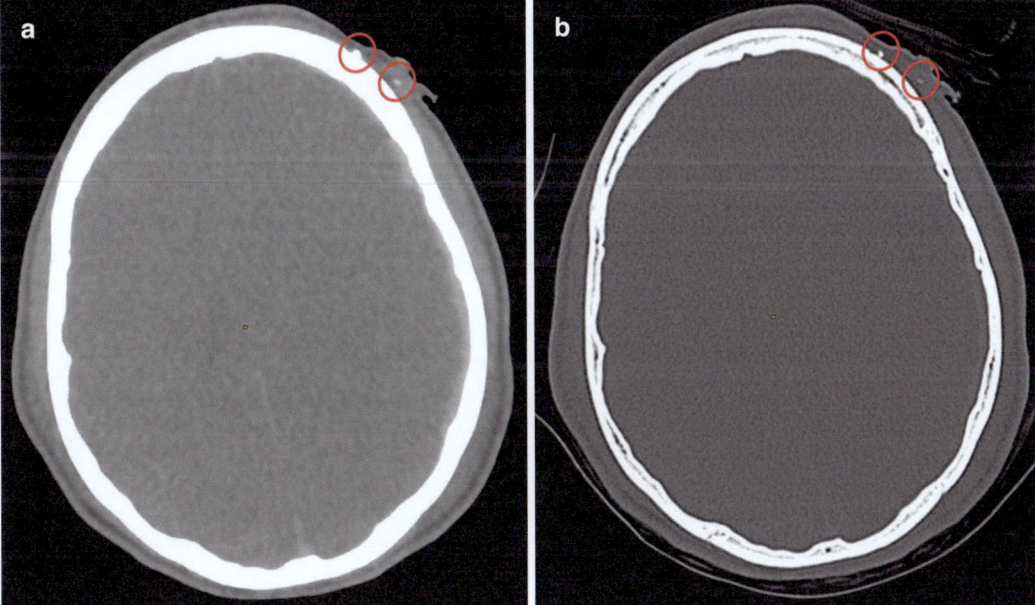

Fig. 6.17 Pedestrian hit by a car with impact on the windshield with the left frontal side of the head. Axial views of a MDCT of the head in soft tissue (**a**) and bone (**b**) window illustrating two foreign bodies in the subcutaneous tissue of the scalp of the left frontal side, underneath a skin lesion, compatible with glass fragments (red circles)

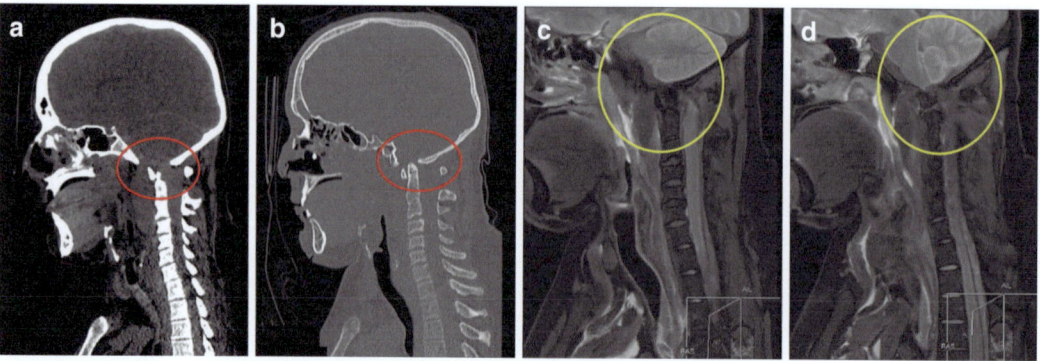

Fig. 6.18 Pedestrian hit by a car with impact on the windshield with the left frontal side of the head. Sagittal views of a MDCT of the head and neck in soft tissue (**a**) and bone (**b**) window, and of a MRI in T2 Dixon W (**c**, **d**) of the base of the skull and neck with visualization of a displacement of the vertebral spine in (**a**, **b**) (red circles), and a complete section of the upper spinal cord in (**c**, **d**) (yellow circles)

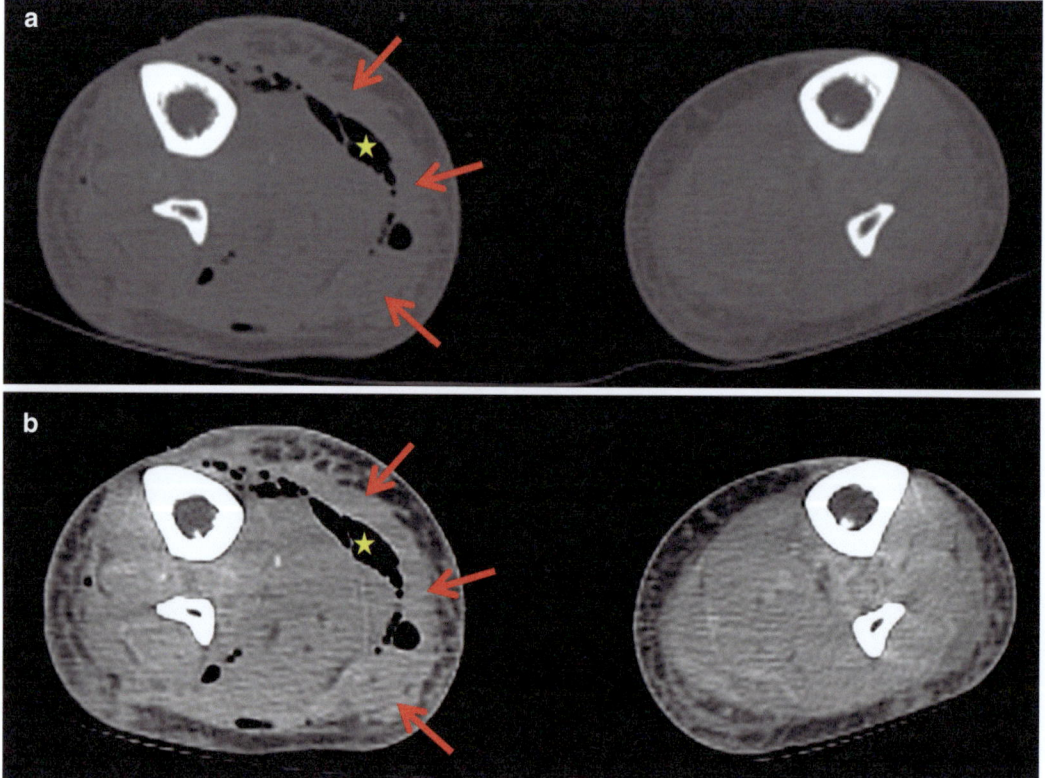

Fig. 6.19 Pedestrian overran by a car at the level of the proximal part of the right leg. Axial views of a MDCT of the lower legs in bone (**a**) and soft tissue (**b**) window illus-trating gas collections (yellow stars) and diffuse infiltra-tion (red arrows) of the soft tissue compatible with a detachment of the soft tissues in case of an overrun

tance for the reconstruction of the accident, if more than one vehicle overran the victim. In the case of a match, it can determine the direction in which the vehicle ran over the body and if several vehicles were implicated, which vehicle ran over the body. Sometimes, it can happen that the pedestrian leave a mark on the vehicle, like make-up residues (Fig. 6.22).

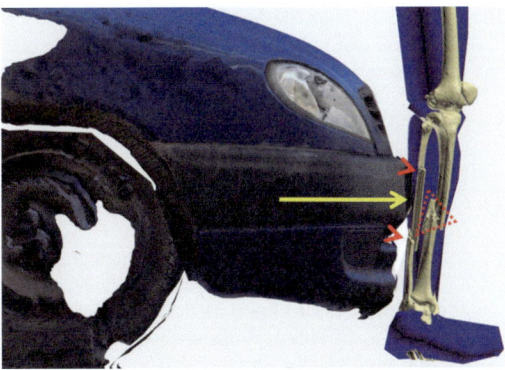

Fig. 6.20 Pedestrian hit by a car in the middle of the night. Reconstruction of the accident. Prominent structures of a car causing a double fracture of the fibula (red arrows' heads) and a Messerer fracture of the tibia (dotted red triangle). The typical triangular-shaped bone fragment of the Messerer fracture shows the direction of the force at the site of the impact (yellow arrow)

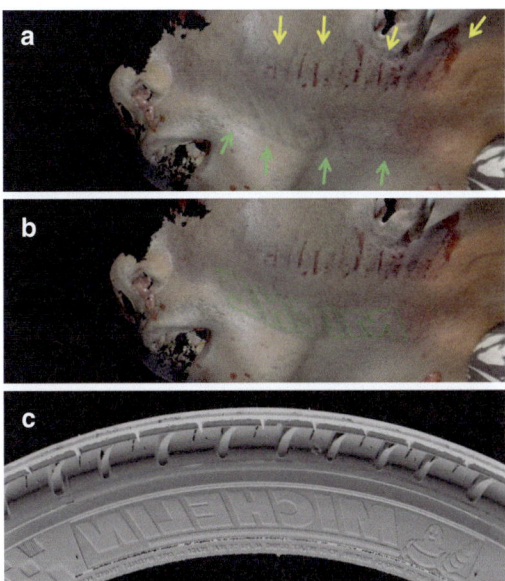

Fig. 6.21 Pedestrian overran by several cars with identification of the vehicle, which overran the head. Textured 3D model of the head and neck showing regular shaped skin lesions (yellow arrows) and dirt impression (green arrows; **a**). Same 3D model with green drawn boundaries to highlight the impressed letters on the skin (**b**). (**c**) 3D model of the tire of the car showing an inscription which letters' size and font correspond to the shaped dirt impression on the skin

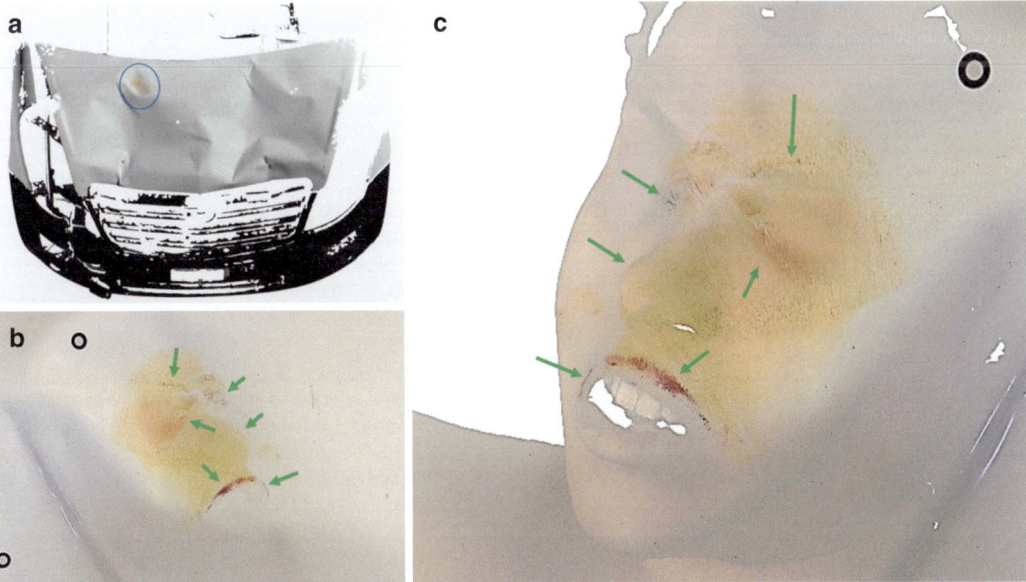

Fig. 6.22 Two pedestrians hit by a transporter on a crosswalk. Reconstruction of the position of the pedestrians during the impact. Face make-up impression on a car hood. (**a**) 3D model of the upper front part of the car with localization of the make-up impression (blue circle) on the hood. (**b**) Enlargement of the make-up trace on the car hood enabling a detailed view of the make-up trace. (**c**) Superposition of the 3D models of the victim's face and of the make-up trace on the car hood. Green arrows (**b, c**) show matches between the make-up trace on the car hood and the different parts of the face

6.5   Conclusion

In summary, the following recommendations can be made for forensic practice:

1. The most suitable imaging modalities for traffic accidents are MDCT combined with angiography and a documentation by 3D-surface scanning.
2. 3D reconstructions permit a detailed analysis and illustration of the injury extent and the reconstruction of a traffic accident victim(s) and implicated vehicle(s).
3. Priority should be given to interdisciplinary work between radiologist, forensic pathologist, the 3D-surface scanner specialist, engineers, and the police because of the complexity of the subject.

References

1. Spitz W. Road traffic victim. In: Spitz WU, Spitz DJ, editors. Spitz and Fisher's medicolegal investigation of death: guidelines for the application of pathology to crime investigation. 4th ed. Springfield, IL: Charles CT; 2006. p. 903–65.
2. Mattern R. Verkehrsunfall. In: Brinkmann B, Madea B, editors. Handbuch gerichtliche Medizin. Springer; 2004. p. 1171–214.
3. Wehner HD, Kernbach-Wighten G. Traffic accidents. In: Madea B, editor. Handbook of forensic medicine. Wiley Blackwell; 2014. p. 1108–39.
4. Saukko P, Knight B. Transportation injuries. In: Knight's forensic pathology. 3rd ed. London: Arnold Publishers; 2004. p. 281–300.
5. Wehner HD. Der Verkehrsunfall. In: Madea B, editor. Praxis Rechtsmedizin. 2nd ed. Springer; 2007. p. 478–94.
6. Karger B, Teige K, Bühren W, DuChesne A. Relationship between impact velocity and injuries in fatal pedestrian-car collisions. Int J Legal Med. 2000;113(2):84–8.
7. Grabherr S, Egger C, Vilarino R, Campana L, Jotterand M, Dedouit F. Modern post-mortem imaging: an update on recent developments. Forensic Sci Res. 2017;2(2):52–64.
8. Jeffery AJ. The role of computed tomography in adult post-mortem examinations: an overview. Diagn Histopathol. 2010;16:546–51.
9. Poulsen K, Simonsen J. Computed tomography as routine in connection with medico-legal autopsies. Forensic Sci Int. 2007;171(2–3):190–7.
10. Dirnhofer R, Thali MJ, Vock P. The virtopsy approach: 3D optical and radiological scanning and reconstruction in forensic medicine. London NW: CRC Press; 2009.
11. Ruder TD, Thali MJ, Hatch GM. Essentials of forensic post-mortem MR imaging in adults. Br J Radiol. 2014;87(1036):20130567.
12. Chevallier C, Doenz F, Vaucher P, Palmiere C, Dominguez A, Binaghi S, Mangin P, Grabherr S. Postmortem computed tomography angiography vs. conventional autopsy: advantages and inconveniences of each method. Int J Legal Med. 2013;127(5):981–9.
13. Grabherr S, Grimm J, Heinemann A. Atlas of postmortem angiography. Springer; 2016.
14. Grabherr S, Cadas H, Riederer BM, Charlier P, Djonov V. Postmortem angiography: a historical review. In: Grabherr S, Grimm J, Heinemann A, editors. Atlas of post-mortem angiography. Springer; 2016. p. 53–70.
15. Vital reactions. In: Dettmeyer RB, Verhoff MA, Schütz HF, editors. Forensic medicine, 1st ed. Berlin: Springer; 2014. p. 97–109.
16. Grabherr S, Lesta Mdel M, Rizzo E, Mangin P, Bollmann M. L'magerie forensique [Forensic imaging]. Rev Med Suisse. 2008;4(164):1609–14. French.
17. Varlet V, Smith F, Giuliani N, Egger C, Rinaldi A, Dominguez A, Chevallier C, Bruguier C, Augsburger M, Mangin P, Grabherr S. When gas analysis assists with postmortem imaging to diagnose causes of death. Forensic Sci Int. 2015;251:1–10.
18. Buck U, Buße K, Campana L, Gummel F, Schyma C, Jackowski C. What happened before the run over? Morphometric 3D reconstruction. Forensic Sci Int. 2020;306:110059. https://doi.org/10.1016/j.forsciint.2019.110059.
19. Buck U, Naether S, Räss B, Jackowski C, Thali MJ. Accident or homicide—virtual crime scene reconstruction using 3D methods. Forensic Sci Int. 2013;225(1–3):75–84.
20. Buck U, Naether S, Braun M, Bolliger S, Friederich H, Jackowski C, Aghayev E, Christe A, Vock P, Dirnhofer R, Thali MJ. Application of 3D documentation and geometric reconstruction methods in traffic accident analysis: with high resolution surface scanning, radiological MSCT/MRI scanning and real data based animation. Forensic Sci Int. 2007;170(1):20–8.
21. Thali MJ, Braun M, Buck U, Aghayev E, Jackowski C, Vock P, Sonnenschein M, Dirnhofer R. VIRTOPSY—scientific documentation, reconstruction and animation in forensic: individual and real 3D data based geo-metric approach including optical body/object surface and radiological CT/MRI scanning. J Forensic Sci. 2005;50(2):1–15.
22. Bolliger MJ, Buck U, Thali MJ, Bolliger SA. Reconstruction and 3D visualisation based on objective real 3D based documentation. Forensic Sci Med Pathol. 2012;8(3):208–17.
23. Maeda H, Higuchi T, Imura M, Noguchi K, Yokota M. Ring fracture of the base of the skull and atlanto-

occipital avulsion due to anteroflexion on motorcycle riders in a head-on collision accident. Med Sci Law. 1993;33(3):266–9.

24. Hitosugi M, Fukui K, Takatsu A. Incomplete decapitation of a motorcyclist from hyperextension by inertia: a case report. Med Sci Law. 2001;41(2):174–7.

25. Kraus JF, Rice TM, Peek-Asa C, McArthur DL. Facial trauma and the risk of intracranial injury in motorcycle riders. Ann Emerg Med. 2003;41(1):18–26.

26. Robertson A, Branfoot T, Barlow IF, Giannoudis PV. Spinal injury patterns resulting from car and motorcycle accidents. Spine. 2002;27(24):2825–30.

27. Madro R, Teresiński G. Neck injuries as a reconstructive parameter in car-to-pedestrian accidents. Forensic Sci Int. 2001;118(1):57–63.

28. Miltner E, Wiedmann HP, Leutwein B, Hepp HP, Fischer R, Salwender HJ, Frobenius H, Kallieris D. Technical parameters influencing the severity of injury of front-seat, belt-protected car passengers on the impact side in car-to-car side collisions with the main impact between the front and rear seats (B-pillars). Int J Legal Med. 1992;105(1):11–5.

29. Miltner E, Salwender HJ. Influencing factors on the injury severity of restrained front seat occupants in car-to-car head-on collisions. Accid Anal Prev. 1995;27(2):143–50.

30. Maxeiner H, Hahn M. Airbag-induced lethal cervical trauma. J Trauma. 1997;42(6):1148–51.

31. Klask J. Verletzungen im Hals-Nasen-Ohren-Bereich durch Auto-Airbags. Laryngorhinootologie. 2001;80(3):146–51.

32. Buck U, Zuber S. Wer lenkte den PW? In: Schaffhauser R, editor. Jahrbuch zum Strassenverkehrsrecht. Stämpfli Verlag; 2015. p. 227–48.

33. Geserick G, Krocker K, Wirth I. Über den Messerer-Bruch—eine Literaturstudie [A literature review on the Messerer's fracture]. Arch Kriminol. 2015;235(5–6):145–65. German.

34. Messerer O. Über Elastizität und Festigkeit menschlicher Knochen. Stuttgart: Cotta; 1880.

35. Teresiński G, Madro R. Pelvis and hip joint injuries as a reconstructive factors in car-to-pedestrian accidents. Forensic Sci Int. 2001;124(1):68–73.

36. Teresiński G, Madro R. Ankle joint injuries as a reconstruction parameter in car-to-pedestrian accidents. Forensic Sci Int. 2001;118(1):65–73.

37. Ishikawa H, Kajzer J, Ono K, Sakurai M. Simulation of car impact to pedestrian lower extremity: influence of different car-front shapes and dummy parameters on test results. Accid Anal Prev. 1994;26(2):231–42.

38. Teresiński G, Madro R. Evidential value of injuries useful for reconstruction of the pedestrian-vehicle location at the moment of collision. Forensic Sci Int. 2002;128(3):127–35.

39. Freund P, Seif M, Weiskopf N, Friston K, Fehlings MG, Thompson AJ, Curt A. MRI in traumatic spinal cord injury: from clinical assessment to neuroimaging biomarkers. Lancet Neurol. 2019;18(12):1123–35.

40. Eli I, Lerner DP, Ghogawala Z. Acute traumatic spinal cord injury. Neurol Clin. 2021;39(2):471–88.

41. Metter D. Das Decollement als Anfahrverletzung. Z Rechtsmed. 1980;85(3):211–9. German.

42. Karger B, Teige K, Fuchs M, Brinkmann B. Was the pedestrian hit in an erect position before being run over? Forensic Sci Int. 2001;119(2):217–20.

43. Maxeiner H, Ehrlich E, Schyma C. Neck injuries caused by being run over by a motor vehicle. J Forensic Sci. 2000;45(1):31–5.

7 Asphyxia

France Evain, Pia Genet, and Christelle Lardi

7.1 Introduction

Asphyxia is defined in the forensic field as a lack of oxygen supply to the brain that can lead to cerebral hypoxic and ischemic lesions as to death [1].

The origin of low brain oxygenation can be multiple, from atmospheric conditions (so-called atmospheric asphyxiation, when oxygen is lacking and/or replaced in ambient air, for example, in high altitude), restriction of the oxygen supply (in cases of strangulation and hanging with compression of the arteries supplying the brain and/or the jugular veins, thoracic compression, and obstruction of the airways), and drowning, to failure in oxygen transportation and cellular impairment of oxygen utilization (e.g., in cases of carbon monoxide and cyanide intoxications) [2]. There are several existing classifications of forms of asphyxia, and the most common one classifies them according to their origin [3].

Asphyxia is a common and important subject in the daily forensic practice. Nowadays, forensic imaging (especially multidetector computed tomography (MDCT) and magnetic resonance imaging (MRI)) is a helpful tool to explore and manage cases of asphyxia, in addition to a complete forensic autopsy or a clinical forensic investigation (in survived victims).

MDCT is the technique of choice to evaluate the bone structure and to detect skeletal fracture. It also permits a three-dimensional reconstruction of the skeleton and soft tissues, providing an iconography, which can be used in Court (especially for an audience that has no knowledge of anatomy). In contrast to MDCT, MRI is a non-irradiant modality that can be used for medicolegal investigation of living victims, without any clinical indication. This imaging technique is the gold standard for the evaluation of soft tissues and the detection of cerebral hypoxic and ischemic lesions related to asphyxia.

In this chapter, we will focus on the advantages and limitations of MDCT and MRI in frequently encountered forms of asphyxia, e.g., cases of strangulation, hanging, drowning, obstruction of the airways, and thoracic compression. Atmospheric asphyxia will not be discussed since it leaves no detectable nor specific signs at imaging and autopsy.

F. Evain (✉) · C. Lardi
Unit of Forensic Medicine, University Center of Legal Medicine Lausanne-Geneva, University and University Hospital of Geneva, Geneva, Switzerland
e-mail: France.Evain@hug.ch; christelle.lardi@hug.ch

P. Genet
Unit of Forensic Imaging and Anthropology, University Center of Legal Medicine Lausanne-Geneva, University of Lausanne, University Hospital of Vaud, Lausanne, Switzerland
e-mail: Pia.Genet@chuv.ch

© The Author(s), under exclusive license to Springer Nature Switzerland AG 2024
S. Grabherr et al. (eds.), *Forensic Imaging of Trauma*, https://doi.org/10.1007/978-3-031-48381-3_7

7.2 Strangulation and Hanging

Strangulation and hanging are forms of asphyxia characterized by the compression of the blood vessels and/or airways of the neck as a result of an external cervical pressure.

7.2.1 Evaluation of Survived Victims

The forensic physician often faces victims of strangulation who survived the alleged assault. Here, the central question will be whether the victim's life was endangered according to the severity and duration of the strangulation. To this end, the medical history will focus on local symptoms (neck pain, voice changes, difficulty to swallow and/or breath) as well as signs of cerebral hypoxia and/or ischemia such as loss of consciousness, sphincter relaxation (urine and feces loss), and visual/auditory impairment [4]. However, these are subjective elements. For this reason, the research of objective indicators of a neck compression by means of a clinical examination is mandatory. Typical clinical signs include local cutaneous blunt trauma (bruises, abrasions, hematomas, strangulation marks) on the neck as well as petechiae of the facial skin, behind the ears, the conjunctiva, and the oral mucosa [4–8].

Obviously, the clinical examination doesn't allow the evaluation of subcutaneous soft tissues (fatty and muscle tissues) that may be crucial for the evaluation of the victim, particularly if skin lesions are minimal or absent. To address this issue, as additional injury assessment, MDCT and MRI can be used to detect hemorrhagic infiltration and edema of deep soft tissues (subcutaneous fatty and muscular tissues, vocal cords, lymph nodes, salivary glands) of the neck and submandibular regions [4, 6, 9–14]. As explained above, in the context of a purely forensic investigation, MRI should be the technique of choice for its non-irradiating property. If possible, a laryngoscopy (provided by a specialized physician) can also be considered to assess laryngeal structures, especially the vocal cords. MDCT can be used during the medical care to detect laryngeal and hyoid bone fracture (Figs. 7.1 and 7.2) [4].

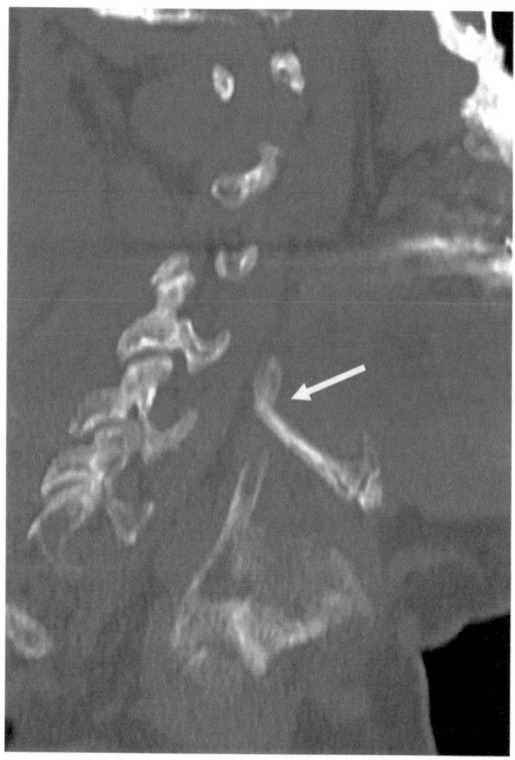

Fig. 7.1 MDCT in MIP (maximum intensity projection) with sagittal view of the skeleton of the neck in a victim of survived strangulation. Fracture of the right great horn of the hyoid bone (white arrow)

Angio-MDCT can also detect cerebrovascular injuries, especially carotid artery dissection (eventually complicated by thrombosis and embolism), in survived prolonged strangulation or hanging cases. Such traumatic carotid artery dissection is secondary to a local mechanical compression and traction of the vessel against cervical bone structures, with damage of the vascular intima and/or media [15–17]. Vascular lesions secondary to strangulation and hanging are, however, extremely rare [8, 17–25].

A prolonged strangulation or hanging can lead to brain hypoxic and ischemic injuries [26–29]. The cerebral MRI is the modality of choice to assess such damages. In these cases, pathological changes are mostly symmetrical and affect the most sensitive regions of the brain such as the hippocampus and the central nuclei (Fig. 7.3). Note that only few changes related to ischemic or hypoxic lesions are detected on cerebral MRI

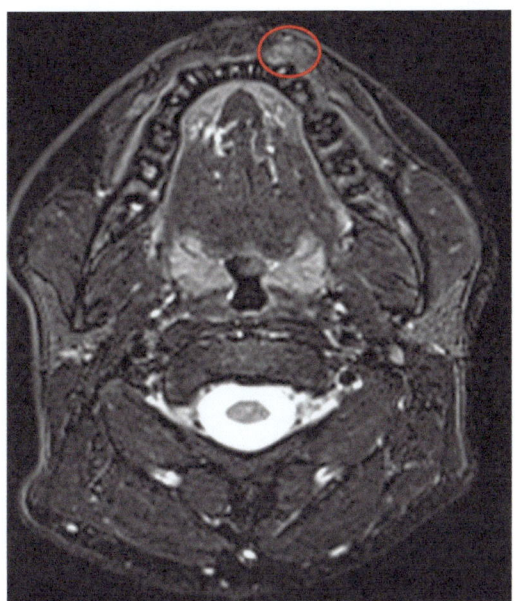

Fig. 7.2 MRI of the neck of a victim of survived strangulation. Acquisition in 2D T2 DIXON with axial view of the neck with visualization of a subcutaneous infiltration of submandibular region (red ellipse)

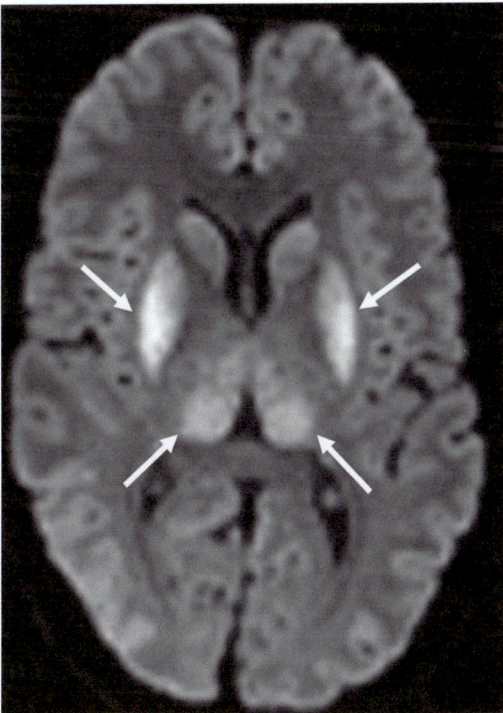

Fig. 7.3 Cerebral diffusion-weighted MRI, 5 days after a survived hanging. Ischemic brain injury with an enhanced signal in central nuclei (white arrows)

before 24 h of survival [30]. The systematic use of cerebral MRI for every victim of strangulation is not indicated, especially without neurological symptoms [8].

7.2.2 Postmortem Evaluation

Typical findings during postmortem external examination in cases of strangulation and hanging include, as for living victims, local cutaneous blunt trauma (bruises, abrasions, hematomas, strangulation, or hanging marks) as well as petechiae of the facial skin, behind the ears, the conjunctiva, and the oral mucosa (congestion). Classical autopsy findings include hemorrhagic infiltration of the neck soft tissues (fatty tissue, muscle, pharyngeal and laryngeal mucosa, lymph nodes, salivary glands), fracture of the laryngeal skeleton (thyroid and cricoid cartilages) and the hyoid bone, as well as subpleural petechial hemorrhages (known as Tardieu spots). Moreover, in cases of hanging, hemorrhagic infiltration of the periosteum of the clavicles, vascular lesions (carotid arteries and jugular veins), as well as anterior intervertebral hemorrhagic infiltrations of the disc or the ligament of the spine (known as Simon's bleedings) can be found [2, 31–35]. Cervical vertebral fracture (Hangman's fracture) is uncommon in nonjudicial hanging [36–42].

Although a conventional autopsy enables detecting most of the classical findings in cases of strangulation and hanging, the use of MDCT and MRI is indicated to assess injury of the soft tissue of the neck and the hyoid bone as the laryngeal skeleton. Imaging is performed before the autopsy. This allows the forensic physicians to raise their suspicion of neck trauma and complete the lesional pattern, especially in cases with minimal or absent external neck lesion [43]. It also permits the collection of images (that could be stored, eventually reviewed, and used in Court) and the prevention of misinterpretation due to artifactual damages during autopsy [33, 43, 44].

MRI is the technique of choice for the evaluation of the soft tissues of the neck (hemorrhage and edema of the fatty tissue, the muscle, lymph nodes, and salivary glands), the ligamentous structures of the cervical spine, and the cervical vessels (depending on their size) [7, 45]. It can also detect edema located around fractures, as well as bone edema which can indirectly indicate a fracture. However, a bone edema often needs a certain survival time to be visible by MRI.

MDCT is the technique of choice for the evaluation of bone structures of the cervical region (hyoid bone, cervical vertebras) (Fig. 7.4) [7, 43]. The laryngeal cartilage can also be evaluated, especially if calcified (Fig. 7.5). Furthermore, MDCT's three-dimensional reconstruction of laryngeal structure and/or cutaneous ligature mark can be useful in Court, as stated above (Figs. 7.6 and 7.7).

Although forensic imaging carries many advantages, MRI and MDCT can miss small fractures and cartilaginous lesions. Hence, radiologists and forensic pathologists should confront and discuss their results to improve the interpretation of their findings.

Finally, not all typical signs of strangulation and hanging (such as petechiae, blunt skin lesion, Tardieu spots, hemorrhagic infiltration of the periosteum of the clavicles, and hemorrhage of the vertebral disc and ligament) can be visualized by MRI and MDCT. Therefore, a complete

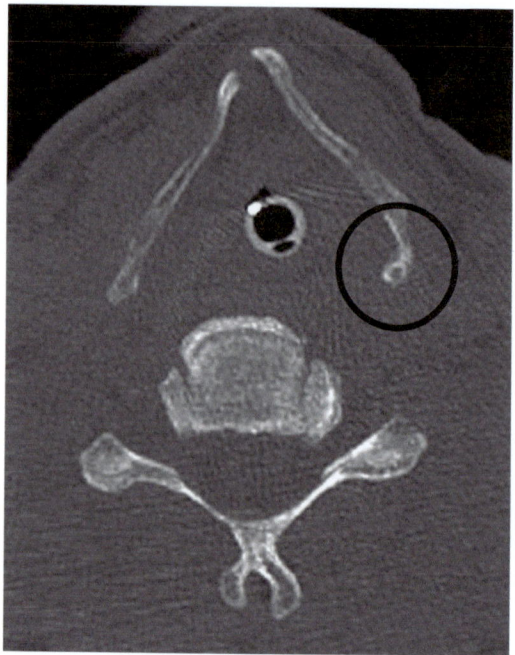

Fig. 7.5 Postmortem MDCT (bone window) with axial view of the skeleton of the neck in a case of hanging. Fracture of the left superior horn of the thyroid cartilage (black circle)

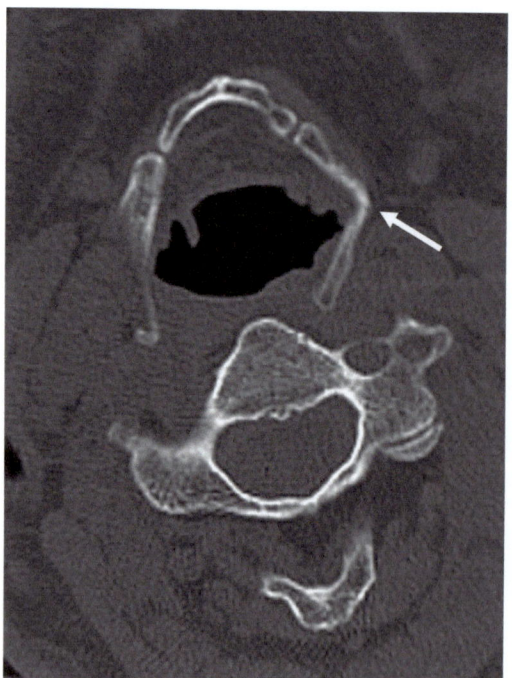

Fig. 7.4 Postmortem MDCT (bone window) with axial view of the skeleton of the neck in a case of hanging. Fracture of the left great horn of the hyoid bone (white arrow)

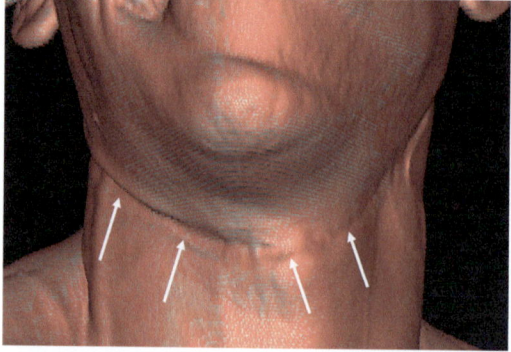

Fig. 7.6 Three-dimensional reconstruction of a postmortem MDCT illustrating the anterior side of the neck with a ligature mark in an autopsy case of hanging (white arrows)

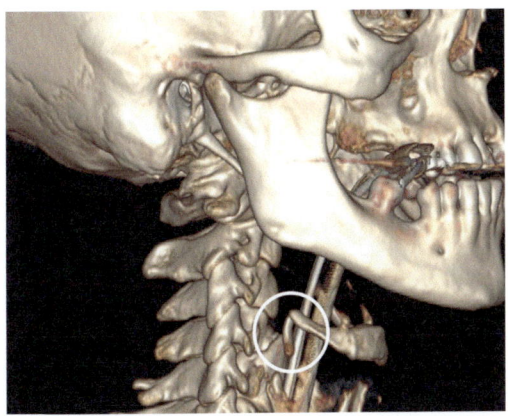

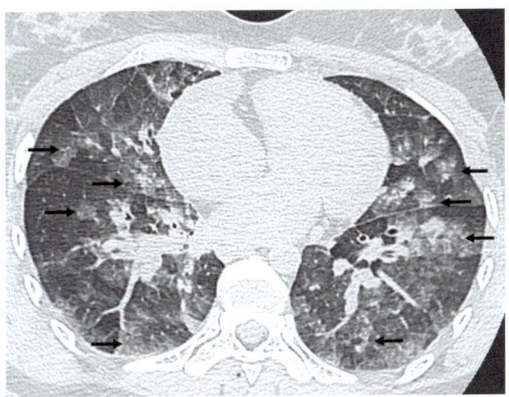

Fig. 7.7 Three-dimensional reconstruction of a postmortem MDCT illustrating the right side of the neck with a fracture of the right great horn of the hyoid bone in an autopsy case of hanging (white circle)

Fig. 7.8 Postmortem MDCT (lung window) with axial view of the lung parenchyma in a case of drowning illustrating diffuse ground-glass opacities (black arrows)

autopsy including a detailed laryngeal examination by an experienced forensic pathologist is still considered as the gold standard.

7.3 Drowning

7.3.1 Evaluation of Survived Victims

In case of survived drowning (near drowning), medical management focuses on the evaluation and treatment of hemodynamic, respiratory, and neurological functions, as well as hypothermia and trauma associated with drowning. Potential origin of near drowning such as natural illness (e.g., acute cardiac event), convulsive crisis, trauma, and intoxication should also be investigated [46, 47].

MDCT and angio-MDCT are the techniques of choice when bone fractures and internal lesions are suspected. It is also indicated in near drowning to evaluate lung injuries after inhalation of liquid (drowning medium) and/or gastric content, both potentially complicated by pneumonia [46–49].

Prognosis of near-drowning victims is mainly based on the extent of hypoxic or ischemic brain damage. If such lesions are suspected, a cerebral MRI should be additionally performed.

7.3.2 Postmortem Evaluation

In the forensic practice, drowning is a diagnosis of exclusion. Therefore, the forensic physician must look for signs supporting the hypothesis of drowning and exclude an alternative cause of death [50]. Classical postmortem findings supporting the diagnosis include froth in the airways (sometimes coming out of the mouth and nostrils), lung overdistension with pulmonary emphysema aquosum (in freshwater drowning) or edema (in saltwater drowning), and subpleural hemorrhages (known as Paltauf spots) [51]. Less specifically, a three-layered gastric content (Wydler's sign), liquid in paranasal sinuses, and hemorrhagic infiltration of the mastoid cells and of the muscles of the neck, the trunk (especially around the scapula), and the upper extremities are described [52, 53].

MDCT can demonstrate frothy liquid in the airways, lung overdistension, and patchy ground glass opacities of the lungs in the context of drowning (Fig. 7.8) [54–59]. However, one must keep in mind that these radiological observations are not specific for drowning as they can also be found in other conditions (e.g., chronic pulmonary emphysema, heart failure, and pneumonia). Liquid level in the paranasal sinuses and in the stomach, muscle hemorrhages (if extended enough), as well as foreign material in the airways (such as sand, among others) can also be detected at MDCT

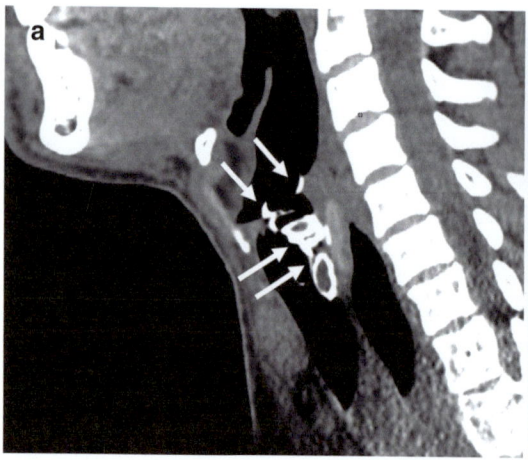
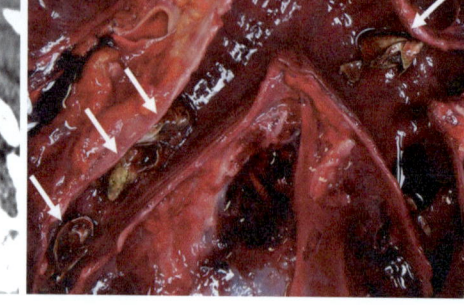

Fig. 7.9 (a) Postmortem MDCT (mediastinal window) with sagittal view illustrating unidentified foreign bodies in the trachea (white arrows). (b) Same case as (a), picture of the airways taken during the forensic autopsy. Foreign bodies visible at postmortem MDCT turned out to be small mussels (white arrows)

(Fig. 7.9a, b) [55, 56, 59–63]. Once again, the final diagnosis must be made according to complete postmortem investigations in such cases.

Postmortem angiography can be helpful in cases of drowning to complete cardiac investigations when a sudden cardiac death is suspected to be the origin of the drowning [56].

7.4   Obstruction of the Airways

An obstruction of the airway is a form of asphyxia by interruption of air passage induced by an external obstruction of the mouth and the nose, but also by a foreign body located in the mouth, the larynx, the trachea, and/or the bronchi.

Obstruction of the mouth and the nose (for example, by hands, soft covering, or other objects) doesn't usually leave any specific mark on the body. However, the external examination sometimes reveals skin lesions (such as abrasions and bruises) of the face, the neck, and the labial mucosa. During autopsy, soft tissue hemorrhage of the face and the neck may be present. Postmortem imaging such as MDCT and MRI have a limited interest for the detection of these findings. However, soft tissue hemorrhage (depending on their size) may be visible by MRI rather than at MDCT (except for important hemorrhage that could be visible by MDCT).

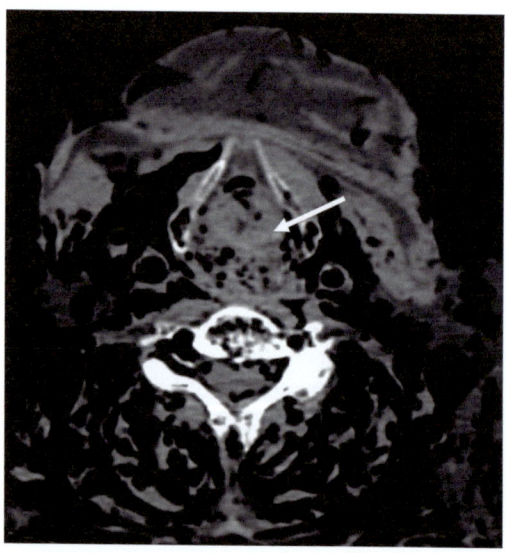

Fig. 7.10 Postmortem MDCT (mediastinal window) with axial view showing laryngeal obstruction by an unidentified foreign material (white arrow)

In cases of obstruction of the superior and/or inferior airways, MCDT and MRI prior to autopsy offer useful images to localize the obstructive material and visualize the level and degree of the obstruction before dissection (Figs. 7.10 and 7.11). However, foreign material may also be too small to be detected by imaging. For example, tissue fibers, which could be found in the airways during autopsy, could be too small

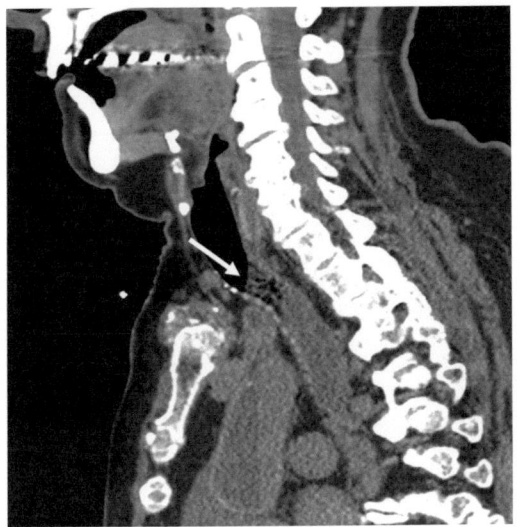

Fig. 7.11 Postmortem MDCT (mediastinal window) with sagittal view showing tracheal obstruction by an unidentified foreign material (white arrow)

to be radiologically visible [64–66]. Note that imaging can't provide information about the exact nature of the obstructive material.

Finally, overdistension of the lungs (as seen in acute pulmonary emphysema) and a frothy material in the airways can be found at autopsy in cases of obstruction of respiratory orifices and airways. Both findings can also be detected on MDCT.

7.5 Compression of the Thoracic Cage

Thoracic compression leads to asphyxiation due to the limitation of respiratory movements. Such scenario can happen, for example, in traffic accident, crush by heavy and large object, crowd movement, landslide, and avalanche. Postmortem findings include skin lesions (depending on the origin of the compression), intense congestion of the skin and soft tissues (fatty tissue and muscles) of the upper part of the body, cutaneous petechiae, as well as traumatic injuries of the thorax and/or abdomen (hemorrhages of the soft tissue and muscles, fractures of the sternum and/or the ribs, tears of thoracic/abdominal organs).

The added value of imaging is limited in cases of compression of the thoracic cage. MDCT can detect bone fractures and large hemorrhagic infiltrations of soft tissues, even though MRI remains the modality of choice for the assessment of such hemorrhages. MDCT prior to autopsy can also assist the forensic pathologist with the detection of hemopneumothorax (and its potential lethal consequences such as mediastinal shifting and compression) and inner organ lesions (such as lung contusions).

7.6 Conclusion

Asphyxia is a major topic in forensic medicine. Forensic imaging, such as MDCT and MRI, is a useful tool to investigate and document these cases on a daily routine. MDCT is the method of choice to detect skeletal lesions, and MRI is recommended for the evaluation of soft tissues (even though hemorrhagic infiltration of soft tissue may not be visible). Both techniques can guide the forensic pathologist during the postmortem investigation and can be useful to complete forensic clinical examinations. During postmortem evaluation, imaging can rule out major traumatic lesion and detect foreign bodies. However, the gold standard in cases of asphyxia remains the complete forensic autopsy and the clinical examination of living victims.

We also would like to highlight the importance of a multidisciplinary collaboration between radiologist and forensic pathologist. Both specialists should confront and discuss their results to improve the accuracy of their final diagnosis.

References

1. Spitz W, Spitz D. Asphyxia. In: Spitz and Fischer's medicolegal investigation of death: guidelines for the application of pathology to crime investigation. 4th ed. Charles C Thomas; 1994. p. 783–845.
2. Saukko P, Knight B. Suffocation and 'asphyxia'. In: Knight's forensic pathology. 3rd ed. Arnold; 2004. p. 353–97.

3. Madea B. Injuries due to asphyxiation and drowning. In: Handbook of forensic medicine. Wiley; 2014. p. 367–450.

4. Yen K, Vock P, Christe A, et al. Clinical forensic radiology in strangulation victims: forensic expertise based on magnetic resonance imaging (MRI) findings. Int J Legal Med. 2007;121(2):115–23.

5. Christe A, Oesterhelweg L, Ross S, et al. Can MRI of the neck compete with clinical findings in assessing danger to life for survivors of manual strangulation? A statistical analysis. Legal Med (Tokyo, Japan). 2010;12(5):228–32.

6. Christe A, Thoeny H, Ross S, et al. Life-threatening versus non-life-threatening manual strangulation: are there appropriate criteria for MR imaging of the neck? Eur Radiol. 2009;19(8):1882–9.

7. Yen K, Thali MJ, Aghayev E, et al. Strangulation signs: initial correlation of MRI, MSCT, and forensic neck findings. J Magn Reson Imaging. 2005;22(4):501–10.

8. Heimer J, Tappero C, Gascho D, et al. Value of 3T craniocervical magnetic resonance imaging following nonfatal strangulation. Eur Radiol. 2019;29(7):3458–66.

9. Bruguier C, Genet P, Zerlauth J-B, et al. Neck-MRI experience for investigation of survived strangulation victims. Forensic Sci Res. 2019;5(2):113–8.

10. Zabel TA, Slomine B, Brady K, Christensen J. Neuropsychological profile following suicide attempt by hanging: two adolescent case reports. Child Neuropsychol. 2005;11(4):373–88.

11. Kalita J, Mishra VN, Misra UK, Gupta RK. Clinicoradiological observation in three patients with suicidal hanging. J Neurol Sci. 2002;198(1–2):21–4.

12. Singhal AB, Topcuoglu MA, Koroshetz WJ. Diffusion MRI in three types of anoxic encephalopathy. J Neurol Sci. 2002;196(1–2):37–40.

13. Matsuyama T, Okuchi K, Seki T, et al. Magnetic resonance images in hanging. Resuscitation. 2006;69(2):343–5.

14. Plattner T, Bolliger S, Zollinger U. Forensic assessment of survived strangulation. Forensic Sci Int. 2005;153(2–3):202–7.

15. Malek AM, Higashida RT, Halbach VV, et al. Patient presentation, angiographic features, and treatment of strangulation-induced bilateral dissection of the cervical internal carotid artery. Report of three cases. J Neurosurg. 2000;92(3):481–7.

16. Hori A, Hirose G, Kataoka S, Tsukada K, Furui K, Tonami H. Delayed postanoxic encephalopathy after strangulation. Serial neuroradiological and neurochemical studies. Arch Neurol. 1991;48(8):871–4.

17. Sethi PK, Sethi NK, Torgovnick J, Arsura E. Delayed left anterior and middle cerebral artery hemorrhagic infarctions after attempted strangulation: a case report. Am J Forensic Med Pathol. 2012;33(1):105–6.

18. Molacek J, Baxa J, Houdek K, Ferda J, Treska V. Bilateral post-traumatic carotid dissection as a result of a strangulation injury. Ann Vasc Surg. 2010;24(8):1133.e9–11.

19. Zuberi OS, Dixon T, Richardson A, Gandhe A, Hadi M, Joshi J. CT angiograms of the neck in strangulation victims: incidence of positive findings at a level one trauma center over a 7-year period. Emerg Radiol. 2019;26(5):485–92.

20. Fabian TC, Patton JH, Croce MA, Minard G, Kudsk KA, Pritchard FE. Blunt carotid injury. Importance of early diagnosis and anticoagulant therapy. Ann Surg. 1996;223(5):513–22; discussion 522–5.

21. Rajz G, Simon D, Bakon M, Goren O, et al. Traumatic carotid artery dissection. Israel Med Assoc J. 2009;11(8):507–8.

22. De Boos J. Review article: Non-fatal strangulation: hidden injuries, hidden risks. Emerg Med Australas. 2019;31(3):302–8.

23. Crissey MM, Bernstein EF. Delayed presentation of carotid intimal tear following blunt craniocervical trauma. Surgery. 1974;75(4):543–9.

24. Kiani SH, Simes DC. Delayed bilateral internal carotid artery thrombosis following accidental strangulation. Br J Anaesth. 2000;84(4):521–4.

25. Vilke GM, Chan TC. Evaluation and management for carotid dissection in patients presenting after choking or strangulation. J Emerg Med. 2011;40(3):355–8.

26. Prosser DD, Grigsby T, Pollock JM. Unilateral anoxic brain injury secondary to strangulation identified on conventional and arterial spin-labeled perfusion imaging. Radiol Case Rep. 2018;13(3):563–7.

27. Imamura K, Akifuji Y, Kamitani H, Nakashima K. [Delayed postanoxic encephalopathy with visual field disturbance after strangulation: a case report]. Brain Nerve Shinkei Kenkyu No Shinpo. 2010;62(6):621–4.

28. Miyamoto O, Auer RN. Hypoxia, hyperoxia, ischemia, and brain necrosis. Neurology. 2000;54(2):362–71.

29. Groenendaal F, de Vries LS. Fifty years of brain imaging in neonatal encephalopathy following perinatal asphyxia. Pediatr Res. 2017;81(1–2):150–5.

30. Maurya VK, Ravikumar R, Bhatia M, Rai R. Hypoxic-ischemic brain injury in an adult: magnetic resonance imaging findings. Med J Armed Forces India. 2016;72(1):75–7.

31. Chevallier C, Doenz F, Vaucher P, et al. Postmortem computed tomography angiography vs. conventional autopsy: advantages and inconveniences of each method. Int J Legal Med. 2013;127(5):981–9.

32. Maiese A, Gitto L, dell'Aquila M, Bolino G. When the hidden features become evident: the usefulness of PMCT in a strangulation-related death. Legal Med (Tokyo, Japan). 2014;16(6):364–6.

33. Kempter M, Ross S, Spendlove D, et al. Post-mortem imaging of laryngohyoid fractures in strangulation incidents: first results. Legal Med (Tokyo, Japan). 2009;11(6):267–71.

34. Castiglioni C, Baumann P, Fracasso T. Acute pulmonary emphysema in death by hanging: a morphometric digital study. Int J Legal Med. 2016;130(5):1281–5.

35. Brinkmann B, Fechner G, Püschel K. Identification of mechanical asphyxiation in cases of attempted masking of the homicide. Forensic Sci Int. 1984;26(4):235–45.

36. Rayes M, Mittal M, Rengachary SS, Mittal S. Hangman's fracture: a historical and biomechanical perspective. J Neurosurg Spine. 2011;14(2):198–208.

37. Hayashi T, Hartwig S, Tsokos M, Oesterhelweg L. Postmortem multislice computed tomography (pmMSCT) imaging of hangman's fracture. Forensic Sci Med Pathol. 2014;10(1):3–8.

38. James R, Nasmyth-Jones R. The occurrence of cervical fractures in victims of judicial hanging. Forensic Sci Int. 1992;54(1):81–91.

39. Nokes LD, Roberts A, James DS. Biomechanics of judicial hanging: a case report. Med Sci Law. 1999;39(1):61–4.

40. Spence MW, Shkrum MJ, Ariss A, Regan J. Craniocervical injuries in judicial hangings: an anthropologic analysis of six cases. Am J Forensic Med Pathol. 1999;20(4):309–22.

41. Amadasi A, Buschmann CT, Tsokos M. Complex fracture patterns in hanging associated with a fall from height. Forensic Sci Med Pathol. 2020;16(2):359–61.

42. Töro K, Kristóf I, Keller E. Incomplete decapitation in suicidal hanging—report of a case and review of the literature. J Forensic Legal Med. 2008;15(3):180–4.

43. Gascho D, Heimer J, Tappero C, Schaerli S. Relevant findings on postmortem CT and postmortem MRI in hanging, ligature strangulation and manual strangulation and their additional value compared to autopsy—a systematic review. Forensic Sci Med Pathol. 2019;15(1):84–92.

44. Peschel O, Szeimies U, Vollmar C, Kirchhoff S. Postmortem 3-D reconstruction of skull gunshot injuries. Forensic Sci Int. 2013;233:45–50.

45. Deininger-Czermak E, Heimer J, Tappero C, Thali MJ, Gascho D. Postmortem magnetic resonance imaging and postmortem computed tomography in ligature and manual strangulation. Am J Forensic Med Pathol. 2020;41(2):97–103.

46. Hausser J, Niquille M. La noyade. Rev Med Suisse. 2007;121:1834–8.

47. Papa L, Hoelle R, Idris A. Systematic review of definitions for drowning incidents. Resuscitation. 2005;65(3):255–64.

48. Ender PT, Dolan MJ. Pneumonia associated with near-drowning. Clin Infect Dis. 1997;25(4):896–907.

49. Cerland L, Mégarbane B, Kallel H, Brouste Y, Mehdaoui H, Resiere D. Incidence and consequences of near-drowning–related pneumonia—a descriptive series from Martinique, French West Indies. Int J Environ Res Public Health. 2017;14(11):1402.

50. Schneppe S, Dokter M, Bockholdt B. Macromorphological findings in cases of death in water: a critical view on "drowning signs". Int J Legal Med. 2021;135(1):281–91.

51. Armstrong EJ, Erskine KL. Investigation of drowning deaths: a practical review. Acad Forensic Pathol. 2018;8(1):8–43.

52. Lin C-Y, Yen W-C, Hsieh H-M, et al. Diatomological investigation in sphenoid sinus fluid and lung tissue from cases of suspected drowning. Forensic Sci Int. 2014;244:111–5.

53. Püschel K, Schulz F, Darrmann I, Tsokos M. Macromorphology and histology of intramuscular hemorrhages in cases of drowning. Int J Legal Med. 1999;112(2):101–6.

54. Christe A, Aghayev E, Jackowski C, Thali MJ, Vock P. Drowning—post-mortem imaging findings by computed tomography. Eur Radiol. 2008;18(2):283–90.

55. Van Hoyweghen AJL, Jacobs W, Op de Beeck B, Parizel PM. Can post-mortem CT reliably distinguish between drowning and non-drowning asphyxiation? Int J Legal Med. 2015;129(1):159–64.

56. Vander Plaetsen S, De Letter E, Piette M, Van Parys G, Casselman JW, Verstraete K. Post-mortem evaluation of drowning with whole body CT. Forensic Sci Int. 2015;249:35–41.

57. Aghayev E, Thali MJ, Sonnenschein M, et al. Fatal steamer accident; blunt force injuries and drowning in post-mortem MSCT and MRI. Forensic Sci Int. 2005;152(1):65–71.

58. Hyodoh H, Terashima R, Rokukawa M, et al. Experimental drowning lung images on postmortem CT—difference between sea water and fresh water. Legal Med (Tokyo, Japan). 2016;19:11–5.

59. Lo Re G, Vernuccio F, Galfano MC, et al. Role of virtopsy in the post-mortem diagnosis of drowning. Radiol Med (Torino). 2015;120(3):304–8.

60. Levy AD, Harcke HT, Getz JM, et al. Virtual autopsy: two- and three-dimensional multidetector CT findings in drowning with autopsy comparison. Radiology. 2007;243(3):862–8.

61. Oshima T, Ohtani M, Mimasaka S. Muscular hemorrhages around the scapula resulting from excessive upper extremity motion in cases of fatal drowning: autopsy findings for insights on manner of death. Forensic Sci Int. 2019;300:82–4.

62. Onitsuka D, Nakamae T, Katsuyama M, et al. Epidemiological analysis of intramuscular hemorrhage of respiratory and accessory respiratory muscles in fatal drowning cases. PLoS One. 2021;16(12):e0261348.

63. Raux C, Saval F, Rouge D, Telmon N, Dedouit F. Diagnosis of drowning using post-mortem computed tomography—state of the art. Arch Med Sadowej Kryminol. 2014;64(2):59–75.

64. Schmeling A, Fracasso T, Pragst F, Tsokos M, Wirth I. Unassisted smothering in a pillow. Int J Legal Med. 2009;123(6):517–9.

65. Schyma C, Madea B. Comments on unassisted smothering in a pillow. Int J Legal Med. 2011;125(1):155–6.

66. Keil W, Berzlanovich A. Ersticken durch weiche Bedeckung. Rechtsmedizin. 2010;20(6):519–28.

Hypothermia

8

Grzegorz Teresiński and Grzegorz Staśkiewicz

8.1 Introduction

Hypothermia is clinically defined as the decrease of the core temperature below 35 °C. For obvious reasons, this essential sign of hypothermia (the only one, sufficient for the clinical diagnosis) is completely useless in diagnosis of fatal cases of cold exposure. In a forensic setting, it is important to identify other diagnostic criteria, which will indicate the excessive loss of the body heat as the cause of death, rejecting other possible causes.

Fatal hypothermia may induce several typical morphological and biochemical changes; however, none of the identified markers of hypothermia is pathognomonic. Furthermore, cases of fatal hypothermia with no external or internal signs of cold exposure are relatively common. Frequency of specific signs is variable in different reports. This also results from different settings and causes of cooling down, external temperature, and length of exposure (rate of hypothermia and degree of activation of physiological mechanisms of prevention of heat loss),

as well as accompanying factors such as trauma, drug or alcohol influence, etc. [1–3]

8.2 Pathophysiology

In the setting of postmortem diagnosis, most frequently we face the cases of primary hypothermia (accidental) due to environmental exposure to cold; less frequently secondary hypothermia due to disturbed thermoregulation in chronic diseases, in intoxicated patients, or due to specific drugs (e.g., benzodiazepines, phenytoin of valproic acid) can be encountered [4].

Cooling rate (i.e., time since the beginning of exposure to cold until the time of death) depends most significantly on the type of hypothermia and the external temperature [1, 5, 6]. Accidental hypothermia may be classified regarding the circumstances into:

- Acute hypothermia (so-called wet)—immersive type (immersion in cold water)
- Subacute (so-called dry)—due to exhaustion (atmospheric condition influence)
- Chronic—urban type (slow cooling of elderly or diseased person in insufficiently heated accommodation)

The rate of decrease of core temperature is the highest in cases of immersion hypothermia (hypothermia level of 35 °C is reached approximately

G. Teresiński (✉)
Department of Forensic Medicine, Medical University of Lublin, Lublin, Poland
e-mail: grzegorz.teresinski@umlub.pl

G. Staśkiewicz
Department of Radiology, Medical University of Lublin, Lublin, Poland
e-mail: grzegorz.staskiewicz@umlub.pl

after 1 h of immersion in water of 5 °C, 2 h at 10 °C, and 3–6 h at 15 °C, as measured in laboratory conditions in adults wearing outdoor clothing, during head-out immersion, while in real setting, death may occur even within the first hour), while for atmospheric exposure it widely estimated between 0.15 and 4.1 °C/h (even faster in newborns) [1, 5, 6]. Decrease of temperature is faster in females and lean persons (adipose tissue is a thermal insulator).

Cooling of the body induces processes which reduce loss of heat and increase its production [7, 8]:

- Adaptative and behavioral reactions:
  - Sympathetic activation: tachycardia, narrowing of peripheral blood vessels, and cardiovascular centralization

- Behaviors which protect against cold: covering, crouching, and seeking shelter
- Shivering thermogenesis:
  - Uncontrolled, uncoordinated contractions of fibers of skeletal muscles
- Non-shivering thermogenesis (chemical):
  - Increased basic metabolism
  - Hormonal activation (Fig. 8.1)

While hypothermia progresses, gradual changes in metabolism occur [9, 10]:

- Initially utilization of glucose and hepatic glycogen
- In shivering phase utilization of muscular glycogen (no release of glucose into blood due to lack of glucose-6-phosphatase in muscles)

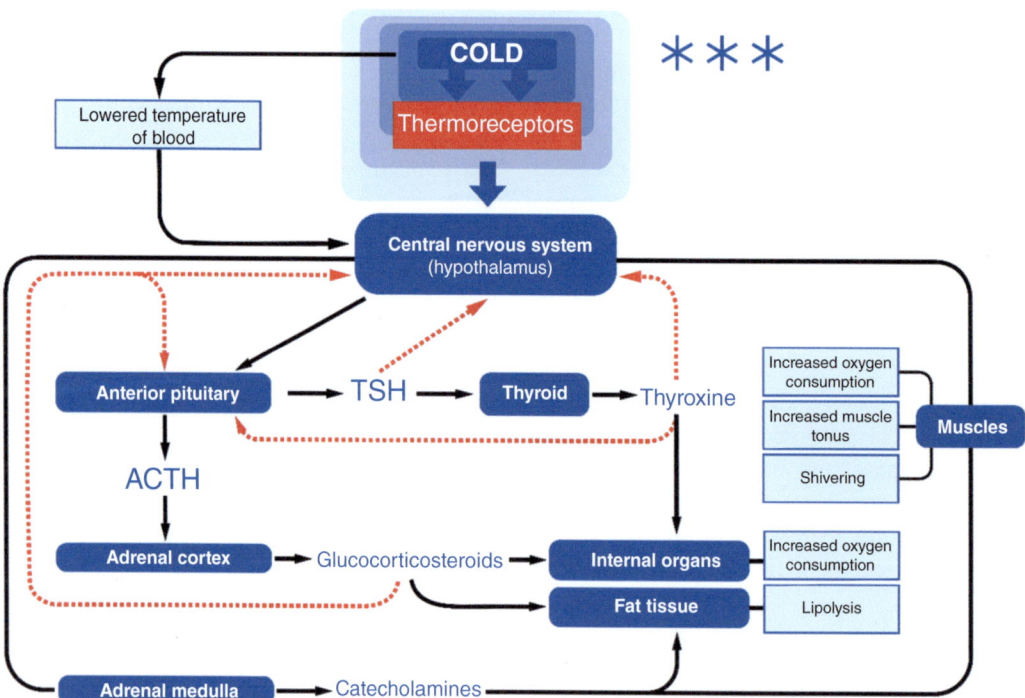

Fig. 8.1 Hormonal reactions due to exposure to low temperature of the body. Solid line, stimulation; dotted line, inhibition

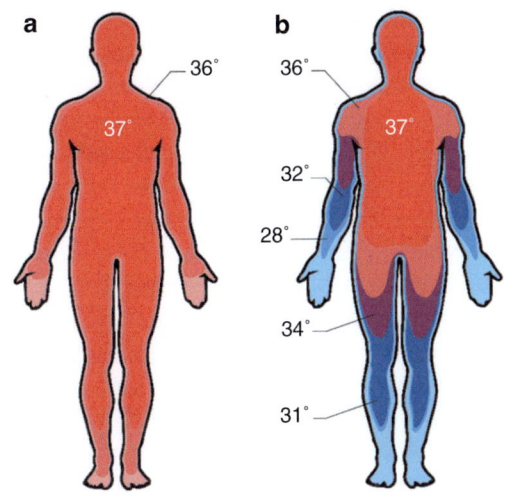

Fig. 8.2 Distribution of temperature in warm environment (**a**) and during exposure to cold (**b**). (Adapted from Witzmann, 2009 [7])

- Hormonal activation of hypothalamic-adrenal axis:
  - Lipolysis of adipose tissue and mobilization of free fatty acids (FFA), which are used by some tissues (e.g., heart, muscles, and kidneys) as energetic substrate
  - Hepatic gluconeogenesis—transformation of glycerol released during lipolysis and maintaining glycemia in glucose-dependent tissues
  - Hepatic ketogenesis—ketone bodies become the main energetic substrate in advanced hypothermia

The cooling body attempts to maintain internal core temperature, which is why the decrease of temperature of distal body parts is much faster

Table 8.1 Clinical signs of disturbed metabolism depending on severity of hypothermia (signs in bold may produce macroscopic findings postmortem)

| | Hypothermia | | |
	Mild	Moderate	Severe (deep)
Range of core temperature	35–32 °C	32–28 °C	<28 °C
Central nervous system	Disturbed speech, loss of coordination, ataxia	Rigidity, dilation of pupils, hallucination	Coma, relaxation, rigid pupils, isoelectric EEG line
Respiratory system	**Increased ventilation rate**—Hyperventilation	Decreased ventilation rate	Apnea (<24 °C), **pulmonary edema**
Circulatory system	Tachycardia, atrial fibrillation, arrhythmia	Bradycardia, ventricular arrhythmia	Hypotension, ventricular fibrillation, asystolia (<20 °C)
	Blood thickening, **coagulopathy**		
Acid-base balance	Respiratory alkalosis	Respiratory acidosis	Metabolic acidosis
Metabolism	Tremor, increased basic metabolic rate, increased oxygen consumption, hyperglycemia	Decreased basic metabolic rate, decreased oxygen consumption, loss of tremor	Decreased basic metabolic rate, minimal thermogenesis
Urinary system	**Cold diuresis**	**Cold diuresis**	Decreased filtration, oliguria
Digestive system	**Pancreatitis, gastric mucosal erosions**, loss of hepatocyte function, **ileus**		

already in the early phase of cold exposure, before hypothermia develops (Fig. 8.2) [7, 8]. Risk of death is proportional to the decrease of core temperature, which determines pathophysiological processes occurring during the cooling of the body (Table 8.1).

8.3 Macroscopic Results of Cold Exposure

Exposure to cold may lead to local and general consequences. Local signs on the skin result from direct thermal injury and secondary consequences of adrenergic activation (significant decrease in blood flow in peripheral vessels) which leads to edema, ischemia, and progressive tissue necrosis [4]. In clinical setting, external signs of this process depend on time of exposure and degree of thermal injury:

- Acute consequences—frostbite:
  - I°—reversibly disturbed circulation: initially pale, next red-blue with painful swelling of the skin
  - II°—blisters filled with serous contents
  - III°—bloody discoloration of fluid in the blisters and superficial skin necrosis
  - IV°—deep necrosis and defects of peripheral parts of the body (distal toes and fingers, nose, ears)
- Consequences of repeated and prolonged vasoconstriction of submaximal severity—chronic inflammatory process:
  - Chilblains (perniosis, perniones)—"dry" form due to exposure to cold and moist air
  - Immersion foot (trench foot)—"wet" form due to prolonged compression and exposure to cold and humidity

In forensic settings, cooling of blood flowing through cold parts of the body results with hemolysis of red blood cells, which produces characteristic red-bluish hemolytic discolorations in typical (particularly exposed) areas of the body—especially the face, hands, elbows, and knees (Fig. 8.3). This process is more severe in cases of breakdown of protection mechanisms and cessation of vasoconstriction, while circulation is still maintained in pre-agony [11]. Ischemia of the tissues results in rupture of cellular membranes and vascular endothelium, and released inflammatory mediators further promote the destruction of tissues.

Process of hemolysis is most pronounced in the areas where the skin is situated very close to a bone (knees, elbows, anterior areas of the legs, zygomatic areas) with no protective layer of subcutaneous adipose tissue and muscles. Significant thermal conduction of bone tissue results in much faster loss of temperature of superficially located bones, which accelerates hemolysis of blood in superficial blood vessels between the skin and blood. Degradation of erythrocytes results in diffusion of pigment into surrounding tissues—skin, subcutaneous tissue, and synovial membrane (so-called inner knee sign [12]). This also occurs in diploic vessels, which leads to formation of pseudo-hemorrhages visible on the diploic sections (Fig. 8.4).

A similar effect may be produced experimentally by direct application of very low temperatures on the knees of deceased, which indicates indirect effect of sedimentation of ice crystals in tissues, which originally did not show postmortem hemolysis (Fig. 8.5).

Despite cardiovascular centralization, thermic shock disturbs perfusion of internal organs, including the digestive tract. This induces acute stress ulcerations, so-called Wischnewski spots (Fig. 8.6) [13]. Less frequently hemorrhagic foci are observed in other parts of the digestive tract (particularly in the distal part of the large intestine).

Rare consequences of hypothermia include acute pancreatitis (Fig. 8.7), which in hospitalized patients present with increased activity of pancreatic enzymes [14]. These nonspecific changes are usually observed in secondary hypothermia, particularly in elderly people with poorly heated accommodation, at above-zero temperatures [11]. Ischemia of various internal organs and hormonal stimulation may cause nonspecific microscopic and histochemical changes in the heart, kidneys, hypothalamus, and adrenal glands. Among typical histopathological

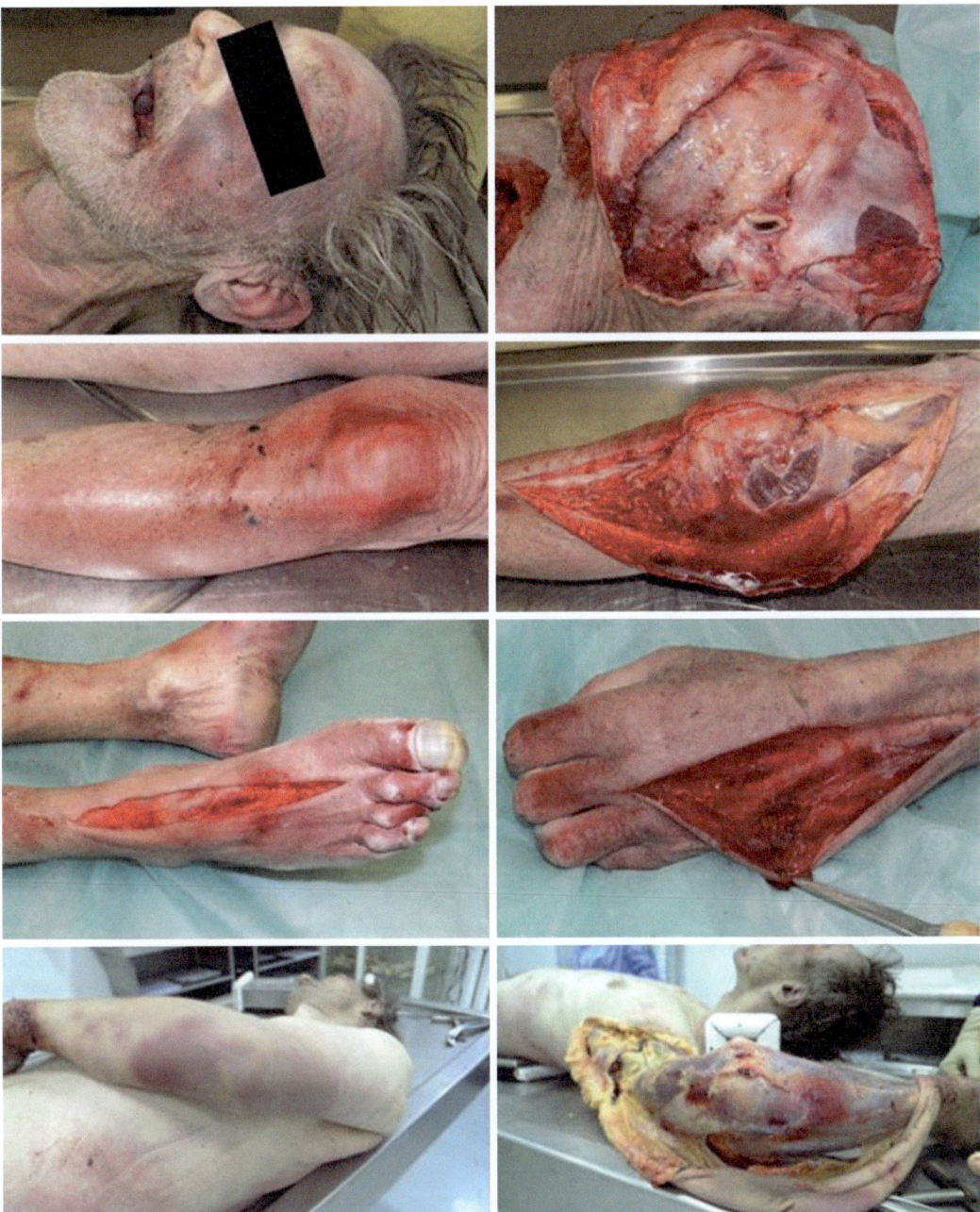

Fig. 8.3 Hemolytic discolorations of the skin and subcutaneous tissue of the face, anterior surface of the knee, foot, hand, and elbow (with no perceptible hemorrhages after dissection of the skin) in victims of fatal hypothermia

findings, there is deficiency of hepatic glycogen in PAS staining (see Sect. 8.6).

In some cases, isolated hemorrhagic foci are observed in deep layer of muscles of the back, chest, pectoral, or pelvic girdle, particularly in the paravertebral muscles, e.g., iliopsoas (Fig. 8.8) [15]. Their formation is attributed to mechanism of intensive shivering in peri-agonal period. This hypothesis resembles explanation of hemorrhages on the ventral surface of the inter-

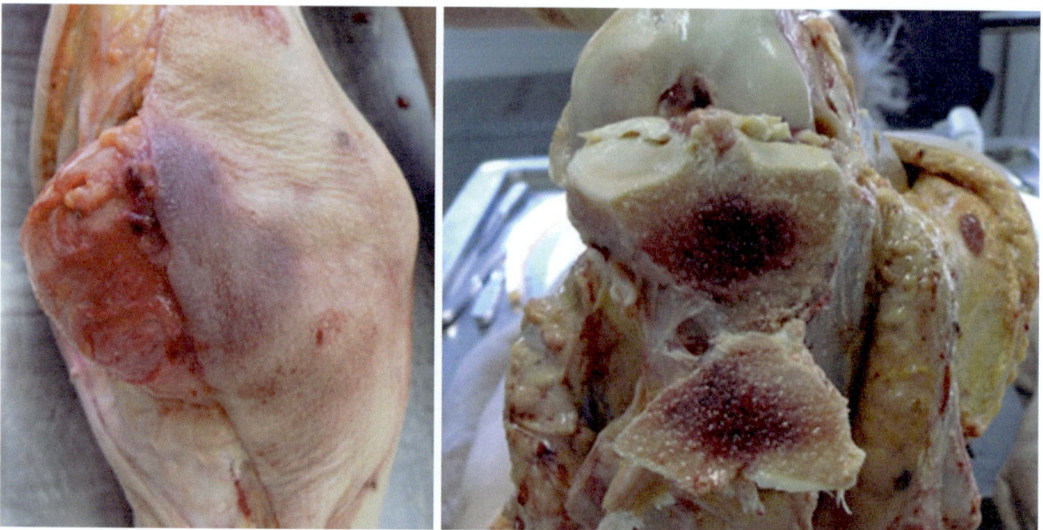

Fig. 8.4 Hemolytic discoloration of the skin, subcutaneous tissue, and section of proximal tibial epiphysis in case of fatal hypothermia (no features of mechanical injury)

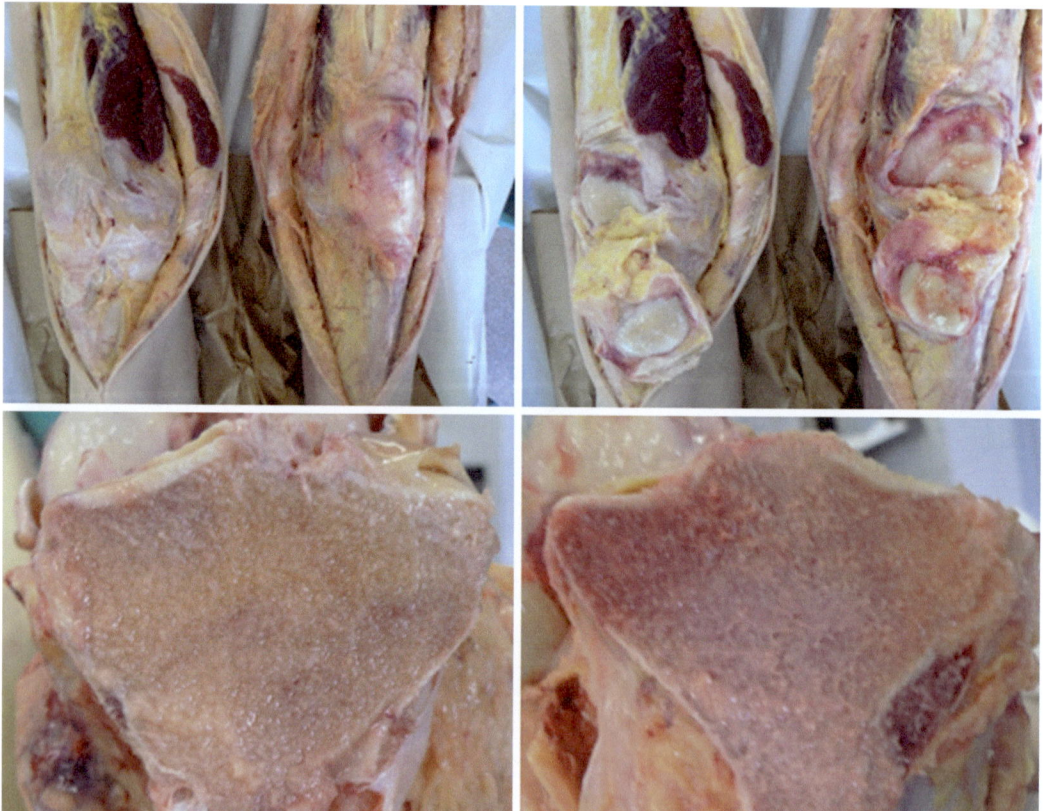

Fig. 8.5 Experimentally induced inner knee sign in case of sudden death not related to hypothermia (left knee packed with dry ice for 24 h)

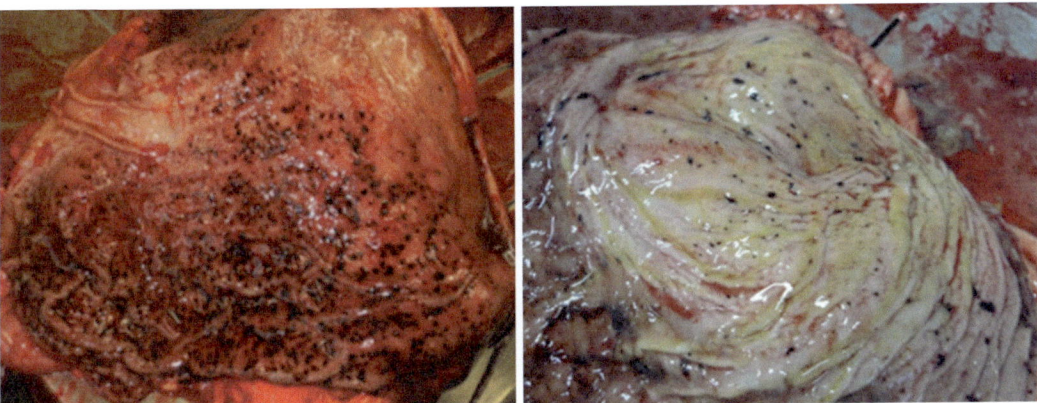

Fig. 8.6 Wischnewski spots in gastric mucosa

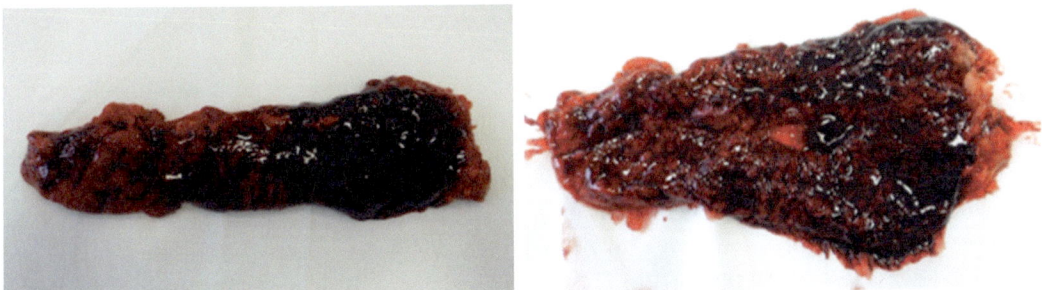

Fig. 8.7 Hemorrhagic pancreatitis in case of fatal hypothermia (isolated organ on the left, dissection on the right)

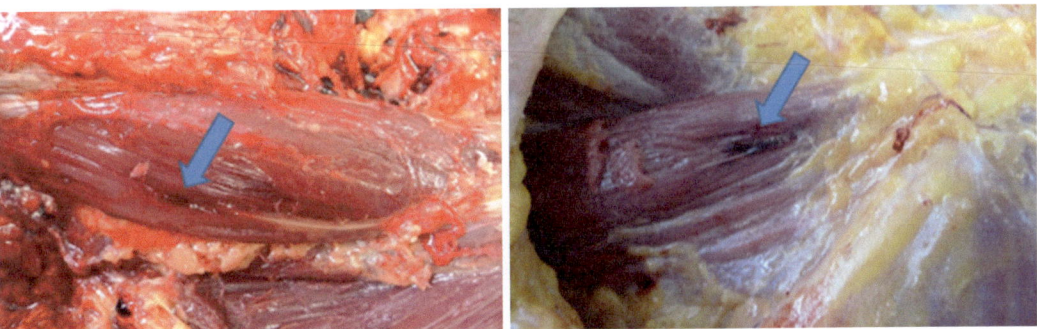

Fig. 8.8 Hemorrhages beneath perimysium of iliopsoas muscles in cases of fatal hypothermia

vertebral disk in the lumbar part of the spinal column (Simon's sign most commonly seen in hanging), which were also occasionally reported in cases of hypothermia [16].

During progression of cooling of external parts of the body, temporary paradoxical relaxation of cutaneous blood vessels occurs (Lewis hunting reaction), which delays irreversible changes in ischemic distal body parts [7, 8].

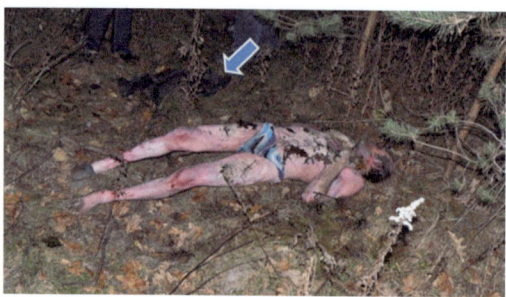

Fig. 8.9 Paradoxical undressing in case of fatal hypothermia—trousers revealed near the body (arrows), red discoloration of knees on the body of the deceased found in a forest in wintertime

Temporary dilation of peripheral vessels may result in perceptible warming and lead to "paradoxical undressing" (Fig. 8.9) [17–19]. Paradoxically percepted warmth may also result from dysfunction of the vasomotor center, as decrease in core temperature reduces protective mechanisms. Primitive protection reactions may also occur in pre-agony (terminal burrowing behavior, hide-and-die syndrome) [20].

8.4 Forensic Imaging in Hypothermia

The main indication for postmortem imaging in suspected fatal hypothermia is to exclude other possible causes of death. In some cases hypothermia may be secondary to traumatic injury (Fig. 8.10):

- Accidental injuries which cause the victim to be unable to move (impaired consciousness due to injuries of central nervous system, fractures of the limbs, etc.)
- Intentional incapacitating injuries in victims left unattended in cold environment
- Climbing injuries (fall during climbing, avalanche accident, hypoxia, and high-altitude pulmonary edema—HAPE)
- Passive infanticide (newborn abandonment)

Postmortem imaging may be useful for diagnosis of pathologies, which indirectly lead to the cooling of the body. Awareness of concomitant

burden may explain the circumstances, which lead to fatal hypothermia. This refers both to accidental exposure to atmospheric conditions (lost in the woods, confused patient leaving ward or care facility, etc.) and relatively frequent cases of chronic city-type hypothermia, e.g.:

- Disabled or infirm person with chronic diseases of musculoskeletal system
- Additional, infective pathology (e.g., pneumonia), which decompensates a relatively efficient person living alone
- Mistakes in pharmacotherapy of chronic diseases (e.g., diabetic hypothermia) or additional influence of treatment on disorders of thermoregulation

The capabilities of postmortem imaging for direct diagnosis of fatal cold exposure are limited. Only nonspecific markers have been identified, which in typical settings may support the hypothesis of hypothermia, while none is pathognomonic. Several published studies focus on two modalities: postmortem computed tomography (PMCT) and postmortem magnetic resonance imaging (PMMRI, PMMR) [21, 22].

8.4.1 PMCT in Diagnosis of Hypothermia

PMCT allows for identification of the following signs suggestive of hypothermia:

- Diffuse hyperaeration with decreased vascularity of the lungs (diminished hypostatic opacification)
- Blood clotting in the heart and big vessels
- Urine retention in the bladder

Relatively most frequently reported radiological marker of fatal hypothermia is low lung attenuation which could be helpful for screening purposes [23]. Explanation of this sign is decreased perfusion of the lungs (Fig. 8.11), which next may lead to lack of typical hyperemia in dependent parts of the lungs in PMCT. Pulmonary hypostasis is significantly less frequently reported and significantly less pro-

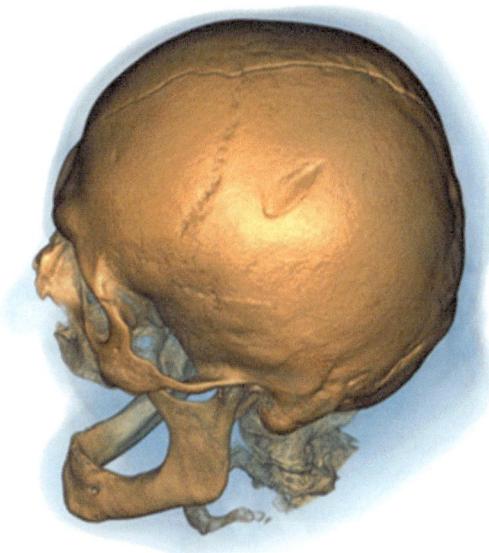
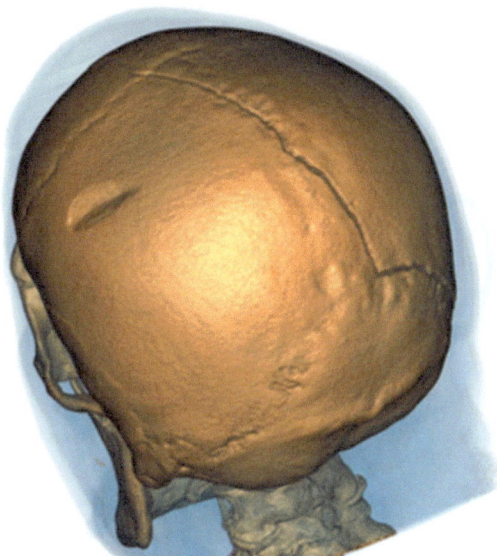

Fig. 8.10 Fracture of calvaria along the sagittal suture, due to fall with hitting the back of the head against a hard surface with secondary hypothermia (two competitive causes of death characterized by prolonged agony: mas-sive epidural hemorrhage and low temperature exposure). Smooth outlined, oblong indentation in the left parietal area after previous injury in chronic alcoholic addiction

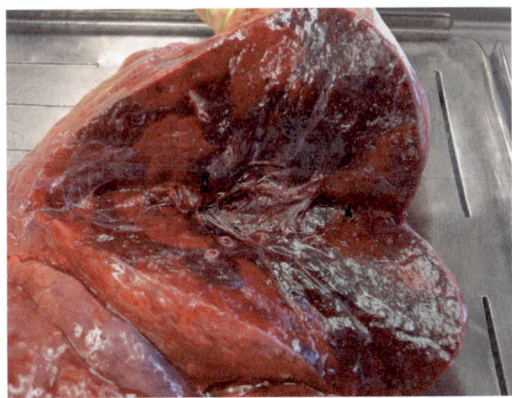

Fig. 8.11 Bright red areas of decreased perfusion on the dissected lung (focal acute emphysema)

nounced in fatal hypothermia cases as compared with other causes of death [24]. The association between hypothermia and low PMCT attenuation of the lungs exhibits a dose-effect relationship (degree of pulmonary aeration is the more pronounced the lower was the temperature of the environment at the time of death). According to Hyodoh et al. [25], hypothermia is very likely to be the cause of death if the percentage of aerated lung (%ALV) is greater than 70%. According to Schweitzer et al. [26], a 90% probability for fatal hypothermia exists for PMCT lung attenuation of less than −780 HU (Hounsfield units).

Published studies are based on rather short series of victims with detailed description missing (most significantly blood alcohol concentration (BAC), possible drug misuse) as well as setting of the event (e.g., indoor/outdoor, minimal temperature of the environment, height above the sea level, etc.). Attempts of application of these findings in our own routine forensic casework were unequivocal. Serial analysis of PMCTs in hypothermia victims showed no cases which would precisely fit the abovementioned criteria (fatal hypothermia cases in Poland are mainly city type or accidental hypothermia in lowland environment, in cases of alcohol intoxication). Furthermore, lowered PMCT attenuation of the lungs can be found in other situations such as suffocation, strangulation, as well as obstructive, mechanical, or positional asphyxia, so it is not specific for fatal hypothermia. Various degrees of hyperaeration visible on PMCT are also a radiological sign of pulmonary emphysema (Fig. 8.11), which is a common marker of acute respiratory distress of different etiologies (e.g., asphyxia deaths, obstructive pulmonary disease, starvation, etc.).

Furthermore, simultaneous intoxications of various etiologies usually induce hyperemia of internal organs (including lungs). Among victims of accidental city or suburban type of hypothermia (not related to climbing or hiking), concomitant alcohol intoxication dominates. In such cases, signs of hyperemia are usually observed, while areas of acute emphysema are limited to peripheral, subpleural areas of the parenchyma.

Also two other signs considered to be markers of hypothermia (blood clotting and urine retention) are closely related with alcohol intoxication [24]. Alcohol consumption increases diuresis, and ethanol is well known for influence on the coagulation status (inhibition of fibrinolysis), and clotted blood is considered a sign of alcohol intoxication (Fig. 8.12) [27].

8.4.2 PMMR in Diagnosis of Hypothermia

Application of MRI in postmortem diagnosis of hypothermia is mainly focused on detection of isolated hemorrhages in deep layers of muscles of the back and iliopsoas muscles [28]. There are no results of systematic studies on larger groups of cases, which would allow to assess diagnostic performance of these signs. In autopsies of victims of hypothermia, hemorrhagic foci within

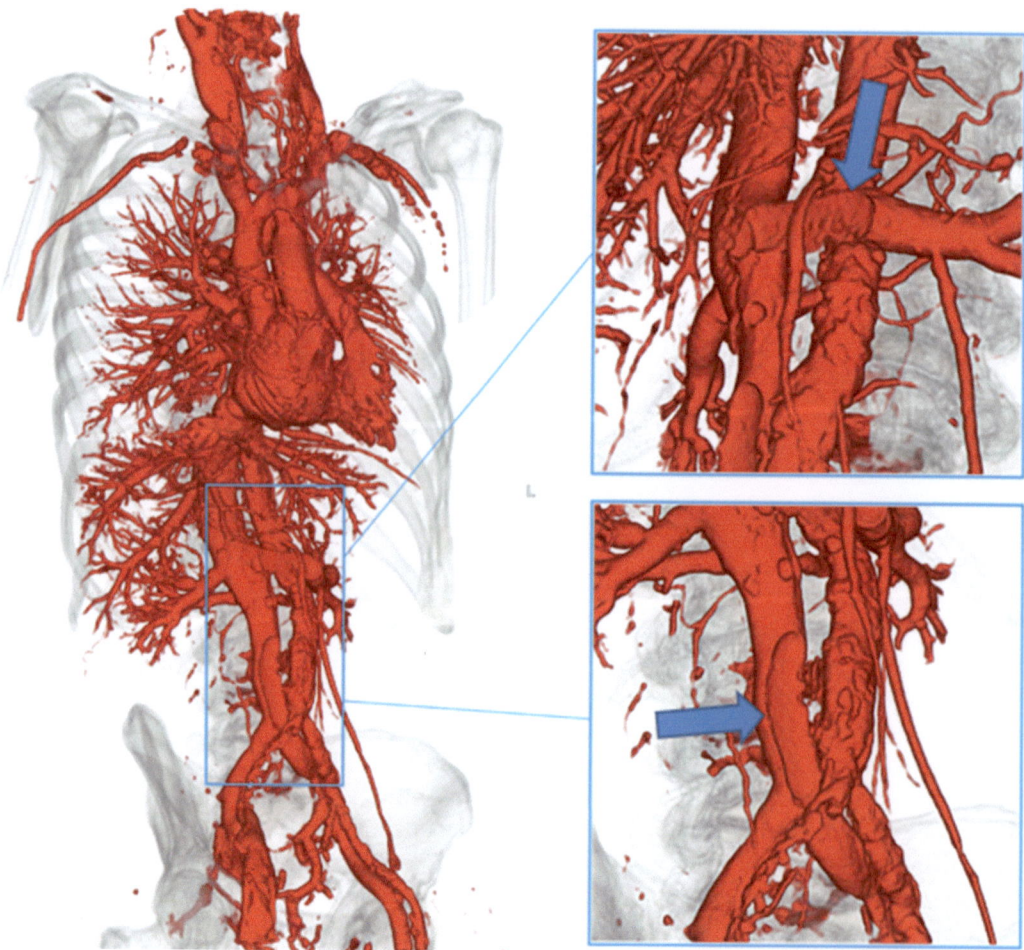

Fig. 8.12 Contrast-filling defects caused by blood clots in PMCT angiography

large paravertebral muscles or accessory respiratory muscles were also only occasionally observed. This may result from the fact that these regions are not routinely dissected in lack of major trauma features, as well as from the size of the foci—approximately of 1–2 cm. For these purposes, screening MRI may improve detection of single, dispersed hemorrhages, which may be missed with routine autopsy technique (detection of single foci of about 1 cm size requires meticulous layer-by-layer preparation with dense incisions of specific muscle bundles).

On the other hand, similar findings are observed in other conditions related with hyperventilation or sudden initiation of extremely forceful respiration (e.g., while drowning, obstruction of the airways with fragments of food, mechanical asphyxia, staying in confined spaces, collapse accidents, etc.). Hemorrhagic foci in deep layers of muscles of pectoral girdle which serve as accessory respiratory muscles show the following identification features (Fig. 8.13):

- Isolated hemorrhages in the deep layers of muscles
- No extension into superficial tissues (particularly subcutaneous fat)
- Extension along muscle fibers without crossing fascial layers (perimysium)
- Specifically confined to muscles supporting respiration (inspiration)

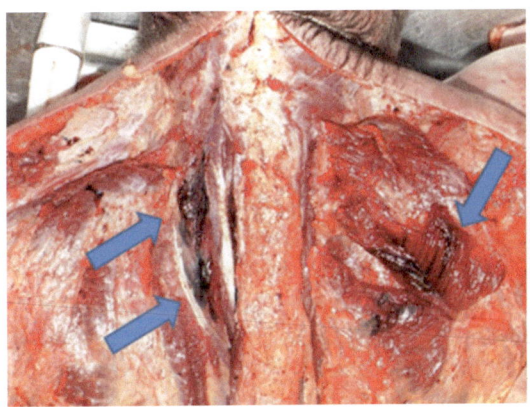 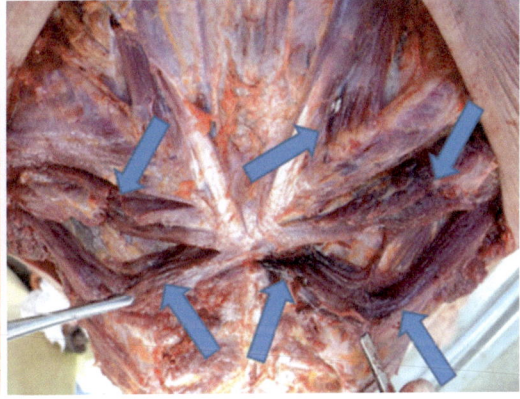

Fig. 8.13 Isolated hemorrhages in accessory respiratory muscles of the back and pectoral girdle (with no hemorrhages in subcutaneous tissue and superficial muscles in drowning (on the left), and trapping in the confined space (hide-and-die syndrome—on the right)

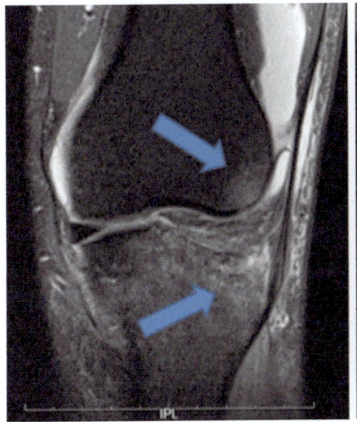 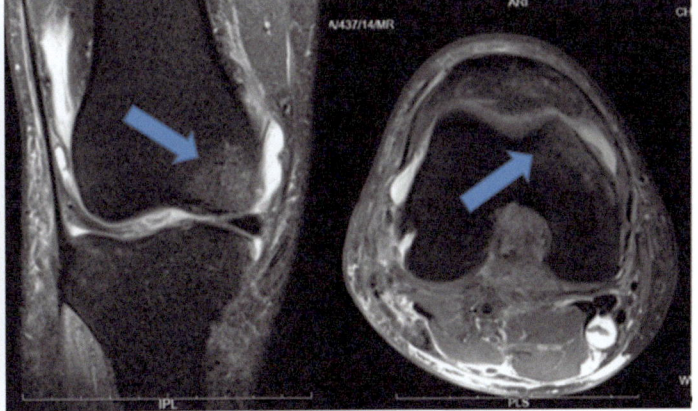

Fig. 8.14 Marrow edema in the medial condyle of the femur, lateral condyle of the tibia, and proximal epiphysis of tibia (arrows)

- Localized close to attachments of muscles on scapulae, clavicles, and ribs

PMMR is the only type of noninvasive studies, which allows for detection of hemorrhagic foci in the bone tissue (Fig. 8.14), frequently observed in epiphyseal cross-sections of knees in post-mortem examinations of traffic accident victims [29]. So far there are no reports on its application for identification of bone bruises in the epiphyses of bones of the knee in victims of hypothermia.

Even so advanced imaging modality does not allow for identification of hemorrhagic foci within the mucosa of the stomach (Wischnewski spots) due to insufficient resolution of typical MRI scanners.

8.4.3 Ultrasonography

As opposed to clinical applications, ultrasound (US) did not become popular in postmortem imaging, although resolution of contemporary scanners allows for intravital detection of abnormal echogenicity <1 mm with high-frequency probes. Resolution improves with increasing frequency of the sound wave, but depth of penetration decreases—which makes ultrasound particularly useful in imaging of superficial structures. Some pathologies in subcutaneous tissue, muscles, or superficial joint structures are more easily visualized with US than with computed tomography. Suggillations are ultrasonographically characterized by local change of echogenicity of subcutaneous tissue with formation of hypoechoic layers or compartments (Fig. 8.15). This technique may be particularly useful in people with dark skin. Local edema of subcutaneous tissue produces even more visible ultrasonographic signs.

Few attempts of application of ultrasound in forensic imaging were related with, among others, postmortem detection of hemorrhages in superficial tissues [30]. Therefore, there is a theoretical basis for application of this modality for supplementary assessment of hemorrhagic lesions in the muscles of the back, as well as analysis of changed echogenicity of periarticular soft tissues and synovial membrane of the knees (Fig. 8.16). Low temperature of the cadaver changes transmission and reflection of ultrasound wave, leading to decrease in difference of echogenicity of different tissues, which is why quality of US imaging significantly improves several hours after the removal of the body from the cold chamber. Significant limitation of postmortem US is presence of decay gas in the tissues, which produces artifacts and disturb penetration of tissues by sound waves. Differences of postmortem echogenicity may also produce false-positive findings like edema and inflammation [31].

US scanners are theoretically more affordable than CT or MR scanners (or even digital radiography scanners), however in postmortem imaging are used mostly as supplementary method for minimally invasive procedures—transcutaneous biopsy or vascular cannulation. US navigation may facilitate collecting samples for additional examinations, also in the field of postmortem

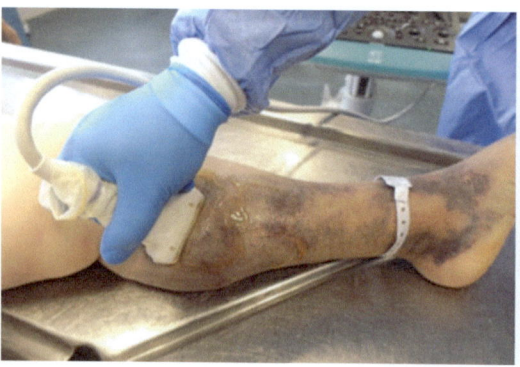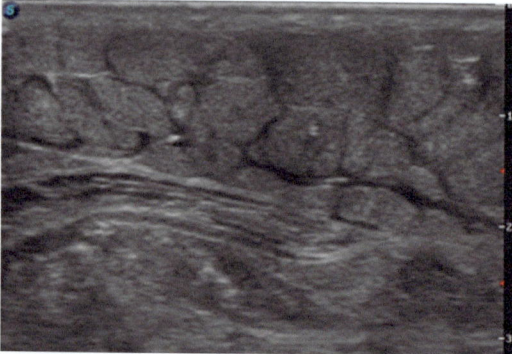

Fig. 8.15 Postmortem US of superficial structures with linear high-frequency probe—abnormal echostructure of subcutaneous tissue within suggillation of the leg

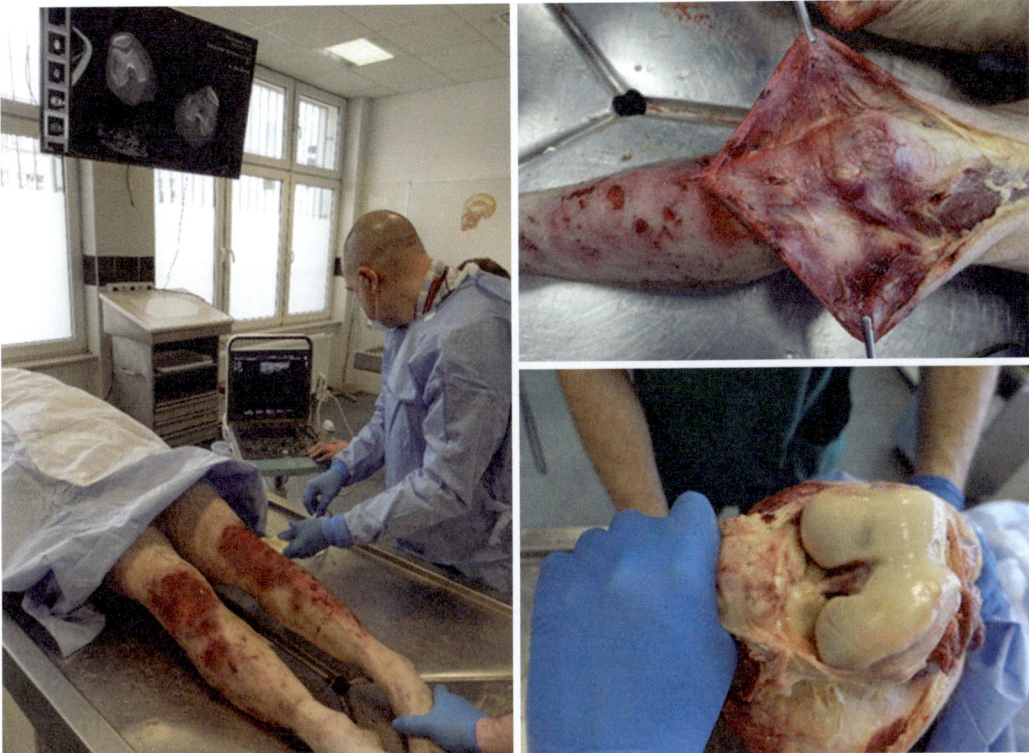

Fig. 8.16 Examination of knee areas in fatal hypothermia victim in search for the so-called inner knee sign (hemolytic discoloration of infrapatellar synovial membrane and anterior cruciate ligament)

diagnosis of hypothermia. US navigation may be useful for visualization of superficial vessels, pleural cavities, pericardium, peritoneal cavity, urinary bladder, or gallbladder and collecting samples for histological, biochemical, toxicological, or microbiological studies [32].

This modality becomes significant, when postmortem angiography is planned. US-guided cannulation reduces range of incision of the skin (which may be important in view of family or prosecutor objections against violation of integrity of the body). It allows for precise cannulation and contrast (positive or negative) administration for selective angiography of specific organ, with no dissection of vessels as well as separate enhancement of arterial and venous vessels—which allows for multiphase angiography. Postmortem visualization of femoral or carotid vessels is usually simple; however, even in clinical settings misidentification may occur (Fig. 8.17).

8.4.4 Other Modalities

Imaging modalities utilized in hypothermia may include analysis of heat-infrared radiation (infrared thermography (IRT), thermal imaging). Thermographic cameras allow for registration of heat waves emitted by physical objects in the range of mid and far infrared (wavelength from 3 to 15 μm) with no need of additional light exposure, as well as measurement of temperature of such objects. Thermographic methods are rarely used in forensic medicine, for example, in contactless measurement of cooling rate or for identification of hidden remains (heat release as an effect of putrefaction).

Limitation of the use of thermographic cameras in routine medicolegal practice is the fact that their capability of measurement is restricted to the surface. Indeed, measurement of temperature of internal organs requires their earlier exposure (Fig. 8.18). The process of cooling is starting

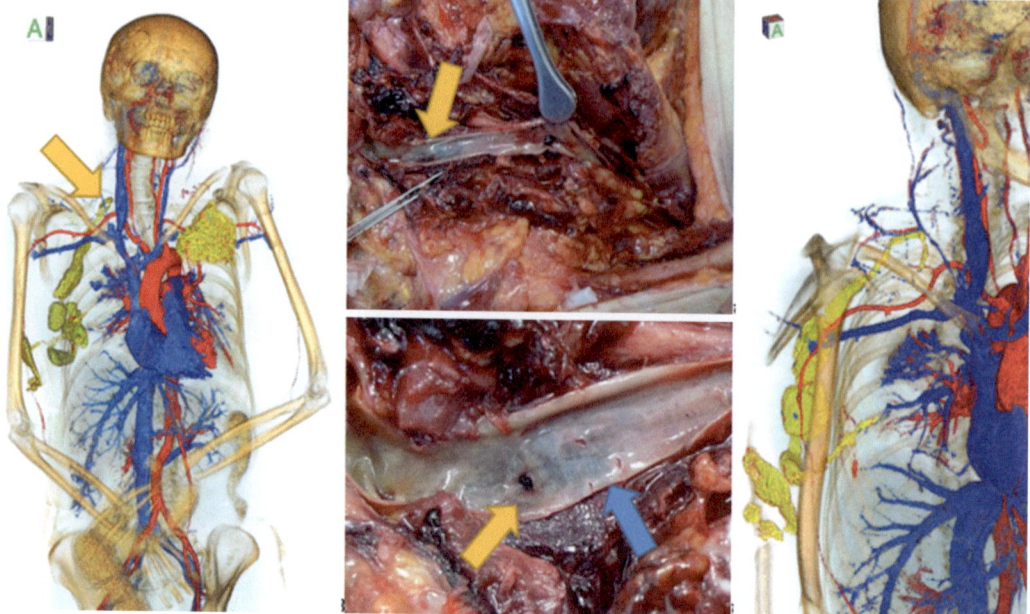

Fig. 8.17 Case of failed cannulation of subclavian vein in clinical setting (artery mistaken with vein while US-guided cannulation)—preautopsy, postmortem CT angiography (phase subtraction visualization: arterial phase, red color; venous, blue; extravascular blood collections, yellow. PMCTA visualized perforation site in right subclavian artery (orange arrows), and nearby three minor intimal injuries (blue arrow)

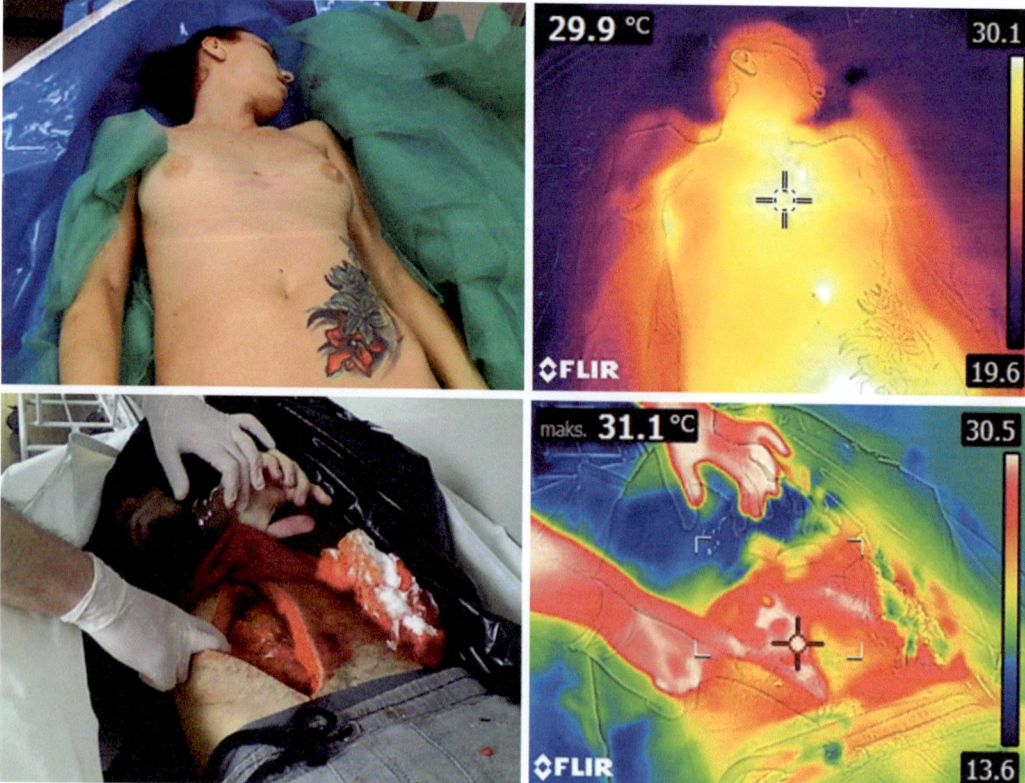

Fig. 8.18 Properties of thermal imaging in postmortem studies: homogenous decrease in temperature of superficial structures (upper row), increased temperature of internal organs can be shown after their exposure (lower row)

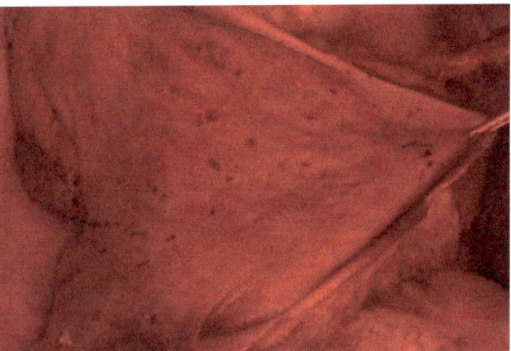

Fig. 8.19 Examples of near-IR use for assessment of putridly transformed mucosa of the stomach (photos taken with modified digital camera, where standard filter which cuts off IR was replaced with filter removing most of vis-ible light spectrum). On the left, course of submucosal blood vessels, on the right: disseminated ulcerations of mucosa

proximal and is much faster on the surface than in internal organs (Fig. 8.2); therefore, control of skin temperature may be only used for initial screening, with no chance of preliminary diagnosis.

Charge-coupled device (CCD) matrix of digital cameras has the capability of recording invisible parts of the spectrum of light within so-called near-infrared light with wavelength 0.75–1.5 μm (Fig. 8.19). This range may be isolated using additional filters (only modified devices allow for direct IR photography) with need of additional processing of images recorded in RAW format [33–35]. Using this feature is a kind of substitute of thermographic camera (due to limited range of detection compared to a thermal camera, need of modification of digital camera) but may significantly improve visualization of some of changes important for medicolegal and criminal aspects:

- Poorly visible suggillations and bloody infiltrations (IR penetrates into subcutaneous or submucosal layers up to few millimeters)
- Some identification features (poorly visible tattoos on decayed or dried bodies)
- Traces of removed tattoo or tattoo masking
- Hemorrhagic foci in decaying tissues

Application of alternative sources of light seems legit in case of widely decayed bodies, as IR photography allows for visualization of hemorrhagic foci (Wischnewski spots) within putridly discolored mucosa of the stomach, after removal of stomach contents and avoiding mechanical injury of easily peeling mucosa [36].

Additionally, in some cases of hypothermia, 3D scanning can be a useful tool where identification is needed (see Chap. 1).

8.5 Special Issues

8.5.1 Pulmonary Edema

Literature data on frequency of pulmonary edema in hypothermia are contradictory. This finding is frequently listed in textbooks and reviews on hypothermia, both clinical and forensic. However, in the published series of CT studies of hypothermia victims, it was observed relatively rarely. Pulmonary edema is a typical sign of acute left ventricular dysfunction, although there may be also a negative-pressure pulmonary edema (post-obstructive pulmonary edema, noncardiogenic pulmonary edema) that occurs after intense inspiratory effort against an obstructed airway, e.g., laryngospasm. Among possible etiologies there is also high-altitude pulmonary edema (see Sect. 8.5.3).

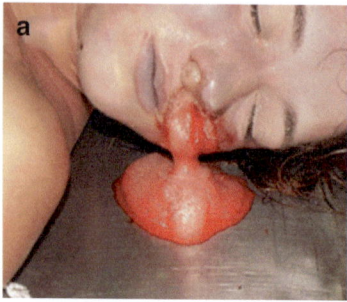 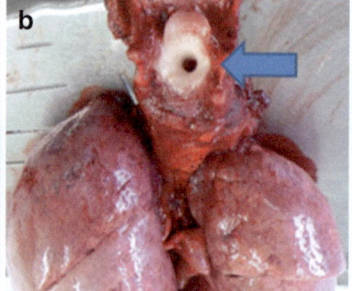 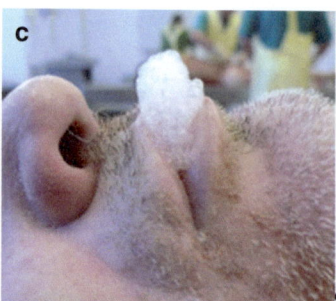

Fig. 8.20 Foamy contents of the airways as macroscopic sign of pulmonary edema—pink-reddish thin foam suggests cardiogenic or high-altitude pulmonary edema (**a**); thick, dense whitish foam is typical for foamed surfactant in cases of drowning (**b, c**)

Variable frequency of pulmonary edema is also reported in fatal alcohol intoxication, which may result from concomitant cardiovascular diseases and degree of intoxication (similarly to hypothermia). In cases of deaths supposedly related to hypothermia, pulmonary edema is observed more frequently macroscopically than in PMCT (postmortem radiography has not been evaluated for this purpose). Therefore, this finding is not considered a reliable marker of hypothermia, as it may also result from aspiration of water into the airways (Fig. 8.20). In the forensic practice, cases of submersion accompanied by cooling of the body (wet hypothermia) are not uncommon.

8.5.2 Immersion Hypothermia or Drowning in Winter Setting

In medicolegal opinions there may be need of distinguishing hypothermia from other causes of death, when the body was revealed in conditions suggestive of possible effect of low environmental temperature. This is particularly valid for cases of unwitnessed death of functional nature with no perceptible morphological changes (nonstructural), e.g., sudden cardiac arrest due to cardiac rhythm disturbances (e.g., inherited arrhythmia syndromes—channelopathies, arrhythmogenic cardiomyopathies), acute diabetic hypoglycemia, sudden death in epileptic patient, etc.

In the autumn/winter time, one frequently has to identify the cause of death in deceased found in water reservoirs, frequently in shallow water. In such cases it is necessary to distinguish drowning from acute hypothermia of immersion type. The so-called wet hypothermia, as opposed to cases of "dry," atmospheric cooling, usually does not produce typical external discolorations with features of frostbite and hemolytic diffusion. Then, the only perceptible external sign is bright lividity; however, this sign is unspecific, and commonly observed in cadavers exposed to cold (independent of cause of death). It may be even artificially produced in cadavers stored in a refrigerator room by lowering the temperature [11]. This sign (just like light red shade of lung tissue) results from left shift of an oxygen dissociation curve which results in an increased hemoglobin's O_2 saturation.

Differential diagnosis between hypothermia and drowning may be challenging [37, 38], as acute pulmonary immersion emphysema (emphysema aquosum) may sometimes appear similar to acute emphysema observed in victims of hypothermia, or in cases of mechanical asphyxia (Fig. 8.21). Furthermore, signs of pulmonary edema observed in some cases of acute hypothermia [39] may mimic signs of foaming of surfactant typical for drowning—immersion pulmonary edema (Fig. 8.26). Typical external foam collection is less frequently observed in winter conditions.

Hypothesis of drowning should be supported by signs detected in PMCT—presence of fluid in sphenoid sinuses and hemorrhages in air cells of pyramids of temporal bones (Fig. 8.22).

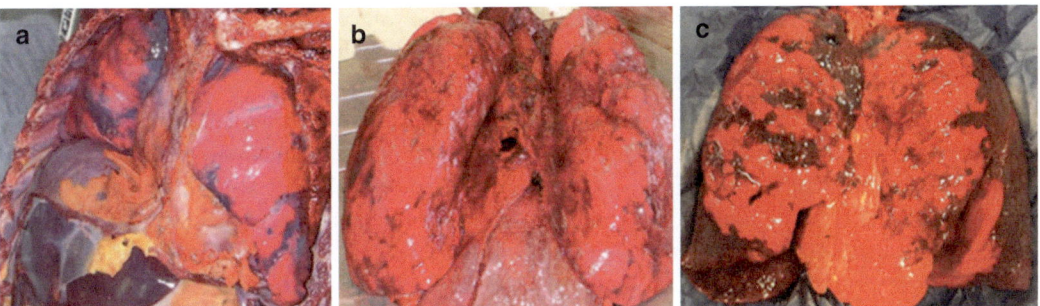

Fig. 8.21 Light red areas of acute subpleural emphysema in fatal hypothermia (**a**), drowning (**b**), and mechanical asphyxia in the mechanism of chest compression by a vehicle (**c**); part (**a**) courtesy of Dr. Pierre Perich, Service de Médecine Légale, Institut Médico-Légal, Marseille, France

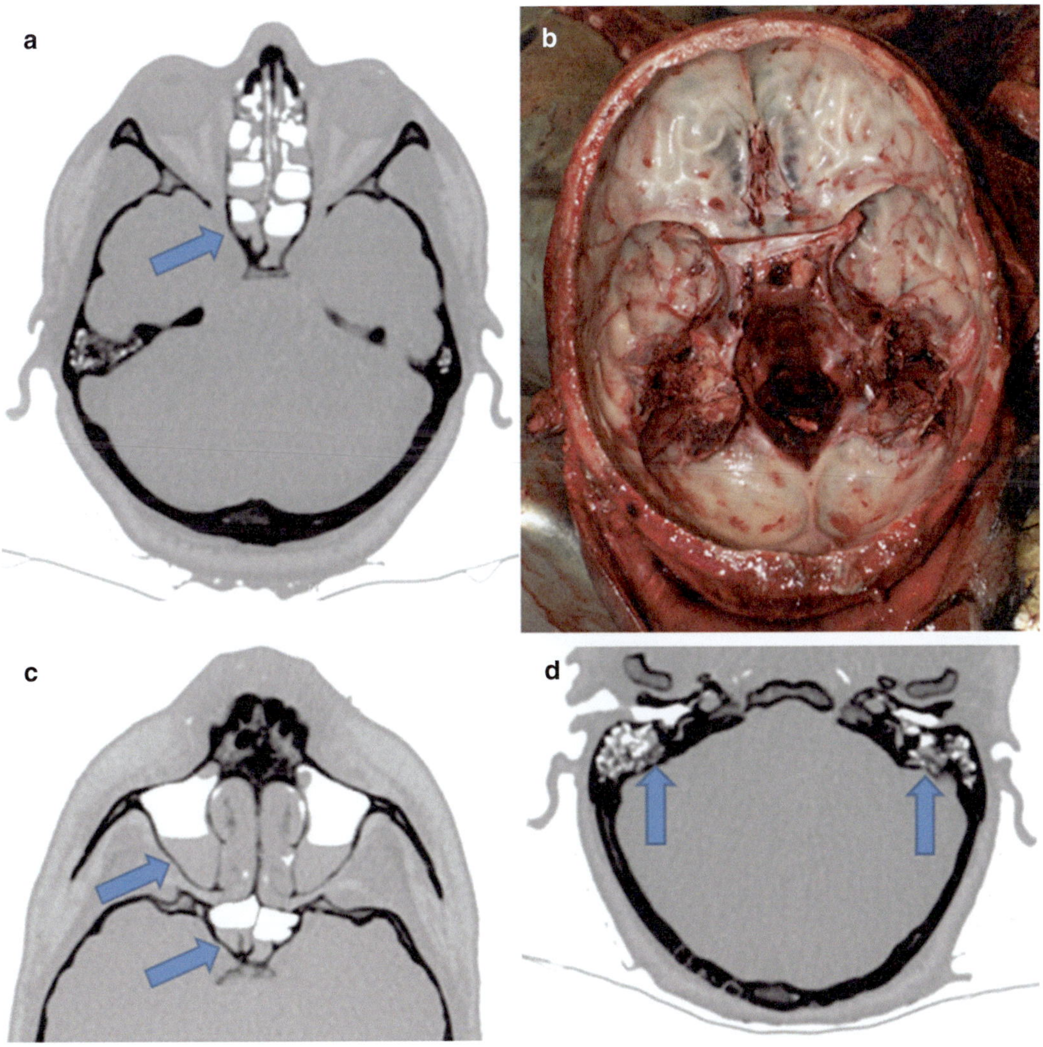

Fig. 8.22 Presence of fluid (**a**, **c**) in sphenoid, maxillary, and ethmoid sinuses (PMCT) and hemorrhages (**b**, **d**) in ethmoid sinuses and air cells of pyramids of temporal bones (chiseled during autopsy) in drowning case

8.5.3 Hypothermia-Related Deaths in Mountains

High-altitude deaths frequently suggest fatal hypothermia, however, should be distinguished from other life-threatening mechanisms. Among them there is HAPE (high-altitude pulmonary edema) syndrome, which is a severe presentation of altitude sickness. It is a form of noncardiogenic pulmonary edema, which affects predisposed people normally living at low altitude who travel to an altitude above 2500 m. One risk factor of HAPE (except cold exposure and low air pressure at high altitudes) is persistent foramen ovale; however, genetic predisposition is also suspected. In postmortem examination in HAPE pink, frothy or frankly bloody sputum is observed. Chest X-ray or CT shows opaque patchy alveolar infiltrates, particularly in the right middle lobe [38, 40, 41].

HAPE may precede other syndrome, HACE (high-altitude cerebral edema), which may develop in the setting of rapid ascent to a high altitude [40, 42]. Pathologically HACE results from vasogenic cerebral edema, which untreated may lead to death due to brain herniation. Intravital radiological diagnosis of cerebral edema is usually uncomplicated. Postmortem identification of cerebral edema in PMCT is more complicated due to postmortem changes. Other signs of HACE are retinal venous dilation and retinal hemorrhages [42], which may be diagnosed postmortem in the fundus of the eyeball, for example, by the use of a mini-endoscope (Fig. 8.23).

Death in the high mountains is characterized by several typical situations, and potential interpretative difficulties. For example, rare cases of skeletal injuries result not from mechanical trauma but deep freezing of the body—classical example is separation of cranial sutures due to freezing of brain, when formation of ice crystals increases the brain volume (Fig. 8.24).

To our knowledge, there are no studies on influence of the altitude to classical markers of hypothermia, particularly to hyperaeration with decreased vascularity of pulmonary tissue.

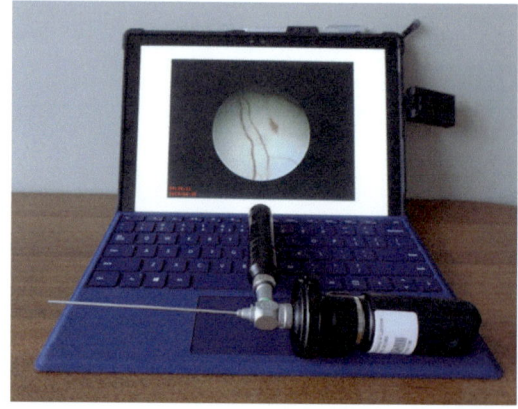

Fig. 8.23 Video arthroscope with source of light, for postmortem analysis of the fundus of the eyeball, with wireless transmission

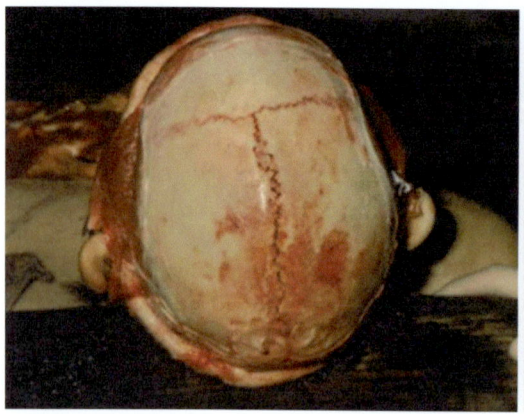

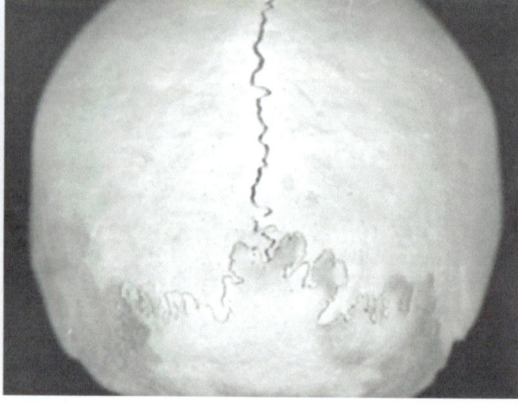

Fig. 8.24 Separation of sagittal suture due to freezing of the brain in case of hanging in secluded forest location in heavy winter conditions; figure courtesy of prof. Anna Niemcunowicz-Janica, Department of Forensic Medicine, Medical University in Bialystok, Poland

Postmortem imaging is extremely useful for differential diagnosis of cause of death in avalanche victims [43–46]. In this population, several groups can be distinguished, according to the pathogenetic cause of the mechanical trauma:

- Mechanical injuries (usually in so-called slab avalanches):
  - Blunt trauma (particularly head) due to hitting by moving fragments of ice or rocks
  - Fall from height
- Asphyxia due to crushing by mass of snow (usually in so-called loose snow avalanches) or mass of soil displaced by avalanche:
  - Compressive asphyxia—immobilization of the chest (suffocation)
  - Obturative asphyxia—blockage of the airways with aspiration (Fig. 8.25)
- Hypothermia—while waiting for rescue:
  - Covering by loose snow with formation of the so-called air pocket
  - Incapacitation trauma
- Drowning—due to dislocation of the victim into a mountain river or lake.

Hypothermia and drowning are the rarest causes of death in avalanche victims; however, such diagnosis can be made after rejection of other causes [47]. In multiple cases, more than one mechanism can be identified (Fig. 8.26). Differential diagnosis between hypothermia, asphyxia, and drowning is particularly difficult due to similar morphological appearance at autopsy (see above). When there are no typical morphological changes, diagnosis of nontraumatic cause of death based only on autopsy results may be extremely difficult or even impossible.

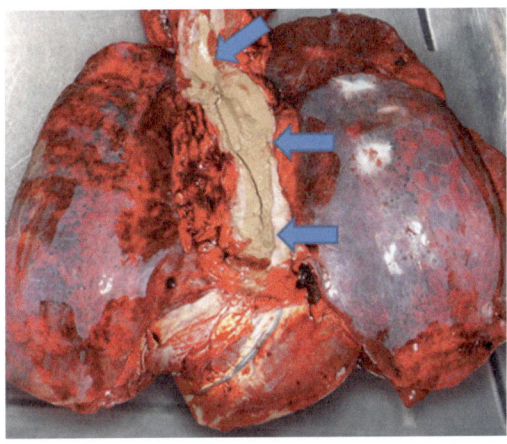

Fig. 8.25 Acute asphyxia due to aspiration of muddy contents into airways and esophagus (arrows) with signs of acute emphysema (pink-red foci on the surface of the lungs) subpleural and subpericardial with disseminated ecchymoses (light red bloody spots on the surface of the lungs)

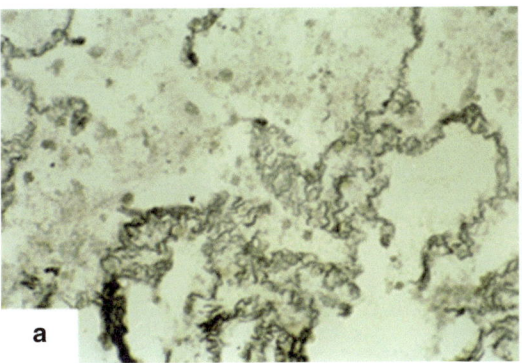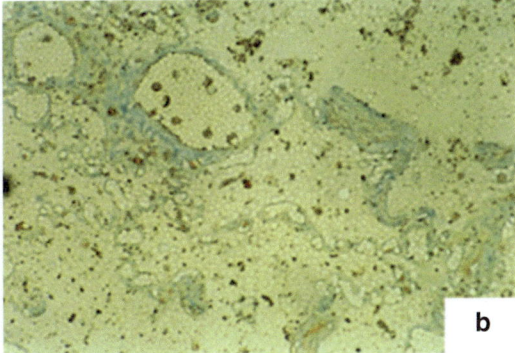

Fig. 8.26 Histochemical specimens of the lung of the avalanche victim—group of tourists was swept by snow masses, which traveled over 1200 m and eventually pushed into a mountain lake (breaking the ice layer), and were found after several months. (**a**) Gomori staining: thickening of interalveolar septa with fragmentation of reticular fibers (typical for IV stage of acute pulmonary emphysema in Reh scale). (**b**) AZAN staining (azocarmine-aniline blue): multiple hemolyzed erythrocytes in the lumen of the vessel and in pulmonary alveoli; stainings courtesy of dr. Rafal Skowronek, Department of Forensic Medicine, Silesian Medical University

8.5.4 Examination of Decomposed Body

Bodies of missing persons revealed in mountains may frequently be revealed after long period, with advanced decomposition. Blurring of tissue architecture due to decay may hinder identification of any morphological features of hypothermia. In some instances, hemorrhagic foci can be visualized within putridly transformed gastric mucosa by infrared photography (see Sect. 8.4.4). Histochemical examination of lung specimens sometimes suggests suffocation as mechanism of death (Fig. 8.26).

Degree of postmortem tissue decay depends on time period between accident and revealing of the body (not uncommonly, after several winter seasons, i.e., multiple freezing and defreezing cycles). Decay further advances in the time required for defreezing of the body before the autopsy. These processes are paradoxically accelerated when additional actions are taken to speed up defreezing—as external layers warm up, decay progresses faster, while the inner structures remain frozen. Therefore, time necessary for defreezing should be used for imaging (see section below).

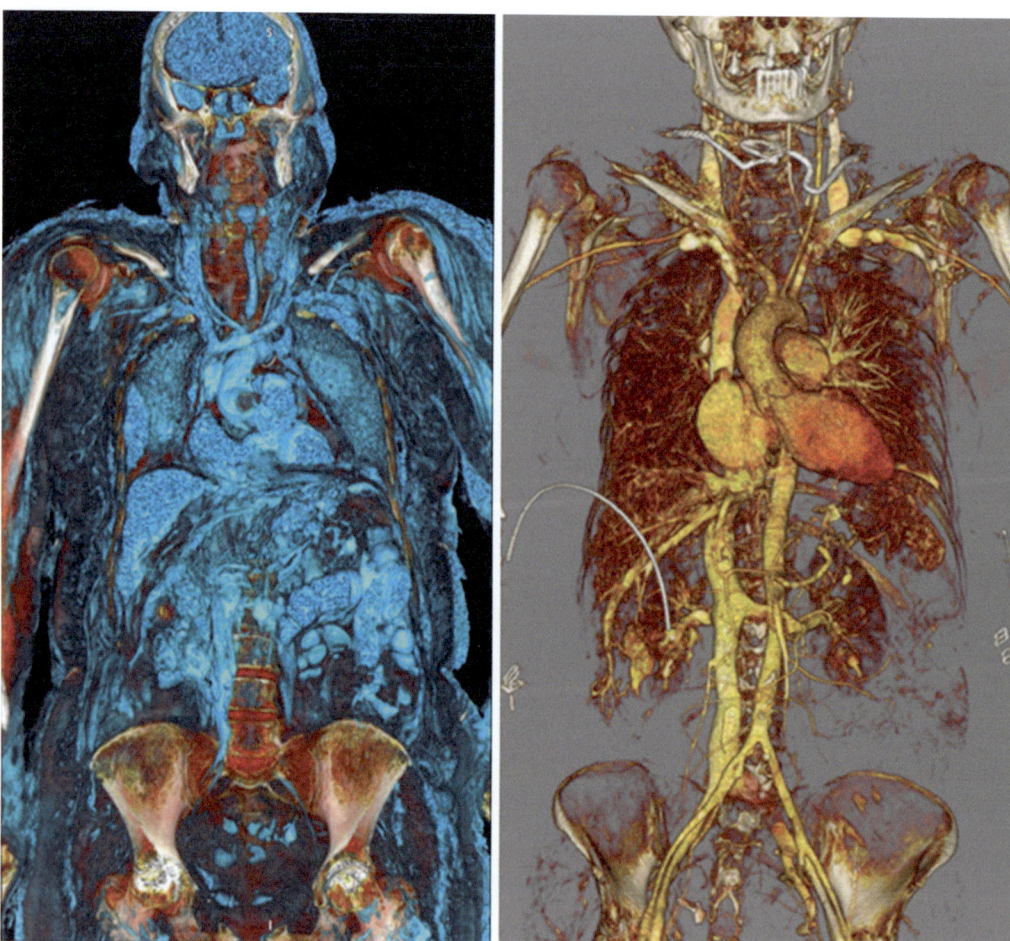

Fig. 8.27 Postmortem CT angiography of remains exhumed 6 months after the death, during severe cold weather—deeply frozen, with extensive putrefaction. Reconstruction of native scan on the left, vascular system partially visualized due to the presence of putrid gases, on the right—vascular reconstruction with contrast in venous and arterial bed

Fig. 8.28 Postmortem imaging of cadaver in metal transport coffin, winter period—virtual fusion of digital radiographs produced with vertical and horizontal exposure, in the bottom—three-dimensional reconstruction of CT (digital radiography and CT performed in Postmortem Imaging Lab at Department of Forensic Medicine, Medical University of Lublin)

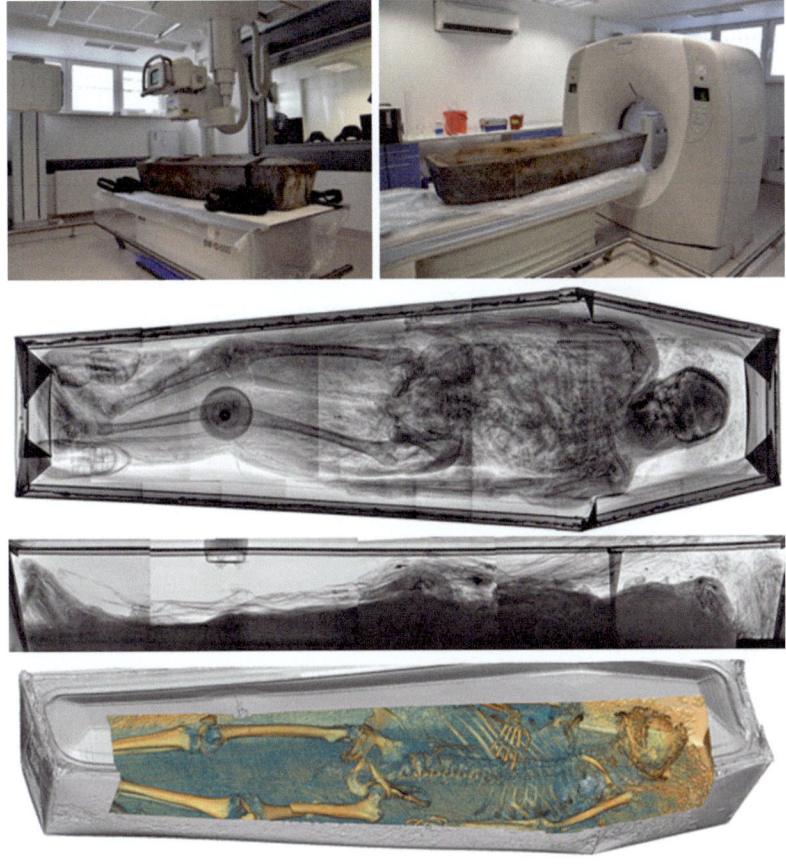

8.5.5 Imaging of Frozen Corpses

Some of the victims revealed in secluded locations after long time since death are referred to forensic medicine departments deeply frozen. Furthermore, as autumn/winter months are standard time of scheduled exhumations, contents of the coffin may present frozen. Freezing of the body hinders immediate autopsy [48], while imaging may be performed at this period [21]. In cases of advanced putrefaction, frozen state of the body allows to visualize outlines of internal organs, as well as course of the main blood vessels, filled with putrid gas, before contrast media administration is even possible (Fig. 8.27). From practical perspective, bodies delivered in coffins may be scanned before their removal, which may be performed already in autopsy room, to avoid contamination of imaging facility (Fig. 8.28). This may be important for departments which share imaging facilities with clinical departments.

8.6 Practice of Investigation of Hypothermic Death

Postmortem diagnosis of hypothermia is still a major challenge in forensic practice, as diagnosis is generally made by exclusion, i.e., when all other evidence is negative (trauma, histopathology, toxicology) except some biochemistry markers [2, 48]. Therefore, a huge panel of examinations is required consisting of both autopsy and additional examinations to exclude other causes of death. Postmortem imaging may play a significant role in this aspect.

The main verification of cause of death bases upon the analysis of the environmental conditions (temperature) after exclusion of other possible causes (trauma, intoxication, disease). Process of cooling the body takes long time (particularly in "city"-type hypothermia), however, is not necessarily accompanied by perceptible macro- or microscopic changes (especially when cooling occurs in above-zero temperatures). Signs identified in such cases are frequently nonspecific and only confirm local effects of cold exposure:

- Effects of cold on the skin:
  - Light red lividity (result of reoxidation of hemoglobin)
  - Discoloration of the skin of extensor side of the limbs, typically knees and elbows (Fig. 8.3: hemolytic discolorations of the skin and subcutaneous tissue of the face, anterior surface of the knee, foot, hand, and elbow (with no perceptible hemorrhages after dissection of the skin) in victims of fatal hypothermia)
  - Frostbite of other, distal or uncovered body parts (hands, feet, face)
  - Hemolytic discolorations of synovial membrane of knee joints (inner knee sign)
- Nonspecific signs of acute multiorgan failure:
  - Cerebral edema, edema or acute emphysema of the lungs, and subpleural petechiae
- Secondary organ lesions:
  - Hemorrhagic erosions of gastric mucosa—Wischnewski spots (Fig. 8.6).
  - Rarely observed hemorrhagic necrosis of other segments of the digestive tract.
  - Acute pancreatitis—usually in slowly progressing hypothermia in elderly patients in unheated accommodation (Fig. 8.7)

- Rarely observed hemorrhages in iliopsoas muscles (Fig. 8.8)
- Microscopic and histochemical changes:
  - Deficiency of hepatic glycogen in PAS staining (Fig. 8.29)
  - Degeneration and necrosis of cardiomyocytes
  - Accumulation of lipids in epithelial cells of proximal tubules in renal cortex
  - Vacuolar degeneration of hypophysis and adrenal medulla
  - Decreased contents of lipids in adrenal cortex and brown adipose tissue cells.
- Lesions diagnosed with postmortem imaging, CT or MR:
  - Increased lung lucency
  - Hemorrhages in paravertebral muscles
- Biochemical consequences of protection mechanisms:
  - Activation of hypothalamus-pituitary-adrenal axis
  - Increased level of catabolic enzymes
  - Markers of activation of lipolysis and ketogenesis
- Behavioral effects:
  - Paradoxical undressing
  - Terminal burrowing

The apparently broad spectrum of diagnostic possibilities does not actually show actual feasibility of markers in real life; indeed there are many aspects that should be considered, such as:

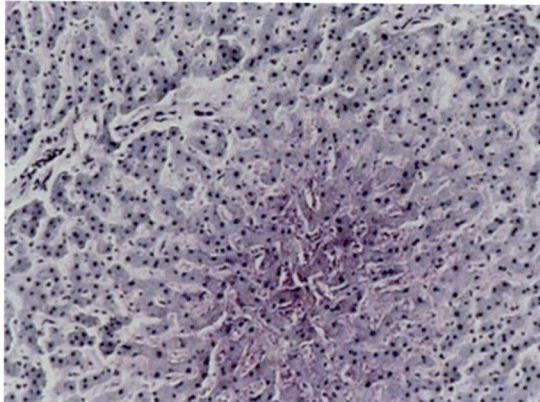
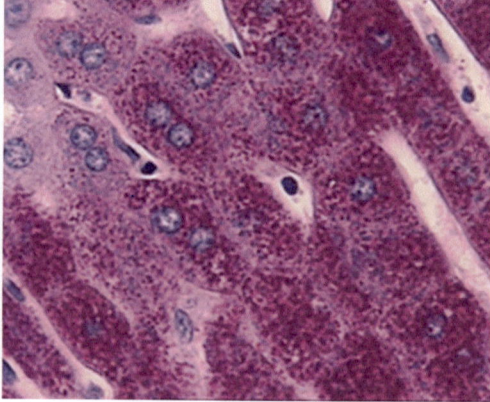
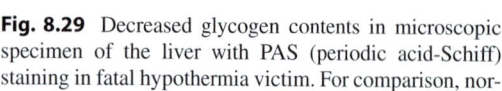

Fig. 8.29 Decreased glycogen contents in microscopic specimen of the liver with PAS (periodic acid-Schiff) staining in fatal hypothermia victim. For comparison, normal glycogen contents in the liver on the right; stainings courtesy of dr. Rafal Skowronek, Department of Forensic Medicine, Silesian Medical University

- Fatal hypothermia may occur in the absence of any classical signs
- Signs of hypothermia are highly variable; some of them occur extremely rarely
- Severity of signs of hypothermia depends on rate of cooling and time of agony
- Most of signs appear after prolonged exposure to cold
- Local effects of exposure to cold occur only when temperature approaches 0 °C
- Most of signs of hypothermia are observed less frequently in alcohol-intoxicated victims
- Signs of hypothermia are unspecific:
  - Wischnewski spots are only one of forms of acute stress ulcerations
  - Similar microscopic changes are observed in several pathologies
  - Red postmortem lividity may occur in carbon monoxide or cyanide poisoning
  - Red postmortem lividity is also observed in freezing of dead body
  - Change of color of postmortem lividity may occur while storage of refrigerated body due to diffusion of environmental oxygen
  - Hemorrhages in perivertebral muscles should not be confused with trauma
  - Paradoxical undressing should not be confused with rape
  - Decreased glycogen contents in the liver may result from cachexia, starvation, alcoholism, and stress
  - Vacuolization and lipid degeneration of epithelium of renal tubules (Armanni-Ebstein sign) may result from diabetes, not hypothermia
  - Postmortem autolysis affects glycogen levels
  - Changes considered to be signs of acute pancreatitis may actually result from autolysis

Basically, microscopic and immunohistochemical studies do not allow yet for reliable diagnosis of fatal hypothermia [11, 49–52].

Even Wischnewski spots considered "classical" sign hypothermia are nonspecific, and are fully formed only after long-lasting agony, when extravasated hemoglobin is transformed into brown hematin by acidic stomach contents. In quick decrease of temperature and more rapid death, gastric ulcerations are less frequent and remain red.

Gradual depletion of energy stores in hypothermia results in transformation of tissue catabolism into glucose-sparing processes. Due to release of insulin-counteracting hormones, free fatty acids are mobilized and ketone bodies are produced in the liver. These substances easily cross cellular membranes and become the main energy substrate in advanced hypothermia. Increased acetonemia is easily detected at routine ethanol analysis by gas chromatography [53]. Ketonemia is usually accompanied by ketonuria, which may be detected during autopsy by means of portable urine analyzer (Fig. 8.30).

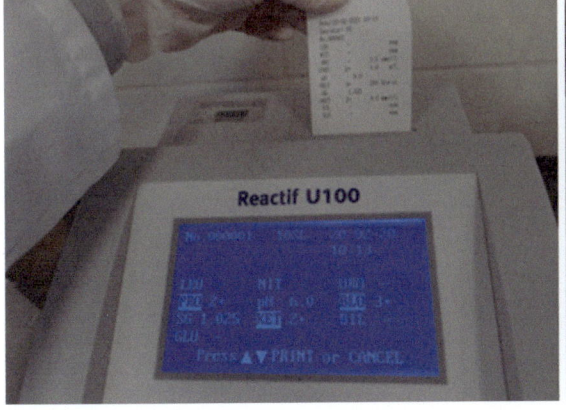 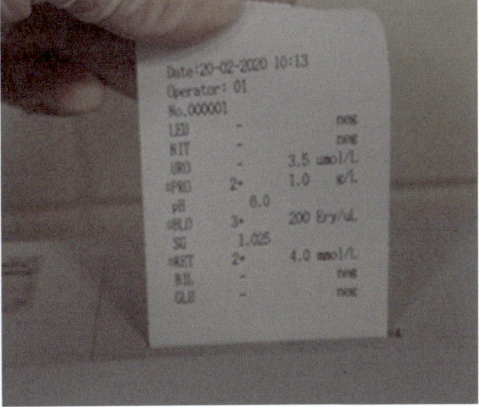

Fig. 8.30 Portable analyzer use for point-of-care assessment of ketonuria in the course of autopsy

Even revealing of the body in a setting suggestive for hypothermia (frozen body covered by snow, or frozen to the ground) does not always lead to confirmation of fatal hypothermia, even in situations of unequivocal earlier alcohol consumption (see section below). In each case, a full autopsy procedure should be conducted, and in lack of clear intravital effects of exposure to cold, broadened toxicological analysis should be performed, to exclude other possible mechanism (trauma, poisoning, perceptible micro- or macroscopic pathologies). Postmortem imaging plays an important role in this field.

In lack of typical morphological signs of hypothermia, analysis using an as broad as possible spectrum of markers should be made, with an increasing role of biochemical analysis (increased level of ketone bodies, free fatty acids, and glucocorticosteroids).

8.7   Diagnosis of Hypothermia in Alcohol Intoxication

Alcohol is frequently detected in victims of fatal hypothermia (vast majority of cases in Poland). Alcohol promotes rapid loss of body heat and shortens agony period [54–56], reducing frequency of classical signs of hypothermia (Table 8.2).

Ethanol does not induce significant thermogenesis—only 10–20% of energy from its oxidation is radiated in the form of heat [9]. Small alcohol doses do not influence significantly loss of heat only in mild exposure to cold [57]. Larger doses combined with exposure to low environmental temperatures lead to rapid decrease of core temperature (poikilothermic effect) due to combination of several actions (Fig. 8.31):

- Dilation of peripheral blood vessels—depletion of basic physiological mechanism protecting against loss of heat
- Relaxation of muscles—blockage of shivering thermogenesis
- Reduced activity of central thermoregulation
- Depressive and analgesic influence to CNS—loss of sensation or increased tolerance of pain (cold induced) and loss of protective mechanisms (protection against cold)
- Behavioral influence—false feeling of heat, undressing, lack of awareness of danger, and seeking protection
- Inhibition of release of catabolic hormones, mainly catecholamines
- Disturbance of adaptation mechanisms on biochemical level—indirect influence of change of redox potential in oxidation of alcohol (increased NADH/NAD ratio)

Table 8.2 Frequency of macroscopic markers of hypothermia depending on sobriety of victims [9]

Marker	Blood alcohol concentration (BAC)	
	≤1‰	>1‰
Red postmortem lividity	60%	36%
Discolorations of knees and elbows	40%	20%
Other location of frostbite	50%	13%
Wischnewski spots	45%	12%
Pulmonary edema	35%	40%
Pancreatitis	10%	0%
Paradoxical undressing	23%	11%

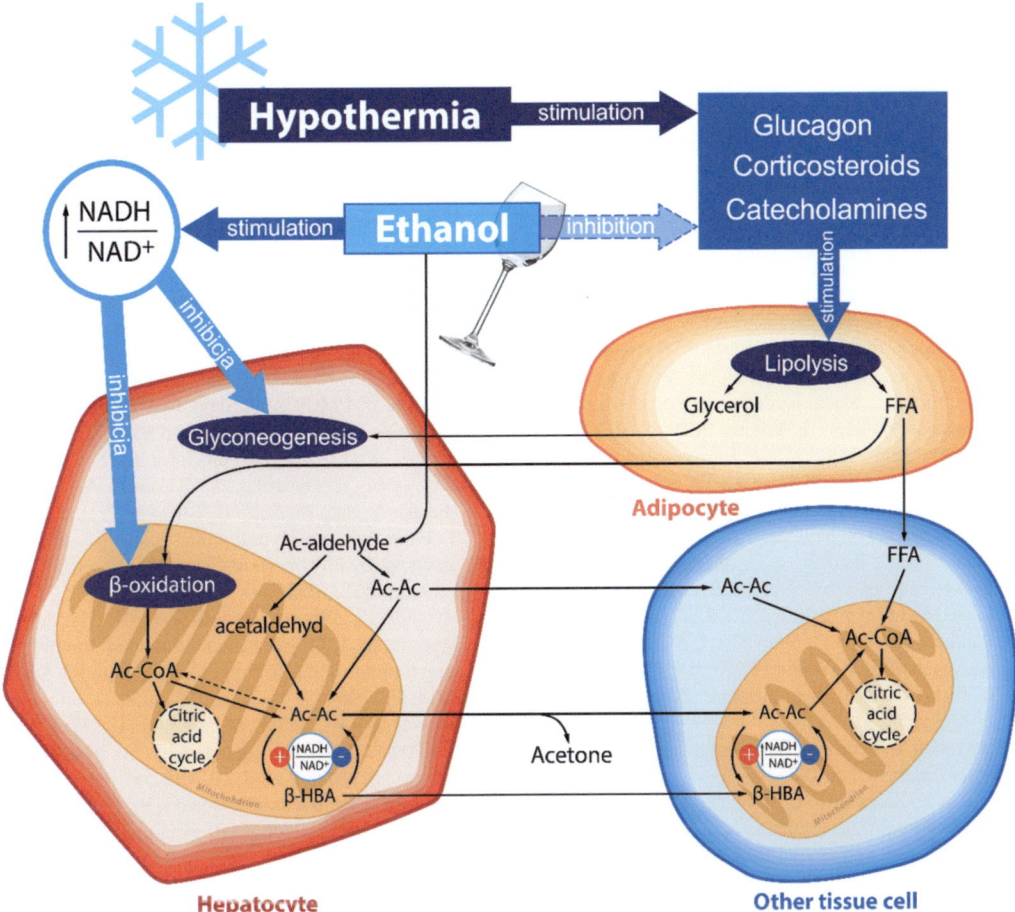

Fig. 8.31 Mechanisms (1–4) of antiketonemic potential of ethanol in hypothermia (*FFA* free fatty acids, *β-HBA* β-hydroxybutyric acid, *Ac-Ac* acetoacetate, *Ac-CoA* acetyl-coenzyme A)

In insobriety and exposure to cold, physiological disturbance of adaptative reactions occurs also on a biochemical level due to inhibition of gluconeogenesis (post-alcohol hypoglycemia), and clearly antiketonemic influence of ethanol (production of ketone bodies in cooling organism is too small compared to tissue needs) [9, 58]. With worsening of insobriety, levels of most of biochemical markers of hypothermia decrease, which is additional difficulty for the diagnostic process of such cases [10, 59]. Except for routine analysis of blood acetone level, other biochemical markers should be included, which are less dependent on simultaneous alcoholemia (glucocorticosteroids, free fatty acids) [60–62].

Acknowledgement Tables and some of the figures have been used in textbook "Medycyna sądowa" [Forensic Medicine] ed. G. Teresiński, volumes 1–3, PZWL Medical Publishing House [in Polish]—with written permission from the Publisher.

References

1. Madea B, Tsokos M, Preuss J. Death due to hypothermia. Morphological findings, their pathogenesis and diagnostic value. In: Tsokos M, editor. Forensic pathology reviews, vol. 5. Humana Press; 2008. p. 3–21.
2. Palmiere C, Teresiński G, Hejna P. Postmortem diagnosis of hypothermia. Int J Legal Med. 2014;128(4):607–14.

3. Türk EE. Hypothermia. Forensic Sci Med Pathol. 2010;6:106–15.
4. Ulrich AS, Rathlev NK. Hypothermia and localized cold injuries. Emerg Med Clin North Am. 2004;22(2):281–98.
5. Lange S, Muggenthaler H, Hubig M, Mall G. The forensic relevance of hypothermia in living persons—literature and retrospective study. Forensic Sci Int. 2013;231(1-3):34–41.
6. Golden FS, Tipton MJ, Scott RC. Immersion, near-drowning and drowning. Br J Anaesth. 1997;79(2):214–25.
7. Witzmann FA. Temperature regulation and exercise physiology, the regulation of body temperature. In: Rhoades RA, Bell DR, editors. Medical physiology: principles for clinical medicine. 3rd ed. Philadelphia: Lippincott Williams & Wilkins; 2009. p. 543–66.
8. Hall JE. Body temperature, temperature regulation, and fever. In: Guyton AC, Hall JE, editors. Textbook of medical physiology. 11th ed. Philadelphia: Elsevier; 2006. p. 889–901.
9. Teresiński G, Buszewicz G, Mądro R. Biochemical background of ethanol-induced cold susceptibility. Legal Med (Tokyo). 2005;7:15–23.
10. Palmiere C, Bardy D, Letovanec I, Mangin P, Iglesias K, Augsburger M, Ventura F, Werner D. Biochemical markers of fatal hypothermia. Forensic Sci Int. 2013;226:54–61.
11. Hirvonen J. Necropsy findings in fatal hypothermia cases. Forensic Sci. 1976;8:155–64.
12. Hejna P, Zátopková L, Tsokos M. The diagnostic value of synovial membrane hemorrhage and bloody discoloration of synovial fluid ("inner knee sign") in autopsy cases of fatal hypothermia. Int J Legal Med. 2012;126:415–9.
13. Bright F, Winskog C, Byard RW. Wischnewski spots and hypothermia: sensitive, specific, or serendipitous? Forensic Sci Med Pathol. 2013;9:88–90.
14. Preuss J, Lignitz E, Dettmeyer R, Madea B. Pancreatic changes in cases of death due to hypothermia. Forensic Sci Int. 2007;166:194–8.
15. Ogata M, Ago K, Kondo T, Kasai K, Ishikawa T, Mikuzami H. A fatal case of hypothermia associated with hemorrhages of the pectoralis minor, intercostals, and iliopsoas muscles. Am J Forensic Med Pathol. 2007;28:348–52.
16. Nikolić S, Zivković V, Juković F, Babić D, Stanojkovski G. Simon's bleedings: a possible mechanism of appearance and forensic importance—a prospective autopsy study. Int J Legal Med. 2009;123(4):293–7.
17. Kitzinger R, Risse M, Puschel K. Kälteidiotie Paradoxes Entkleiden bei Unterkühlung. Arch Kriminol. 1991;187:47–56.
18. Rothschild M. Lethal hypothermia: paradoxical undressing and hide-and-die-syndrome can produce very obscure death scenes. In: Tsokos M, editor. Forensic pathology reviews, vol. 1. Humana Press Inc.; 2004. p. 263–72.
19. Wedin B, Vanggaard L, Hirvonen J. Paradoxical undressing in fatal hypothermia. J Forensic Sci. 1979;24:543–53.
20. Schäfer AT. Human primitive behavior. In: Tsokos M, editor. Forensic pathology reviews, vol. 2. Humana Press; 2005. p. 189–204.
21. Grabherr S, Baumann P, Minoiu C, Fahrni S, Mangin P. Post-mortem imaging in forensic investigations: current utility, limitations, and ongoing developments. Res Rep Forensic Med Sci. 2016;6:25–37.
22. Grabherr S, Egger C, Vilarino R, Campana L, Jotterand M, Dedouit F. Modern post-mortem imaging: an update on recent developments. Forensic Sci Res. 2017;2(2):52–64.
23. Chatzaraki V, Heimer J, Thali M, Dally A, Schweitzer W. Role of PMCT as a triage tool between external inspection and full autopsy—case series and review. J Forensic Radiol Imaging. 2018;15:26–38.
24. Kawasumi Y, Onozuka N, Kakizaki A, Usui A, Hosokai Y, Sato M, Saito H, Ishibashi T, Hayashizaki Y, Funayama M. Hypothermic death: possibility of diagnosis by post-mortem computed tomography. Eur J Radiol. 2013;82:361–5.
25. Hyodoh H, Watanabe S, Katada R, Hyodoh K, Matsumoto H. Postmortem computed tomography lung findings in fatal of hypothermia. Forensic Sci Int. 2013;231:190–4.
26. Schweitzer W, Thali M, Giugni G, Winklhofer S. Postmortem pulmonary CT in hypothermia. Forensic Sci Med Pathol. 2014;10:557–69.
27. Fracasso T, Brinkmann B, Beike J, Pfeiffer H. Clotted blood as sign of alcohol intoxication: a retrospective study. Int J Legal Med. 2008;122:157–61.
28. Aghayev E, Thali MJ, Jackowski C, Sonnenschein M, Dirnhofer R, Yen K. MRI detects hemorrhages in the muscles of the back in hypothermia. Forensic Sci Int. 2008;176:183–6.
29. Teresiński G. Injuries of the thigh, knee, and ankle as reconstructive factors in road traffic accidents. In: Rich J, Dean DE, Powers RH, editors. Forensic medicine of the lower extremity. Forensic science and medicine. Totowa: Humana Press; 2005. p. 311–42.
30. Mimasaka S, Oshima T, Ohtani M. Characterization of bruises using ultrasonography for potential application in diagnosis of child abuse. Legal Med (Tokyo). 2011;14(1):6–10.
31. Charlier P, Chaillot PF, Watier L, Ménétrier M, Carlier R, Cavard S, Hervé C, de la Grandmaison GL, Huynh-Charlier I. Is post-mortem ultrasonography a useful tool for forensic purposes? Med Sci Law. 2013;53(4):227–34.
32. Fariña J, Millana C, Fdez-Aceñero MJ, Furió V, Aragoncillo P, Martín VG, Buencuerpo J. Ultrasonographical autopsy (echopsy): a new autopsy technique. Virchows Arch. 2002;440:635–9.
33. Sterzik V, Bohnert M. Reconstruction of crimes by infrared photography. Int J Legal Med. 2016;130(5):1379–85.

34. Oliver WR, Leone L. Digital UV/IR photography for tattoo evaluation in mummified remains. J Forensic Sci. 2012;57(4):1134–6.

35. Cullip M, Tran VC, Ball CG. Tattoo visualization using cross-polarized lighting and infrared photography. Forensic Sci Med Pathol. 2021;17(2):350–3.

36. Rost T, Kalberer N, Scheurer E. A user-friendly technical set-up for infrared photography of forensic findings. Forensic Sci Int. 2017;278:148–55.

37. Hourscht C, Christe A, Diers S, Thali MJ, Ruder TD. Learning from the living to diagnose the dead—parallels between CT findings after survived drowning and fatal drowning. Forensic Sci Med Pathol. 2019;15(2):249–51.

38. Lindholm P, Swenson ER, Martínez-Jiménez S, Guo HH. From ocean deep to mountain high: similar computed tomography findings in immersion and high-altitude pulmonary edema. Am J Respir Crit Care Med. 2018;198(8):1088–9.

39. Perich P, Tuchtan L, Bartoli C, Léonetti G, Piercecchi-Marti MD. Death from hypothermia during a training course under "extreme conditions": related to two cases. J Forensic Sci. 2016;61(2):562–5.

40. Hackett PH, Luks AM, Lawley JS, Roach RC. High-altitude medicine and pathophysiology. In: Auerbach PS, Cushing TA, Harris NS, editors. Auerbach's wilderness medicine. 7th ed. Philadelphia: Elsevier; 2017. p. 8–29.

41. Yanamandra U, Vardhan V, Saxena P, Singh P, Gupta A, Mulajkar D, Grewal R, Nair V. Radiographical spectrum of high-altitude pulmonary edema: a pictorial essay. Indian J Crit Care Med. 2021;25(6):668–74.

42. Wilson MH, Newman S, Imray CH. The cerebral effects of ascent to high altitudes. Lancet Neurol. 2009;8(2):175–91.

43. Grosse AB, Grosse CA, Steinbach LS, Zimmermann H, Anderson S. Imaging findings of avalanche victims. Skeletal Radiol. 2007;36(6):515–21.

44. Hohlrieder M, Brugger H, Schubert H, et al. Pattern and severity of injury in avalanche victims. High Alt Med Biol. 2007;8:56–61.

45. McIntosh SE, Grissom CK, Olivares CR, et al. Cause of death in avalanche fatalities. Wilderness Environ Med. 2007;18:293–7.

46. Stalsberg H, Albretsen C, Gilbert M, Kearney M, Moestue E, Nordrum I, Rostrup M, Orbo A. Mechanism of death in avalanche victims. Virchows Arch A Pathol Anat Histopathol. 1989;414(5):415–22.

47. Kobek M, Skowronek R, Jabłoński C, Jankowski Z, Pałasz A. Histopathological changes in lungs of the mountain snow avalanche victims and its potential usefulness in determination of cause and mechanism of death. Arch Med Sadowej Kryminol. 2016;66(1):23–31.

48. Dolinak D, Matshes E, Lew E. Hypothermia. In: Forensic pathology. Principles and practice. 1st ed. San Diego: Elsevier Academic Press; 2008. p. 248–9.

49. Byard RW, Zhou C. Erosive gastritis, Armanni-Ebstein phenomenon and diabetic ketoacidosis. Forensic Sci Med Pathol. 2010;6:304–6.

50. Preuss J, Dettmeyer R, Lignitz E, Madea B. Fatty degeneration in renal tubule epithelium in accidental hypothermia victims. Forensic Sci Int. 2004;141:131–5.

51. Tsokos M, Rothschild MA, Madea B, Rie M, Sperhake JP. Histological and immunohistochemical study of Wischnewsky spots in fatal hypothermia. Am J Forensic Med Pathol. 2006;27(1):70–4.

52. Zhou C, Byard RW. Armanni-Ebstein phenomenon and hypothermia. Forensic Sci Int. 2011;206:82–4.

53. Teresiński G, Buszewicz G, Mądro R. Acetonaemia as an initial criterion of evaluation of a probable cause of sudden death. Legal Med (Tokyo). 2009;11:18–24.

54. Huttunen P. Effect of ethanol on the processes of thermoregulation. Acta Physiol Pol. 1990;41:25–31.

55. Huttunen P, Hirvonen J. The effect of ethanol on the ability of Guinea-pigs to survive severe cold. Forensic Sci. 1977;9:185–93.

56. Kalant H, Le AD. Effects of ethanol on thermoregulation. Pharmacol Ther. 1983;23:313–64.

57. Andersen KL, Hellstrøm B, Lorentzen FV. Combined effect of cold and alcohol on heat balance in man. J Appl Physiol. 1963;18:975–82.

58. Teresiński G, Buszewicz G, Mądro R. The influence of ethanol on the level of ketone bodies in hypothermia. Forensic Sci Int. 2002;127:88–96.

59. Palmiere C, Mangin P. Postmortem biochemical investigations in hypothermia fatalities. Int J Legal Med. 2013;127:267–76.

60. Bańka K, Teresiński G, Buszewicz G. Free fatty acids as markers of death from hypothermia. Forensic Sci Int. 2014;234:79–85.

61. Bańka K, Teresiński G, Buszewicz G, Mądro R. Glucocorticosteroids as markers of death from hypothermia. Forensic Sci Int. 2013;229:60–5.

62. Palmiere C, Teresiński G, Hejna P, Mangin P, Grouzmann E. Diagnostic performance of urinary metanephrines for the postmortem diagnosis of hypothermia. Forensic Sci Med Pathol. 2014;10:518–25.

Heat-Related Injuries

9

Claudia Castiglioni, Virginie Magnin,
and Alessia Carminati

9.1 Introduction

Burn injuries are essentially skin lesions, caused by different injury mechanisms, such as the application of heat, cold, electricity, or corrosive chemicals. All skin burns, regardless of the mechanism at their origin, have the same appearance and are therefore classified according to their severity, ranging from first to fourth degree. A first-degree burn only affects the surface layer of the skin, the epidermis, representing a painful red discoloration. Burns of the second degree reach the dermis and are separated in second degree superficial or second degree deep, depending on whether they reach the depth of the dermis. A superficial second-degree burn is red, painful, with the presence of blisters, while a deep second-degree burn is lighter, even white, less painful, without blisters. A third-degree burn consists in the complete loss of the thickness of the skin, down to the subcutaneous adipose tissue, or even deeper (muscles, bones); it looks like "cardboard", white or pink, and is painless because of the loss of the cutaneous nerve endings. A fourth-degree burn represents charring of the tissue.

The severity of the burn injuries is also classified according to the percentage of body area affected, regardless of the depth of the burn. If more than 20% of body area is affected, it is a severe injury.

In the case of death following burn injuries, death may be due to the burns themselves (sometimes with survival and delayed death, particularly because of kidney failure) but also, in the case of exposure to fireplaces, to different gas poisoning because of the inhalation of fumes, including carbon monoxide and cyanide. Another mechanism is the inhalation of heat, leading to burns of the airways. The circumstances of the occurrence of burn injuries can be accidental, suicidal (immolation), or homicidal (to destroy the body post-mortem).

The first step if a burned body has to be investigated is the identification of vitality signs by looking for burns of the respiratory tract and detection of CO with toxicological exams [1, 2].

Up to second-degree burns, the examination of the body in order to detect other traumatic injuries and to identify the cause of death is quite easy. Instead, the examination of a body with third-degree burns or a charred body is

C. Castiglioni (✉) · A. Carminati
Unit of Forensic Medicine, University Center of Legal Medicine Lausanne-Geneva, University of Lausanne, University Hospital of Vaud, Lausanne, Switzerland
e-mail: Claudia.Castiglioni@chuv.ch; Alessia.Carminati@chuv.ch

V. Magnin
Unit of Forensic Imaging and Anthropology, University Center of Legal Medicine Lausanne-Geneva, University of Lausanne, University Hospital of Vaud, Lausanne, Switzerland
e-mail: Virginie.Magnin@chuv.ch

more difficult, as the charring alters some lesions or characteristics. In charred bodies, some characteristics are typically found in the process of charring, for example, the "boxer attitude" or "pugilistic attitude" (due to shortening of the flexor muscles), the thermic epidural coagulated hematoma (due to the retraction of the dura mater), or the thermic fractures with limb amputation (due to the loss of the soft tissues of the joints). These findings are related to the heat and are not vitality signs. Due to the major tissue alterations in charred bodies, imaging is mandatory.

Burn lesions of the soft tissues, if superficial, are usually not visible with standard imaging techniques. The main indications for imaging are the assessment of the presence/absence of radio-opaque foreign bodies and of traumatic lesions, as well as the compatibility between the observed lesions and the circumstances of death. As imaging is limited in the detection of vital signs and can be complicated by the stiffness of the body due to the carbonization, an autopsy must always be performed after the radiological investigations.

9.2 Most Suited Imaging Methods

9.2.1 Standard Radiography

Standard radiography should be used in post-mortem examination of a body, if the CT scanner is not available. This technique permits good visualization of the skeletal system and detection of radio-opaque foreign bodies. The visualization of soft tissues is very limited and the 2D projection creates superimposed images, which are difficult to interpret. In charred bodies, if no other imaging method is available, standard radiography can be used to visualize fractures. Although this technique allows the detection of radio-opaque foreign bodies, their location is often difficult to specify; the charred bodies having to be handled as little as possible, a single incidence is frequently carried out. Moreover, in certain cases

(e.g., road-traffic accidents), many foreign bodies can be found on the body and are responsible for imaging artifacts (Fig. 9.1). In conclusion, when possible, it is better to carry out a CT scanner of the body.

9.2.2 Post-Mortem Computed Tomography (PMCT)

PMCT is the standard imaging technique for investigating cases of charred bodies [3–6]. In burned bodies, the 3D examination of the body surface does not show first- and second-degree burns, but it permits an approximate evaluation of loss of substance of the soft tissues in third-degree burns and charred bodies (Fig. 9.2a, b).

Typical findings of charred bodies, such as the "pugilistic attitude", fractures of the long bones, thermic epidural hematoma, loss of soft tissue with sometimes opening of the chest and/or abdomen, and a "mottled" aspect of the bone marrow, can be observed with PMCT (Figs. 9.3, 9.4, 9.5a, b, 9.6, and 9.7). Due to the "pugilistic" position, exposing essentially the knees (poor in soft tissues), the thermic fractures of the lower limbs usually occur with an amputation at the knee level. It is to note that, in the absence of the limb amputated by fire, it is impossible to determine if the limb was previously traumatized [7].

PMCT is also the standard imaging technique for the assessment of the presence of radio-opaque foreign bodies such as a projectile, or for the assessment of dental work or prosthesis that can be used to identify the deceased (Fig. 9.8a, b). For formal identification, it is necessary to obtain antemortem radiological images (CT scanner or dental radiographies) in order to compare with the post-mortem images. In cases of charred bodies, the dental examination for identification purposes has to be carried out by a forensic dentist.

PMCT is essential for performing an injury assessment, including the thermic fracture distribution. Some fractures are typical for a certain injury mechanism, and, if present, they suggest a

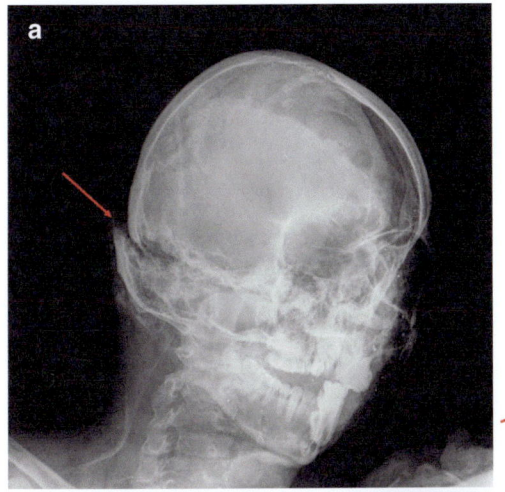
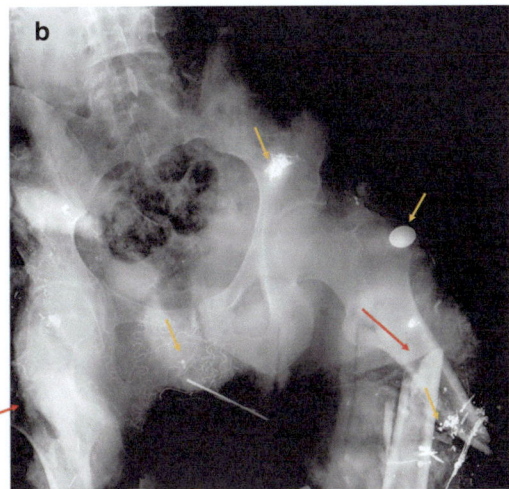
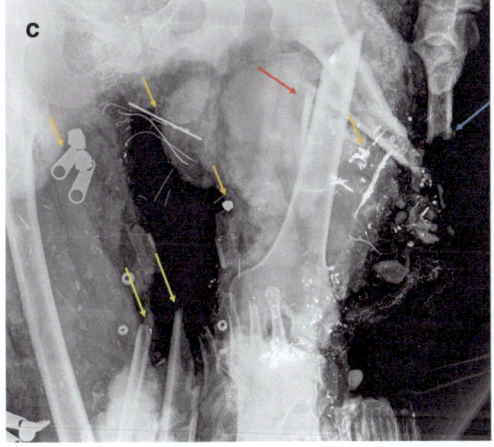

Fig. 9.1 Full-body standard radiographies of a charred body: (**a**) fracture of the right petrous temporal bone (red arrow). (**b**) fracture of the femurs (red arrows) and multiple foreign bodies of unknown etiology and localization (orange arrows). (**c**) fractures of the left femur (red arrow), the left forearm (blue arrow), and right tibia and fibula (yellow arrows), multiple foreign bodies of unknown etiology and localization (orange arrows)

previous trauma. It is interesting to note that antemortem bone fractures (that occurred before the fire) usually resist to the fire, and are still visible on the burned bones [8, 9].

Thermic fractures of the bones show specific characteristics. In anthropology, some different types of thermic fractures are described, for example, "longitudinal" (the most common, parallel to the axis of the long bones); "stairstep" shaped; "transverse"; "flute-mouthpiece" shaped; "patina" (superficial and mosaiclike); "delamination" (layer separation of the bone,

especially the skull); "curved transverse" (due to the shrinkage of the tissues); and "warping" (change in the alignment of the bone) (Figs. 9.9, 9.10, and 9.11) [11, 12]. These fractures are essentially correlated to the temperature and the duration of the fire, and are usually multifragmented, with multiple small fragments scattered around the fracture site. The extremities of the long bones and the ribs/sternum are the first parts to burn (usually until amputation of the long bones), and the scapular/pelvic belts and the vertebrae the last [7, 13].

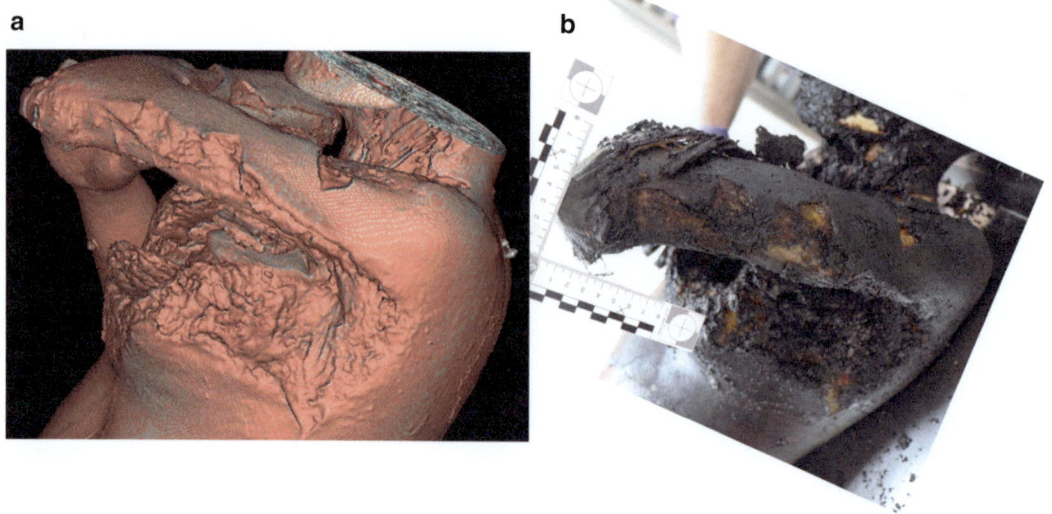

Fig. 9.2 (**a**) 3D reconstruction of the surface of a charred body, left side view. (**b**) In comparison with the external examination

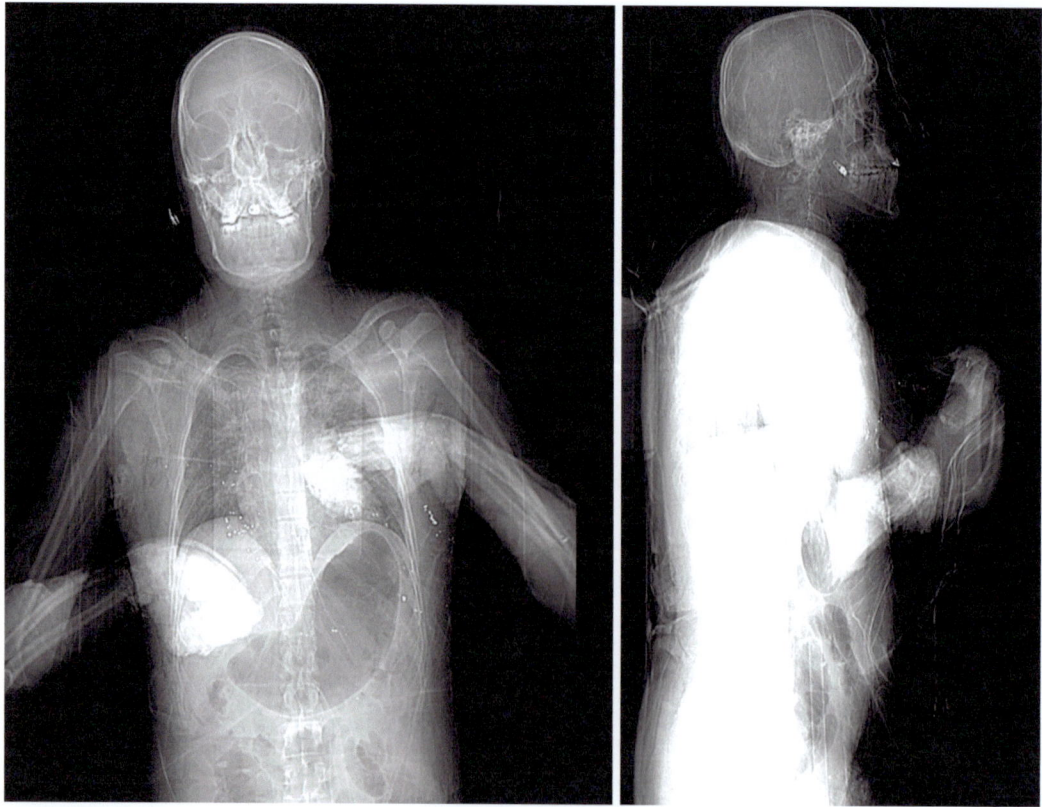

Fig. 9.3 Upper body scout view, face, and right side views of a charred body: typical "boxer attitude" (flexion of the elbows, hands closed)

Some types of fractures, for example, transverse fractures or "stairstep" fractures, can be observed in blunt force trauma of the limbs. Fractures in the unburned areas are suggestive of a previous trauma. Instead, when the fractured bone is burned, it is very difficult or impossible to

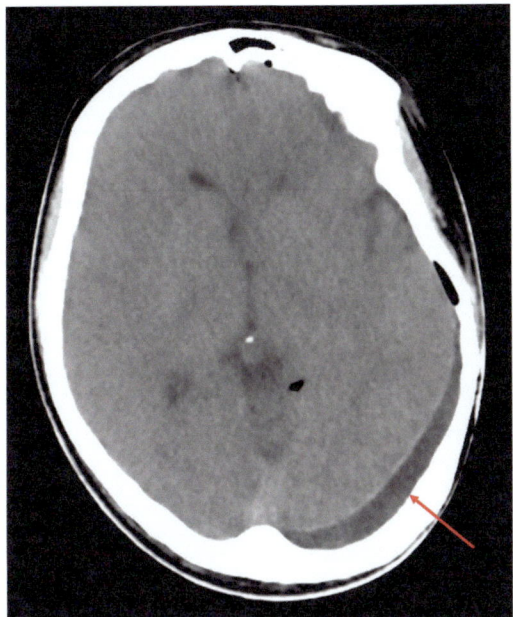

Fig. 9.4 Axial view of the head of a charred body at PMCT: epidural collection of the left convexity (red arrow)

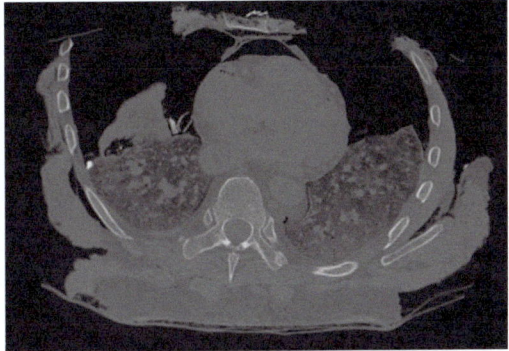

Fig. 9.6 Axial view of the chest of a charred body at PMCT: loss of substance of the soft tissue, with an anterior "opening" of the chest

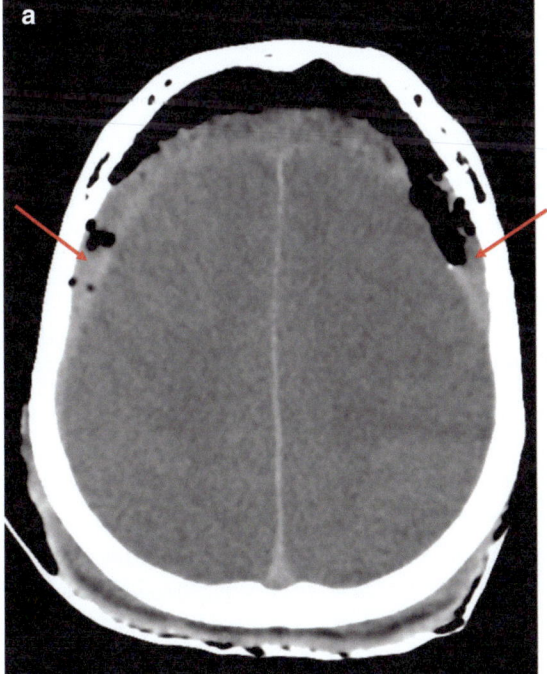

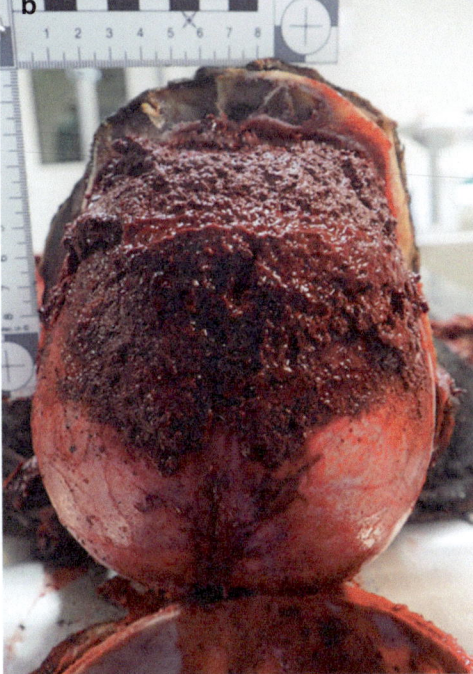

Fig. 9.5 (**a**) Axial view of the head of a charred body at PMCT. (**b**) In comparison with the autopsy: bilateral frontoparietal epidural hematoma (red arrows)

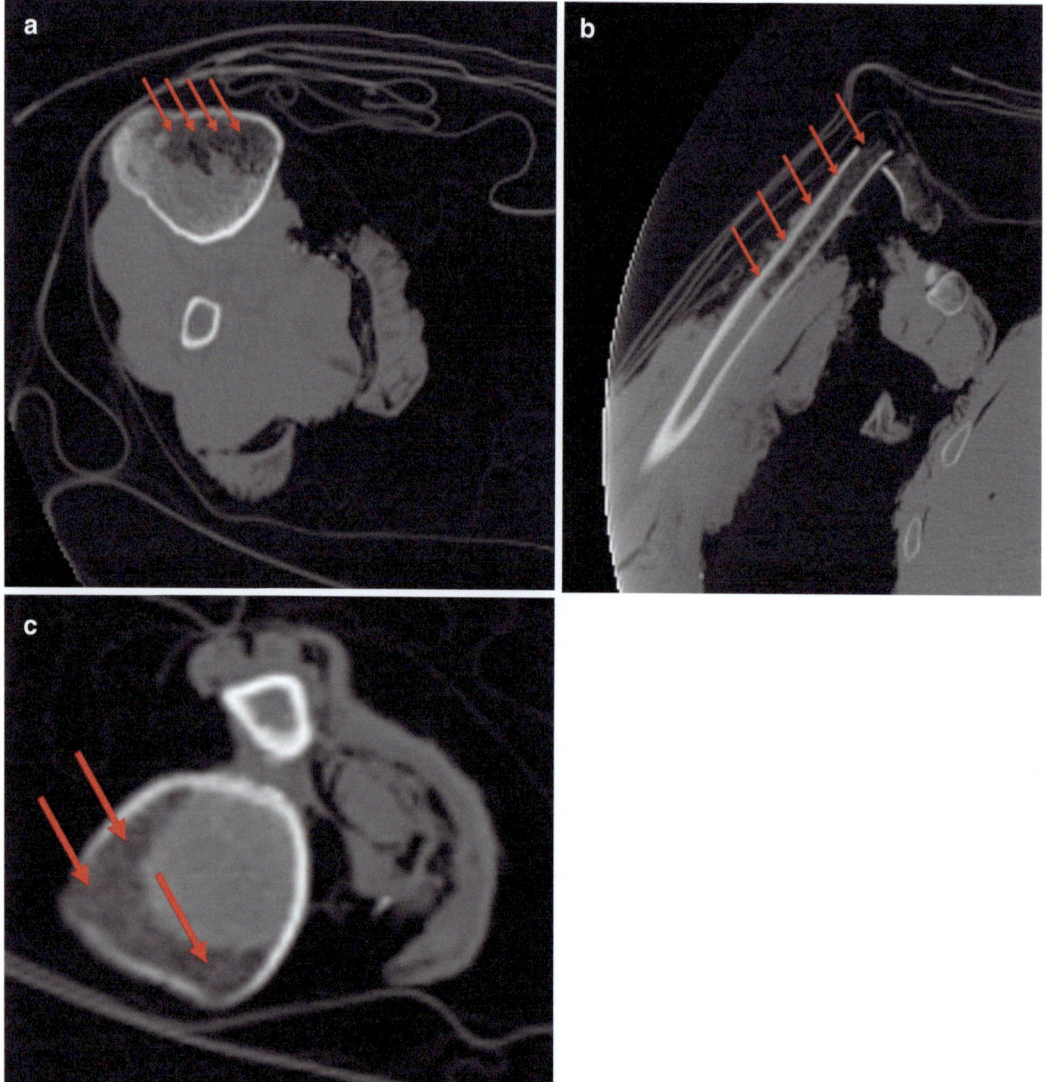

Fig. 9.7 Axial views of the leg (**a**, **c**) and coronal view of the arm (**b**) of a charred body at PMCT: "mottled" aspect of the bone marrow in the long bones (red arrows)

determine whether this fracture is a thermic fracture or another traumatic fracture [14].

Some fractures can show typical characteristics of a traumatic event at PMCT. For example, Messerer's fracture is a comminuted fracture with a triangular bone fragment, typically observed on the long bones of the lower limbs following a blunt force trauma in pedestrian-car accidents (Fig. 9.12). Therefore, the detection of a Messerer's fracture in a charred body can provide important information about the circumstances of death.

Another example is skull fracture. Biomechanics of skull fractures is well known; each different type of trauma generates a well-defined type of skull fracture. Taking into account the difficulties in visualizing the skull fractures during the autopsy in charred bodies, and the risk of creating artifacts during the opening of the scalp, the PMCT is the gold standard to visualize these fractures.

Skull fractures due to blunt force trauma or gunshot are from the outside to the inside, in a "spider web shape" with radiating lines. They

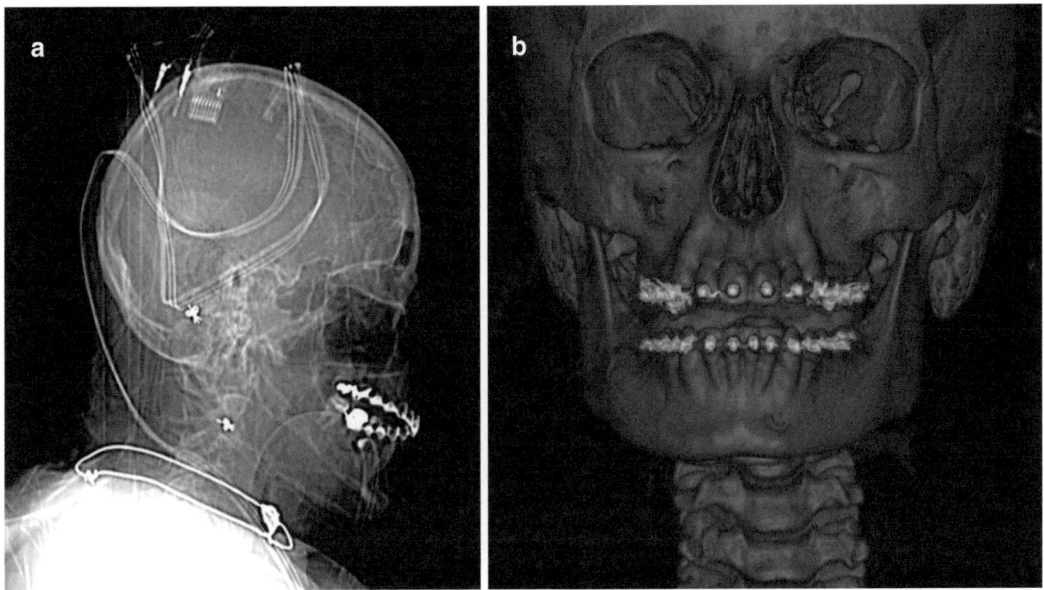

Fig. 9.8 (**a**) Scout view of the head, right side view. (**b**) 3D reconstruction of the facial bones, anterior view: necklace, dental work, and medical equipment

Fig. 9.9 Schematic representation of thermic fractures: (**a**) longitudinal, (**b**) curved transverse, (**c**) transverse, (**d**) patina, (**e**) delamination. (Taken from [10])

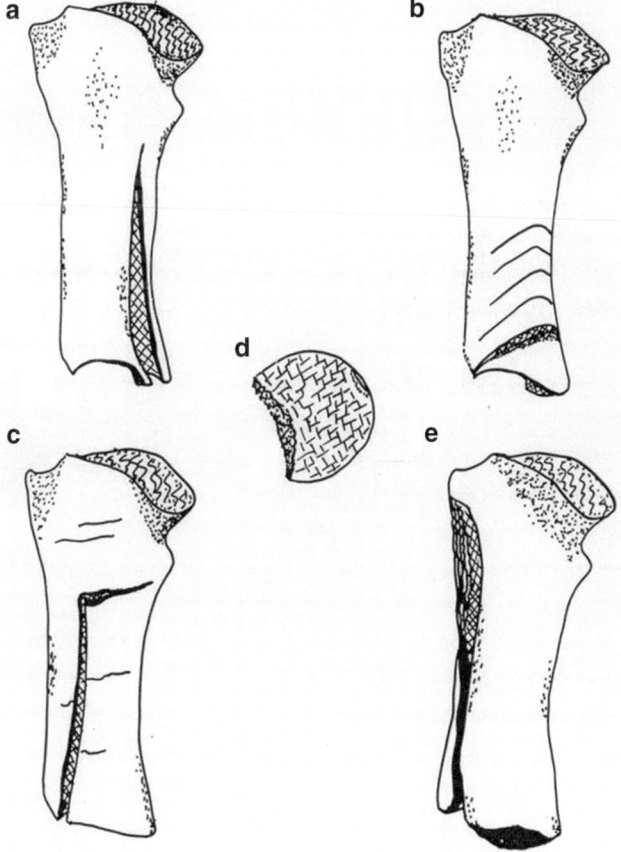

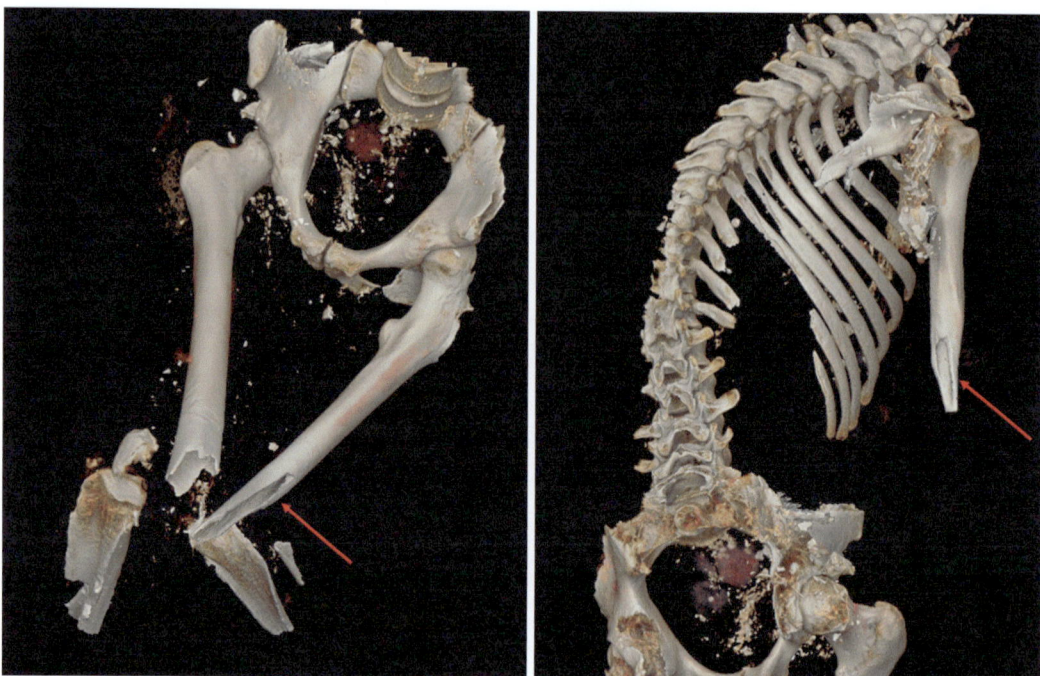

Fig. 9.10 3D reconstruction of a charred body: thermic fractures (multifragmented, in some places "flute-mouthpiece" shaped (red arrows)

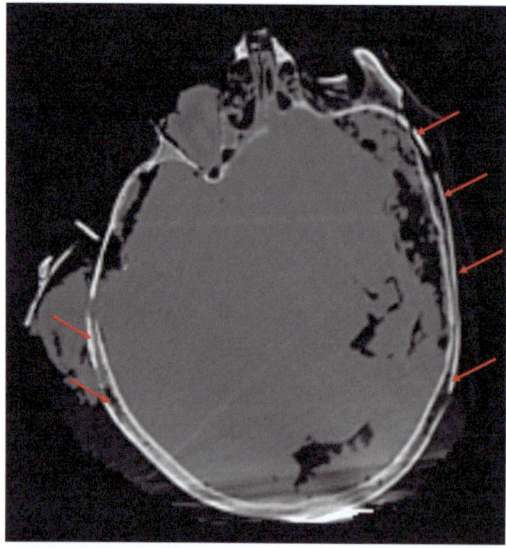

Fig. 9.11 Axial view of the head of a charred body at PMCT: longitudinal trans-diploic fracture of the skull, with delamination (red arrows)

typically show a "depressed" aspect, with a central loss of substance in the case of a gunshot (Figs. 9.13 and 9.14). These fractures stay visible at PMCT even if the skull is burned (Fig. 9.15a, b).

Thermic fractures of the skull are due to the increase of the intracranial pressure due to heat. Typically, there is a loss of bone substance, and the thermic fracture is shaped "from the inside to the outside," next to the skull sutures. The external table of the skull is more injured than the internal table, associated with a delamination between the layers of the skull, a patina of the external table, or a curved aspect of the cranial bone. These characteristics can be easily detected by PMCT. The skull is also affected by other events occurring during the fire, for example, due to debris, and, due to the delamination, the external table

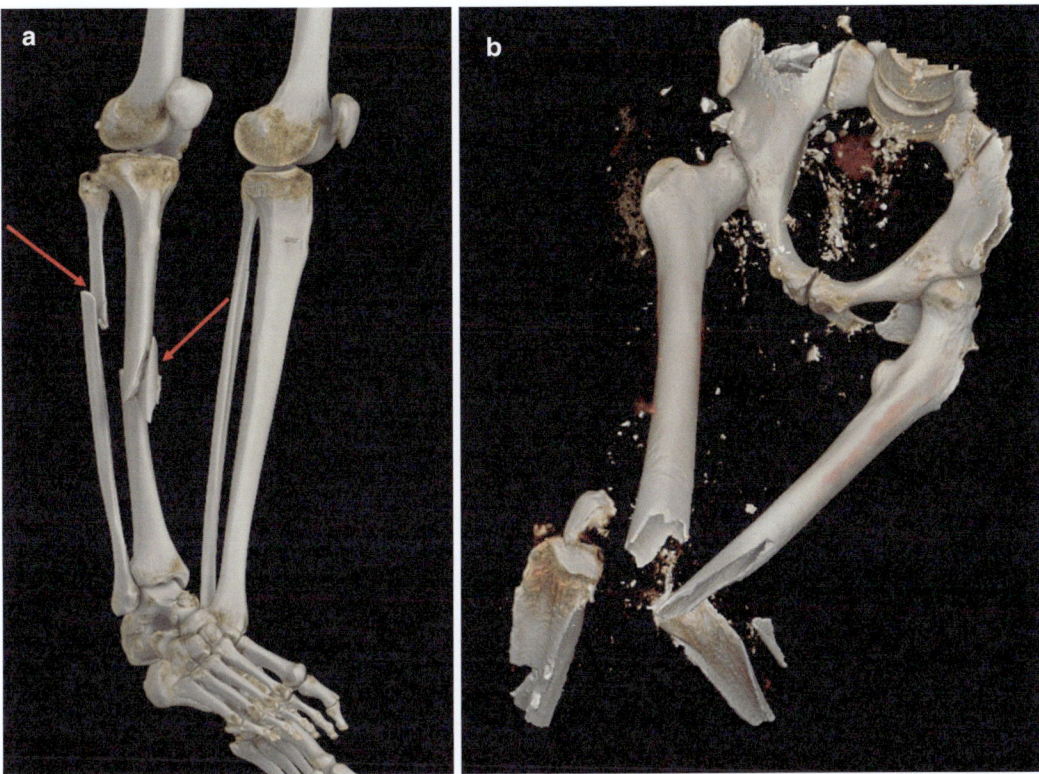

Fig. 9.12 3D reconstruction of the lower limbs: (**a**) Motorcycle—car accident: typical Messerer's fracture of the right tibia and fibula (red arrows); (**b**) charred body: thermic fractures of the lower limbs

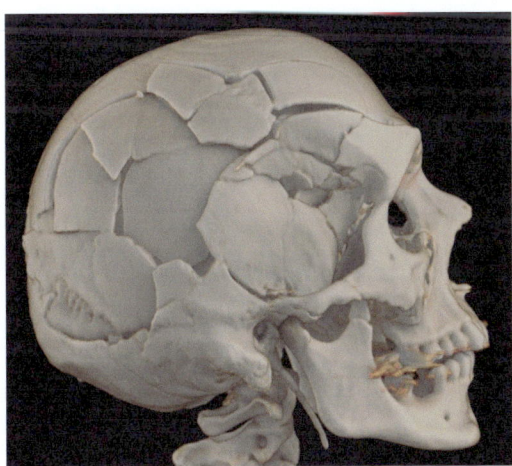

Fig. 9.13 3D reconstruction of the skull, right lateral view: traumatic fracture due to blunt force trauma (here, homicidal)

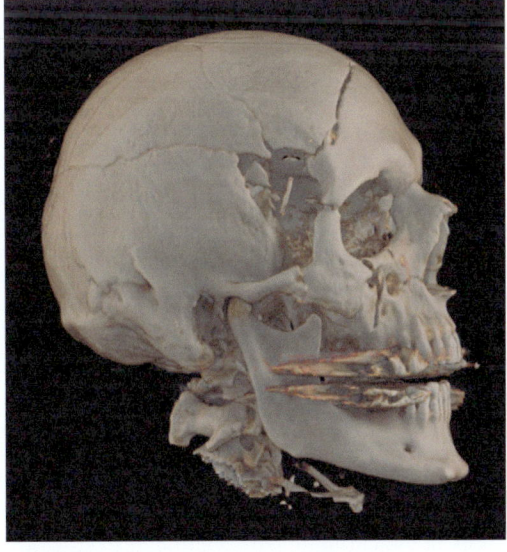

Fig. 9.14 3D reconstruction of the skull, right lateral view: traumatic fracture due to gunshot trauma (here, suicidal)

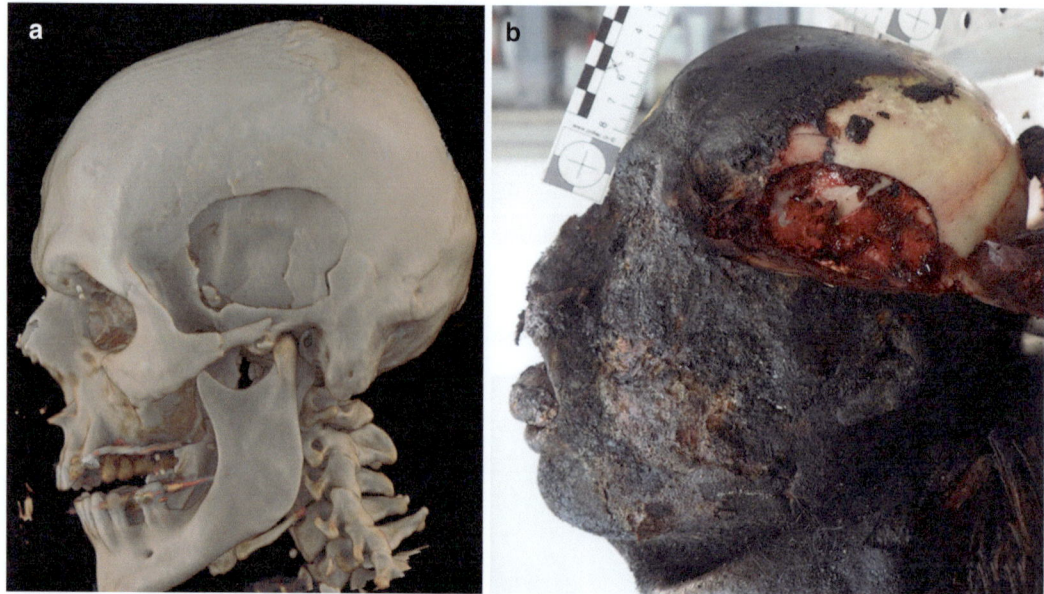

Fig. 9.15 (**a**) 3D reconstruction of the skull, left lateral view. (**b**) In comparison with the autopsy: traumatic fracture due to blunt force trauma with a sledge hammer (here, homicidal, the perpetrator set fire to the body afterward)

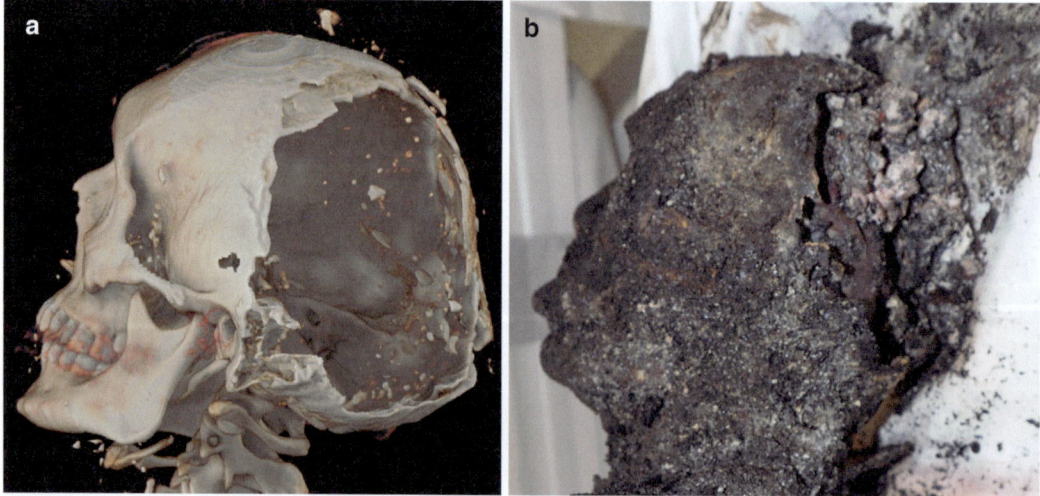

Fig. 9.16 (**a**) 3D reconstruction of the skull (left posterolateral view). (**b**) In comparison with the external examination: thermic fractures

"falls"; these factors create an "exploded" appearance of the skull (Figs. 9.16a, b, 9.17, 9.18, and 9.19a, b) [15]. Other thermic trauma signs in the cephalic part, visible at PMCT, are epidural hematoma and shrinking of the brain in the skull. It is interesting to note that thermic trauma never leads to subdural hematoma or skull-base fractures (as skull base is protected by the rest of the skull, soft tissues of the neck, and the cervical vertebral column). If these are visualized, another trauma or cause has to be suspected [16].

As a medicolegal challenge in charred bodies is to determine whether a bone fracture is related

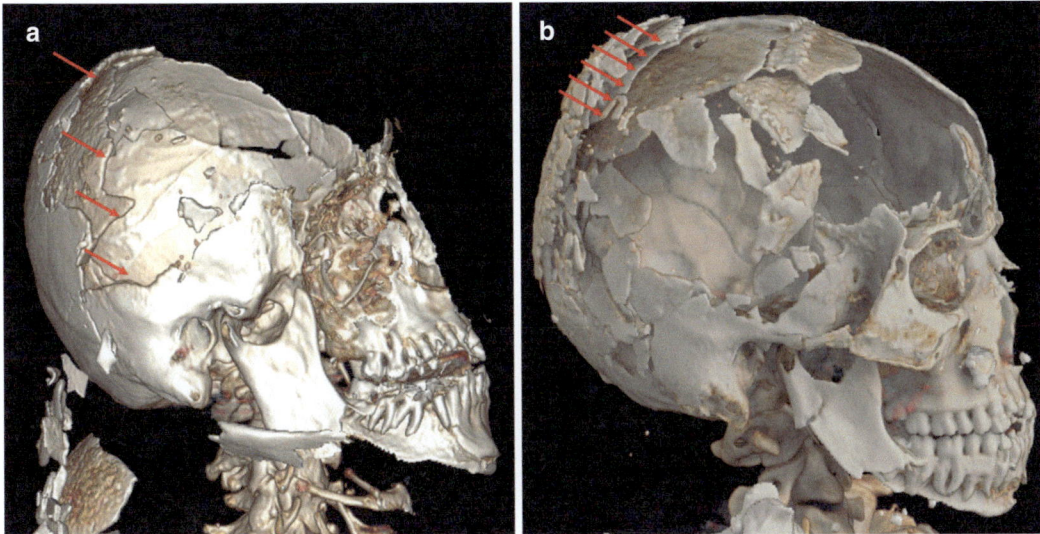

Fig. 9.17 3D reconstruction of the skull (right lateral view) of charred bodies: thermic fractures with (**a**) disappearance of the external table and (**b**) delamination (red arrows)

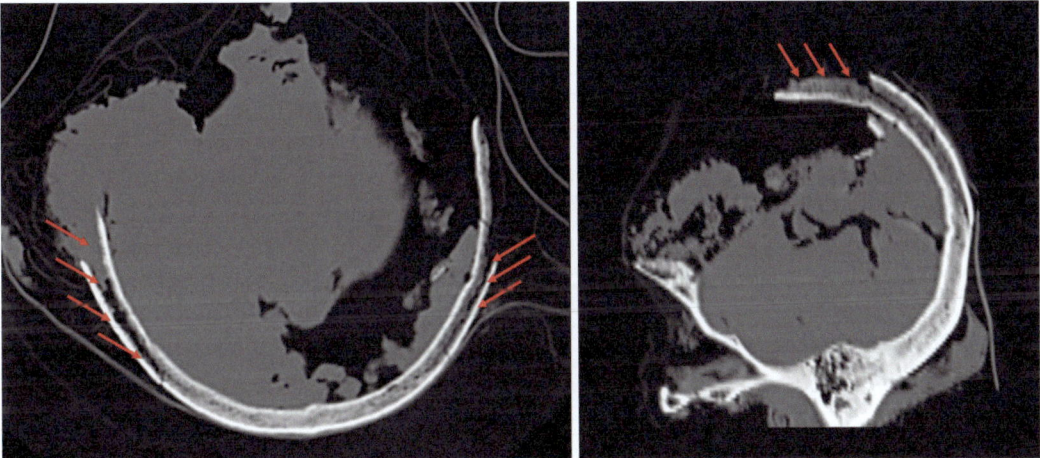

Fig. 9.18 Axial views of the head of a charred body at PMCT: thermic fractures with superficial delamination and disappearance of the external table (red arrows)

to the fire or to a previous trauma, it is important to detect all the fractures and their characteristics, and, to do so, PMCT is the gold standard. It is important too to know the differences between thermic fractures and other traumatic fractures. For this reason, it is recommended that the images are interpreted by a specialist in forensic imaging.

9.2.3 Multiphase Post-Mortem CT Angiography (MPMCTA)

MPMCTA is not the standard for burn trauma. If the burn lesions are too extended or if the body is charred, it is not possible to perform MPMCTA as the vascular access is compromised. In intact bodies, MPMCTA can be used

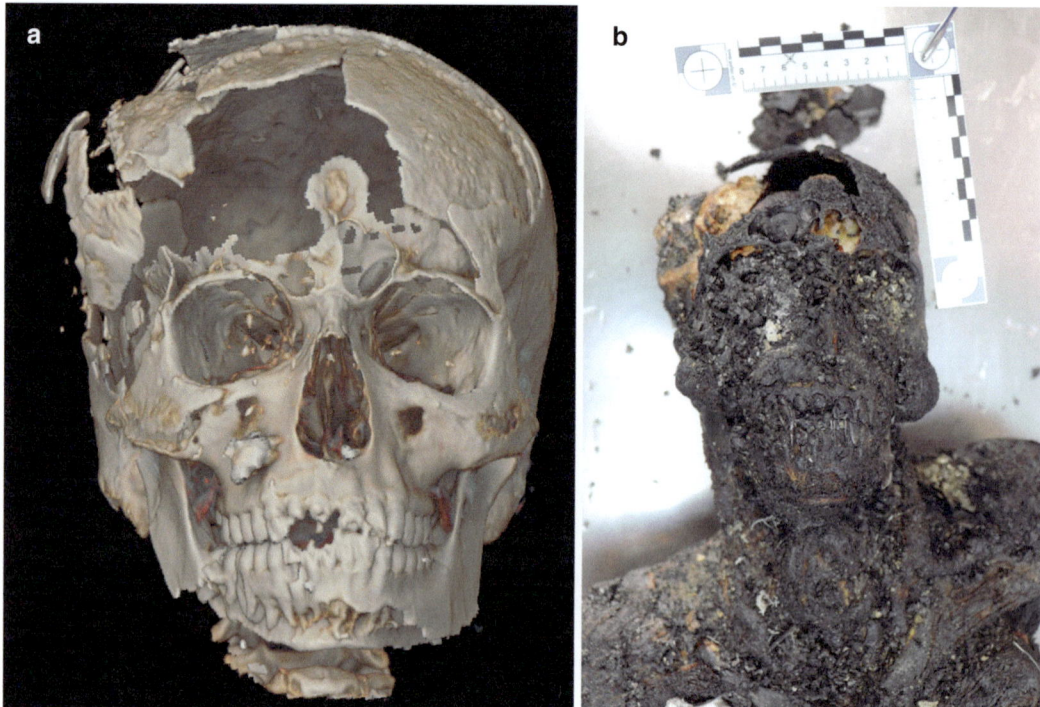

Fig. 9.19 (**a**) 3D reconstruction of the skull (anterior view). (**b**) In comparison with the external examination

to confirm or exclude an ischemic or bleeding pathology that could have occurred before the thermic trauma.

9.2.4 Magnetic Resonance Imaging (MRI)

MRI is rarely used in post-mortem examination of a body. Furthermore, in cases of severely burned or charred bodies, it is contraindicated as metallic fragments can be present on the body, show artifacts, and even damage the machine.

9.3 Conclusion

In summary, the most important medicolegal questions when investigating burned bodies are:

- Was the person alive before it burned?
- Did the person die due to the exposition to fire and its different gases?

The method of choice in forensic imaging to investigate burned bodies is PMCT, if available.

Typical observations that should be known are those that appear in the post-mortem period due to the exposure to fire and that have to be differentiated from vital lesions: the pugilistic attitude, the thermic fractures, and the thermic epidural hematoma.

References

1. Dettmeyer RB, Verhoff MA, Schütz HF. Forensic medicine, fundamentals and perspectives. 1st ed. Berlin: Springer-Verlag; 2014.
2. Madea B. Chap. 22: Injuries due to heat. In: Handbook of forensic medicine. Wiley Blackwell; 2014. p. 451–67.
3. de Bakker H, Roelandt GHJ, de Bakker BS, et al. The value of post-mortem computed tomography of burned victims in a forensic setting. Eur Radiol. 2019;29:1912–21.
4. Cittadini F, Polacco M, Pascali VL, et al. Virtual autopsy with multidetector computed tomography of three cases of charred bodies. Med Sci Law. 2010;50:211–6.

5. Levy AD, Harcke HT, Getz JM, Mallak CT. Multidetector computed tomography findings in deaths with severe burns. Am J Forensic Med Pathol. 2009;30(2):137–41.

6. Coty JB, Nedelcu C, Aubé C, et al. Burned bodies: post-mortem computed tomography, an essential tool for modern forensic medicine. Insights Imaging. 2018;9:731–43.

7. Alunni V, Grevin G, Buchet L, Quatrehomme G. Forensic aspect of cremations on wooden pyre. Forensic Sci Int. 2014;241:167–72.

8. Herrmann NP, Bennett JL. The differentiation of traumatic and heat-related fractures in burned bone. J Forensic Sci. 1999;44(3):461–9.

9. Ubelaker DH. The forensic evaluation of burned skeletal remains: a synthesis. Forensic Sci Int. 2009;183:1–5.

10. Correia PM. Fire modification of bone: a review of literature. In: Haglund WD, Sorg MH, editors. Forensic taphonomy: the postmortem fate of human remains. Boca Raton: CRC Press; 1997. p. 275–86. copyright 2023, reproduced by permission of Taylor & Francis Group LLC (Books) US through PLSclear, license 78426.

11. Quatrehomme G. Chap. 3.2.4: Les os brûlés. Les lésions de carbonisation. In: Traité d'anthropologie medico-légale. De Boeck; 2015. p. 1421–85.

12. Hammarlebiod S, Farrugia A, Willaume T, et al. Thermal bone injuries: postmortem computed tomography findings in 25 cases. Int J Legal Med. 2022;136:219–27.

13. Schmidt CW, Symes SA. The analysis of burned human remains. 2nd ed. Elsevier; 2015.

14. Tutor PM, Benito Sanchez M, Villoria Rojas C. Cut or burnt? Categorizing morphological characteristics of heat-induced fractures and sharp force trauma. Legal Med. 2021;50:101868.

15. Pope EJ, Smith OC. Identification of traumatic injury in burned cranial bone: an experimental approach. J Forensic Sci. 2004;49(3):1–10.

16. Bohnert M, Rost T, Faller-Marquardt M, Ropohl D, Pollak S. Fractures of the base of the skull in charred bodies—post-mortem heat injuries or signs of mechanical traumatization ? Forensic Sci Int. 1997;87(1):55–62.

10

Jean-Loup Gassend, Fabiano Riva, and Virginie Magnin

10.1 Thermal Injuries

Explosions consist of a chemical reaction during which a large amount of heat and gases are generated in a brief time period, causing a rapid increase in local gas pressure and temperature, and therefore a violent displacement of the surrounding medium (e.g., air or water). The intense production of heat during the process is visible in the form of a flame that can cause severe burns and set fire to elements of the environment. High temperatures are usually only produced in close proximity to the explosion, however so will not affect people located out of the immediate vicinity of it (within a few meters). Radiological examinations are not appropriate for the investigation of burn injuries.

10.2 Blast Injuries

Explosions can be subcategorized into high-order explosions (or detonations), during which the expansion of gases occurs at supersonic speeds, or low-order explosions (deflagrations), during which the expansion occurs at subsonic speeds. Explosives used in military explosive devices typically cause a high-order explosion, while gunpowder, gas, and industrial explosions are typically of low-order type. To illustrate the difference between a detonation and a deflagration in an intuitive manner, if one were to replace the gunpowder in a cartridge by a military-grade explosive, when the gun was fired, the rapidity of the explosive combustion would cause the chamber and/or the barrel to explode instead of the bullet being fired.

High-order explosions cause an overpressure blast wave that travels at supersonic speeds. The wounding potential of a blast wave decreases rapidly with range (within a few dozen meters). At very close range, it can blow a person to pieces or cause traumatic amputations. As the range increases, it is mainly hollow air-filled organs such the lungs, ears, and gastrointestinal tract that are subject to overpressure wounds, though other non-hollow organs such as the brain (explosive blast brain injury) and eyes can also be injured [1].

Examples of classical consequences of exposure to a blast wave are lung contusions, air

J.-L. Gassend (✉)
Unit of Forensic Medicine, University Center of Legal Medicine Lausanne-Geneva, University of Lausanne, University Hospital of Vaud, Lausanne, Switzerland
e-mail: Jean-Loup.Gassend@chuv.ch

F. Riva · V. Magnin
Unit of Imaging and Anthropology, University Center of Legal Medicine Lausanne-Geneva, University of Lausanne, University Hospital of Vaud, Lausanne, Switzerland
e-mail: Fabiano.Riva@chuv.ch;
Virginie.Magnin@chuv.ch

© The Author(s), under exclusive license to Springer Nature Switzerland AG 2024
S. Grabherr et al. (eds.), *Forensic Imaging of Trauma*, https://doi.org/10.1007/978-3-031-48381-3_10

embolism, pneumo- and hemothorax, lung parenchymal damage, lung edema, subcutaneous and mediastinal emphysema, tympanic membrane rupture, ossicular dislocation or fracture, and, less frequently, bowel contusion or perforation. The lungs are affected the most commonly, and "blast lung" is reported to be found in approximately half of terrorist explosion fatalities [2]. There may be a delay before some of these blast injuries become apparent. Low-order explosions (deflagrations) are less potent but can cause similar injuries if they are particularly powerful, or if experienced at particularly close range. As fluids are incompressible, they transmit the forces of an explosion with particular lethality, as is illustrated by the infamous deadly effect of underwater explosions during "dynamite fishing." Explosions occurring in enclosed spaces such as a subway, bus, or building are also particularly lethal as the blast waves will reflect off walls and the force of the explosion will be magnified in whatever open areas are available to it [1].

CT is the radiological exam of choice in blast cases, as it can detect the more discreet injuries such as pneumomediastinum, bronchopleural fistulae, air emboli, intraperitoneal free fluid, and gas, as well as injuries to the bowel, as it can demonstrate bowel wall thickening in areas of bowel contusion. The classical radiological appearance of a "blast lung" is that of bilateral infiltrates with a perihilar "butterfly" or "batwing" distribution, corresponding to alveolar rupture and hemorrhage, sometimes accompanied by pneumo- and/or hemothorax (Fig. 10.1) [3].

In limb amputations due to stepping on a mine, there can be a so-called umbrella effect: when the foot is blow off, the more proximal soft tissues of the leg are momentarily peeled away from the bone in a manner resembling that of an opening umbrella. Damage may therefore extend much further proximally than is visible from the outside appearance of the leg. Radiologically, the "umbrella effect" can be apparent in the form of air, fragments, and debris present along the tibial and fibular shafts proximally to the blown off foot [4].

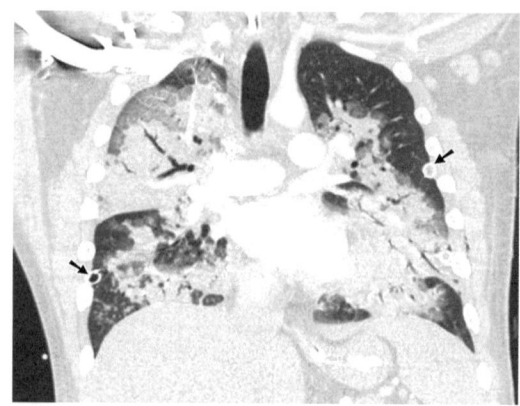

Fig. 10.1 Blast injuries to the lungs. Coronal reformatted image (lung windows) of a soldier exposed to an IED blast in Afghanistan showing multiple areas of consolidation caused by the overpressure blast wave. Note bilateral chest tubes (arrows). (Source: Blast Injuries: From Improvised Explosive Device Blasts to the Boston Marathon Bombing. Singh A. et al. Radiographics. 2016. Used with permission)

The radiological appearance of the various other blast injuries mentioned above (such brain edema, subarachnoid hemorrhages, pneumomediastinum, and free air in the abdomen) has a nonspecific appearance, resembling that when such injuries are caused by other mechanisms [5]. Ossicular fractures or dislocation can be diagnosed by thin-sliced CT of the temporal bone.

10.3 Projection and Blunt Force Injuries

The violent displacement of air caused by an explosion can cause a person to be thrown against part of his environment, resulting in unspecific blunt force trauma. A classic example is the crew of an armored military vehicle sustaining injuries by being projected against prominent pieces of the vehicle's interior when it drives over a mine. People can also be thrown off cliffs bordering a road, off (or onto nearby) rooves or balconies, etc. Large explosions may also cause a building to collapse over a victim, providing another mechanism of blunt force injuries. Blunt force injuries linked to an explosion, such as bone fractures and organ injuries (such as pulmonary contusions or lacerations, splenic lacerations or rupture, liver and kidney lacerations, brain injuries), are easily diagnosed with CT but are unspecific, appearing the same as when they are caused by other traumatic mechanisms (i.e., fall from a great high).

10.4   Fragment Injuries

When an explosion occurs, fragments of the exploding agent, as well as fragments of the environment from its immediate vicinity, are projected away from the center of the explosion at velocities that can reach the order of 2000 m/s, in other words much faster than rifle bullets. However, because the fragments are not stabilized or shaped aerodynamically as bullets are, they quickly lose speed, and their range and penetration capacity is therefore typically inferior to that of bullets [6]. For a typical bomb fragment, for example, loss of roughly 50% of velocity, in other words 75% of energy, occurs within 30 m [7]. Nonetheless, and with few exceptions, fragments are the type of explosion wounding mechanism with the greatest range, being potentially lethal hundreds of meters from the explosion site.

In accidental explosions, fragments are incidental, such as boiler fragments, glass, pebbles, construction materials, etc. Furthermore, as accidental explosions are usually of the low-order type, the fragments will not reach high velocities, and the primary wounding mechanisms in such cases may therefore be burns, blast, and blunt force injuries. In the context of military or terrorist explosions, the opposite is true. Military explosive devices normally consist of a steel envelope meant to fragment (or prefragmented) into hundreds or thousands of pieces (Fig. 10.2), the size of which has been designed for maximum efficiency. Sometimes, as in the case of small mines, lethality is not the primary goal, the reasoning being that a severely wounded soldier

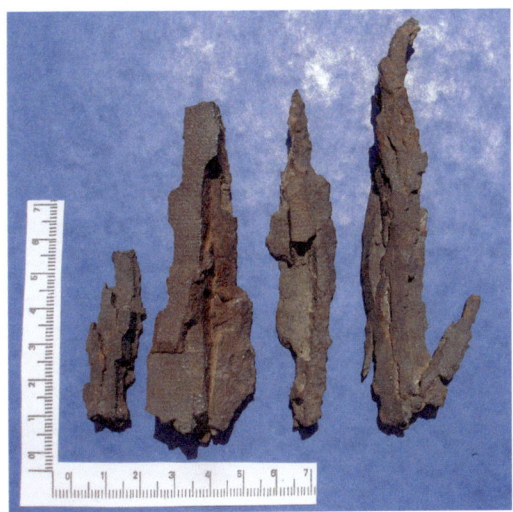

Fig. 10.2 Typical artillery shell fragments, displaying sharp and irregular edges. (Collection Jean-Loup Gassend)

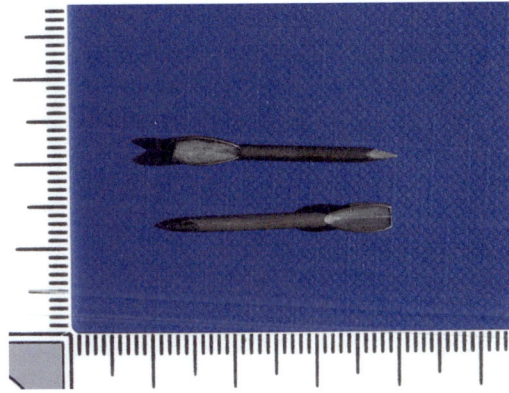

Fig. 10.3 Flechette specimens. These can be included by the thousands in artillery shells. (Collection James Wesley Miller)

will not return to combat and will mobilize costly resources. Terrorists are infamous for including such items as nails and ball bearings in their bombs, and the military has used similar methods such as including flechettes (small darts) (Fig. 10.3) or shrapnel balls (lead balls the size of marbles) into artillery shells. Literally anything can become a fragment when projected at high speed, and people have even been known to be wounded by bone fragments of suicide bombers or of their co-victims [8].

Fragments cause injury by penetrating into the body. If they are traveling with high enough velocity, fragments may cause temporary cavities, just like bullets [9]. When entering the body, classical military artillery or bomb fragments travel with their long axis perpendicular to their direction of travel [10], just as dead leaves oscillate on a roughly horizontal axis as they fall in autumn. This results in less penetration, but also in a greater permanent and temporary cavity diameter and thus in greater damage. The severity of a wound will depend completely on the characteristics (size, mass, shape, velocity, and energy) of a fragment and the anatomical region affected.

When a military or terrorist explosion occurs at close range, the victim can expect to be "peppered" with dozens or hundreds of fragments—including numerous tiny millimetric fragments—as well as soiled with projected dirt and dust [10]. As the range increases, the density of fragments decreases (as they are projected in all directions), and smaller fragments quickly lose their wounding potential. Within a dozen meters of the typical explosion site, a victim can therefore be expected to have only a few fragment wounds. At further ranges, single larger fragments will be the culprits, and there will be no dirt soiling.

Standard radiography and CT are the imaging modalities of choice for the assessment of fragment injuries as fragments are highly characteristic and easily recognizable (Fig. 10.4). In military device explosions, irregular metallic fragments of various shapes and sizes will classically be seen within the body. In terrorist or accidental explosions, more exotic and miscellaneous items including ball bearings, nails, and screws may be seen (Figs. 10.5 and 10.6). Regarding the identification of wound tracks, the same principles described for bullets (see Chap. 5) also apply for fragment wounds. CT scan will quickly differentiate superficial from deep wounds, and postmortem angiography may help highlight wound tracks and identify vascular injuries such as lac-

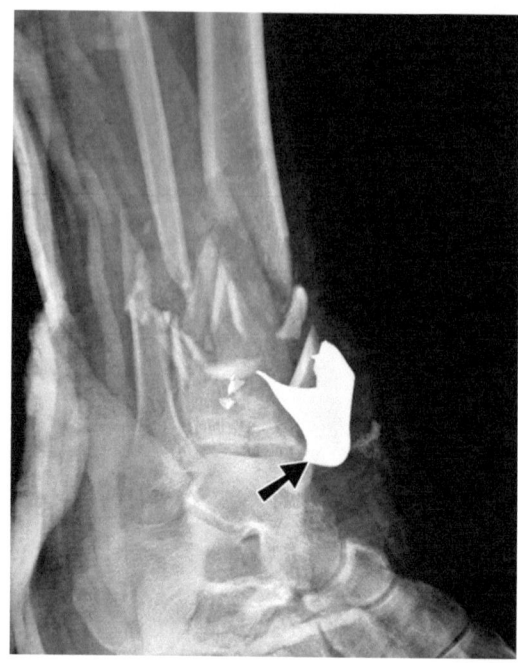

Fig. 10.4 Lateral radiograph of the right leg showing an open comminuted fracture of the distal tibial and fibular shaft caused by a large piece of shrapnel (arrow). (Source: Blast Injuries: From Improvised Explosive Device Blasts to the Boston Marathon Bombing. Singh A. et al. Radiographics. 2016. Used with permission)

erations, pseudoaneurysm, and arteriovenous fistulae.

In the context of terrorist bombings in general, tiny medically insignificant fragments of the explosive device may be of great importance to the police investigation. This is well illustrated by the Lockerbie Pan Am Flight 103 investigation in which two miniscule fragments of a radio-cassette player were instrumental in discovering where the bomb had been hidden [11]. The radiological examination of unsolved terrorist bombing victims is therefore highly advisable. In plane crashes of unknown origin—particularly over the sea where only tiny proportions of the wreckage may ever be recovered—radiological investigation of all the victims in search of possible fragments is of utmost importance, as this may be the only evidence of an explosive device having been present onboard.

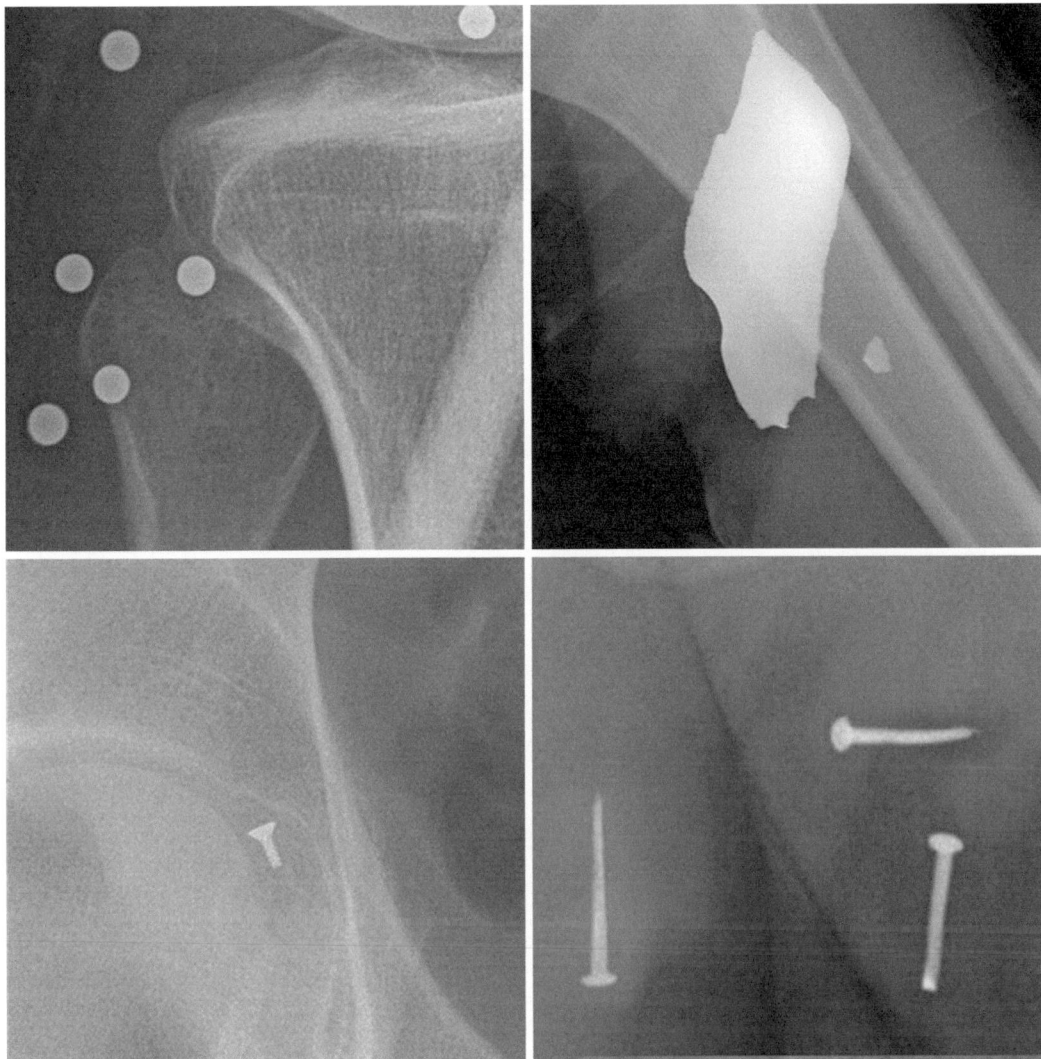

Fig. 10.5 Shrapnel found among Boston Marathon bombing victims, illustrating the heterogeneity that can be expected from terrorist bombs and improvised explosive devices. Radiographic images show the four types of shrapnel found (clockwise from top left): ball bearings, pressure cooker fragments, nails, and screws. (Source: Blast Injuries: From Improvised Explosive Device Blasts to the Boston Marathon Bombing. Singh A. et al. Radiographics. 2016. Used with permission)

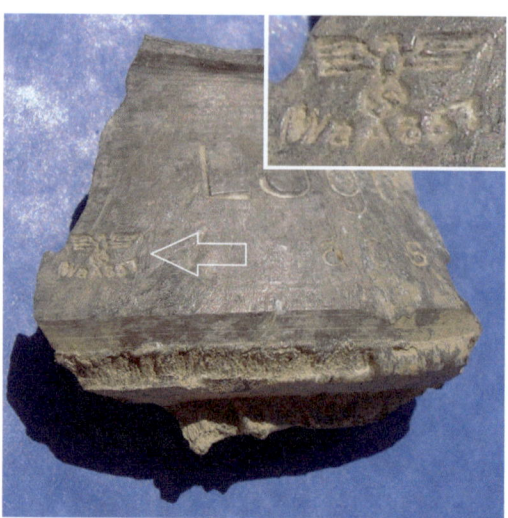

Fig. 10.6 Terrorist explosive devices are not the only ones that may display unusual or surprising characteristics, as is illustrated by this World War II era German shell fragment with an eagle and swastika (arrow and inlay) stamped on its surface. Such markings on fragments can prove invaluable if an investigation is performed. (Collection Jean-Loup Gassend)

10.5   Conclusion

Imaging is of great value in the evaluation of explosion victims and is a useful complement to the autopsy. The choice of the imaging modality depends mostly on the condition of the corpse and on the radiological devices available. Standard radiography enables the detection of foreign bodies and fractures as well as of pneumothorax or pneumoperitoneum. CT is however the technic of choice as it can detect and precisely locate foreign bodies and the accumulation of gas in various anatomic compartments, as well as highlight all the injuries that can be encountered in such cases, including some that may be difficult to see at autopsy, such as facial bone fractures. Moreover, the injection of contrast medium (using the multiphase postmortem CT angiography protocol) [12] can demonstrate the presence of vascular injuries and locate

sources of possible bleeding. MRI is usually contraindicated until the presence of metallic foreign bodies has been ruled out and is in any case a bad screening tool.

References

1. Jorolemon MR, Lopez RA, Krywko DM. Blast injuries. In: StatPearls. Treasure Island, FL: StatPearls Publishing; 2021. Available from https://www.ncbi.nlm.nih.gov/books/NBK430914/. Last accessed: 7 Feb 2022.
2. Frykberg ER, Tepas JJ 3rd. Terrorist bombings. Lessons learned from Belfast to Beirut. Ann Surg. 1988;208(5):569–76. https://doi.org/10.1097/00000658-198811000-00005.
3. Barnard E, Johnston A. Blast lung. N Engl J Med. 2013;368:1045. https://doi.org/10.1056/NEJMicm1203842.
4. Nessen SC, Lounsbury DE, Hertz SP. War surgery in Afghanistan and Iraq: a series of cases, 2003–2007, Textbooks of military medicine. Borden Institute; 2008. p. 292–6.
5. Ling G, Ecklund JM, Bandak FA. Brain injury from explosive blast: description and clinical management. Handb Clin Neurol. 2015;127:173–80. https://doi.org/10.1016/B978-0-444-52892-6.00011-8.
6. Wakabayashi K, Homae T, Ishikawa K, Kuroda E. Fragment velocity measurement of steel container during explosion tests by using high-speed and flash X-ray photography. Sci Technol Energ Mater. 2009;70:94–100.
7. French RW, Callender GR. Ballistic characteristics of wounding agents. In: Heaton LD, editor. Wound ballistics. Washington, DC: Office of the Surgeon General, Department of the Army; 1962. p. 91–132.
8. Aharonson-Daniel L, Klein Y, Peleg K, ITG. Suicide bombers form a new injury profile. Ann Surg. 2006;244(6):1018–23. https://doi.org/10.1097/01.sla.0000225355.06362.0f.
9. Plurad DS. Blast injury. Mil Med. 2011;176(3):276–82. https://doi.org/10.7205/milmed-d-10-00147.
10. Kneubuehl BP, Coupland RM, Rothschild MA, Thali MJ, editors. Wound ballistics: basics and applications. Translation of the revised third German ed. Berlin: Springer Verlag; 2011. ISBN: 978-3-642-20355-8.
11. Syracuse University Libraries. Pan Am Flight 103/Lockerbie Air Disaster Archives. 1990. https://panam103.syr.edu/. Last accessed: 7 Feb 2022.
12. Grabherr S, Doenz F, Steger B, et al. Multi-phase postmortem CT angiography: development of a standardized protocol. Int J Legal Med. 2011;125:791–802.